ERADICATION

Eradication

Ridding the World of Diseases Forever?

Nancy Leys Stepan

Cornell University Press
Ithaca, New York

This book is dedicated to my grandchildren, Isabel, Colin, Helena, Esther, Heloisa, Fiona and Erica

Originally published in Great Britain
in 2011 by Reaktion Books, London.
First published in the United States of America
in 2011 by Cornell University Press.

ISBN 978-0-8014-5058-7 (cloth: alk. Paper)

Printed and bound in Great Britain
by MPG Books Group

Librarians: A CIP catalog record for this book is available
from the Library of Congress.

Cloth printing 10 9 8 7 6 5 4 3 2 1

Contents

Introduction

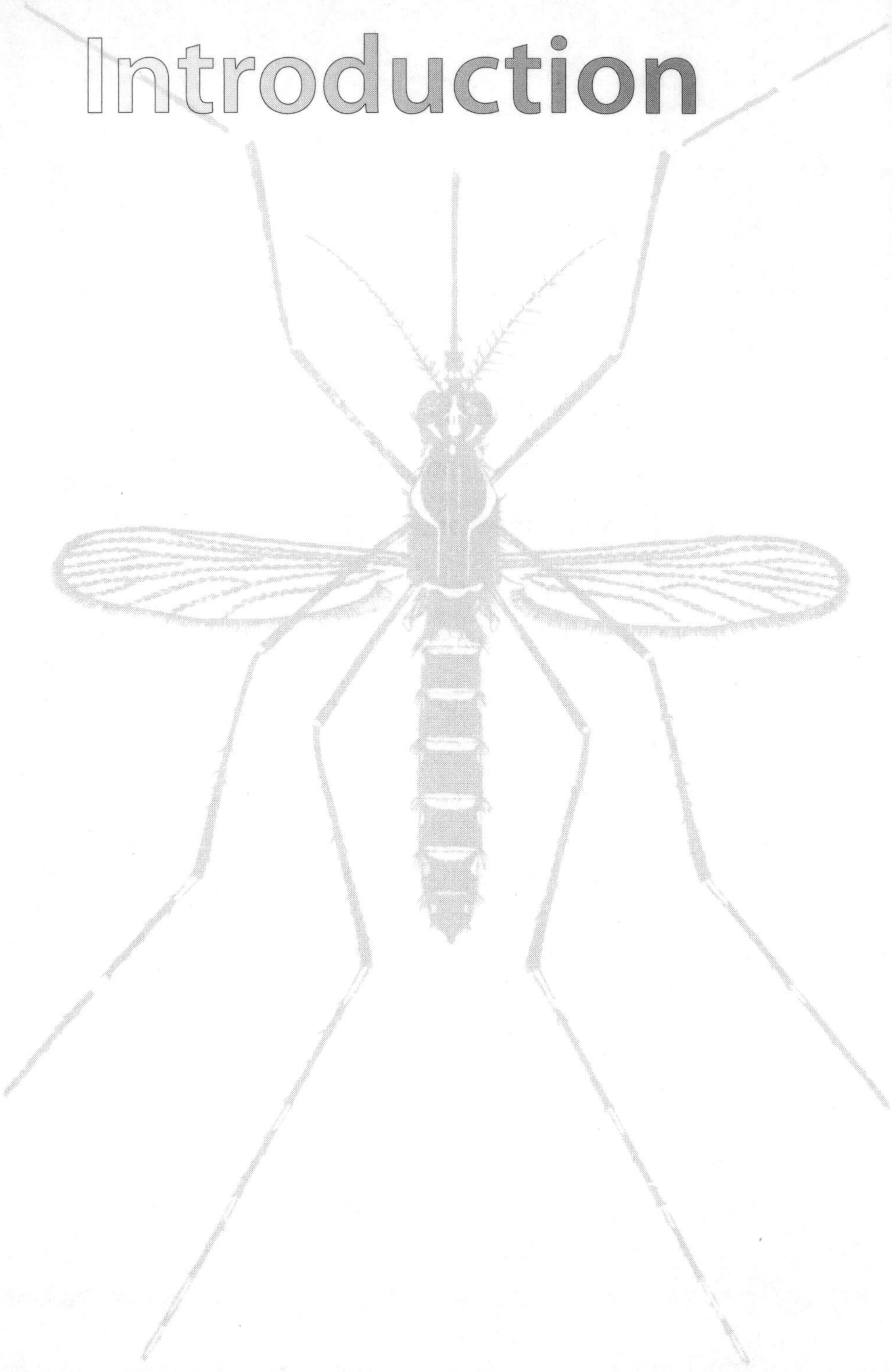

The purpose of this book is to examine the origins, historical development, impact and controversies surrounding disease eradication as a goal in international public health.

We often use the term 'eradication' in a loose way, as when, for example, we talk about eradicating poverty, when what we really mean is that we hope to greatly reduce poverty in the world. In this book, however, I am using the term in its more precise, modern, public health sense to mean the 'reduction of the worldwide incidence of a disease to zero as a result of deliberate efforts'.[1] Eradication is distinguished from disease 'control', which refers simply to the reduction of disease incidence to an acceptable level, without the expectation that we are ridding the world of the disease forever. In eradication, the emphasis is instead on zero disease and purposeful public health intervention. Eradication also sets a deliberate start- and end-date to the project (usually a span of ten to twenty years). Finally, eradication makes an argument about costs; it is argued that although eradication is expensive to carry out, it is cheaper in the long run than disease control because, once the goal of zero disease incidence is achieved, the continued costs of maintaining control measures can be given up forever, without the risk of the disease coming back.

Eradication, in short, stands for an absolute.

Eradication is a modern concept and a modern achievement. Although many diseases (and biological species) have become extinct over the course of human history without deliberate campaigns being waged against them (because of changed environmental conditions or unknown mutations in the genetic makeup of biological organisms), the deliberately aimed-for, complete elimination of a disease is very recent, a product of the twentieth century.[2] The eradication concept was pioneered by the Rockefeller Foundation in campaigns against hookworm disease, yellow fever and malaria before the Second World War. After the war eradication was endorsed by the newly founded World Health Organization (WHO), with eradication campaigns being launched against yaws, yellow fever, malaria and smallpox and, more recently, against poliomyelitis and Guinea Worm Disease (dracunculiasis). These campaigns are among the largest, most logistically complex, and costly initiatives ever undertaken in international public health. They involve the participation and support of numerous national governments, working across the political spectrum, with a degree of cooperation rare in the international arena. They also absorb the resources – political, financial, technical and human – of the most significant international health organizations, such as UNICEF and the WHO, as well as of the major philanthropic organizations of the times, from the Rockefeller Foundation in the pre-Second World War era, to the Bill and Melinda Gates Foundation today. Indeed, eradication campaigns must be counted as some of the most ambitious programmes in international public health history.

The trouble is that, thus far, only one of the eradication campaigns has met its absolutist goal – smallpox.[3]

Perhaps no single disease has killed or disfigured more people in human history than smallpox. The hideous smallpox blisters that covered infected people's faces and bodies are unforgettable to those who saw them before smallpox was finally eliminated. Many people were left not just severely pockmarked, but also blind as a result of the infection. In some populations, up to 70 per cent of those infected died of the disease. The WHO first endorsed eradication in 1958; an intensified programme, starting in 1967, halted transmission ten years later, the last case of naturally occurring smallpox being identified in a Somali man in October 1977. The official announcement that smallpox had truly gone was made in Geneva in 1980 – the first time in human history that a disease had been eliminated throughout the entire world as a result of deliberate human effort.[4] It was a great achievement. As a consequence, routine smallpox vaccinations were eventually stopped (the US had given them up as early as 1972).

This proof in 1980 that eradication was actually feasible came at a critical moment when enthusiasm for eradication had waned in the face of several setbacks and failures. As a result of the smallpox success, two new global eradication campaigns were launched in the 1980s and '90s, along with several regional eradication efforts. Several other diseases (for example, measles) wait in the wings as potential candidates for future eradication efforts.

It is against the background of the disappearance of smallpox as a human affliction, and the renewed enthusiasm for disease eradication campaigns internationally, that we need to assess the impact of the attacks of 11 September 2001 in the United States, and then the events that followed shortly afterwards, when the deliberate spread of spores of the deadly disease anthrax by an unknown person or persons caused five deaths, paralysed for weeks the functioning of fundamental institutions of the federal government, like the post office, and for a while terrified the population.[5] The term 'bioterrorism' entered political discourse. The fear that in the future there might be a deliberate, malicious attempt to use smallpox as a weapon against civilian populations, who lacked any vaccination and therefore any immunity to the disease, changed everything. The long deferred plans to destroy the remaining smallpox virus stocks, originally believed to be held in just two guarded laboratories in the United States and the ex-Soviet Union, were halted; smallpox vaccine was put hastily into production once again.[6] Decisions now have to be made about whom to vaccinate and when; the attendant risks of fatalities and side effects caused by vaccination itself have to be weighed against the assessed risk of infection from a potential bioterrorist smallpox attack.[7]

The dramatic story of smallpox eradication underlines the continued relevance, but also the problematic status, of eradication as a public health philosophy and goal. On the one hand, who could deny that the complete eradication of a disease is a positive achievement? On the other hand, who can deny that complete eradication thus far is very rare, and that there may be unforeseen consequences to eradication, such as the lack of defence against rogue infections?

Looking at eradication from a larger, less immediate perspective, many public health experts have asked whether the pursuit of the eradication of specific human diseases, one by one, is the best way to improve health in the international arena. Is eradication worth the intense effort it takes to achieve? Is complete eradication the best way to achieve human health, especially in poor countries where most eradication campaigns are carried out? What are the costs as well as the benefits of eradication? Are there alternative and more effective approaches to disease that are overlooked or marginalized by the intense concentration on eradication? Is the concept of the complete extinction of a biological agent or a disease in some kind of tension or even in contradiction with modern environmentalism and ecology? Has eradication become 'eradicationism', a faith, or a utopian dream, rather than a practical solution to ill health in human populations?

Given the historical record, it is perhaps understandable that many historians of public health and medicine view the concept of absolute disease eradication negatively. They point especially to the Malaria Eradication Programme (the MEP, led by the World Health Organization from 1955 to 1969), the largest eradication campaign of them all, which ended in failure and which they judge to have been based on insufficient scientific knowledge, false analogies and Western hubris.

But is this judgement entirely right? There are those who disagree, who think that the malaria eradication campaign deserves a more positive assessment. In a letter to *Science* in 2008, for example, Dr Timothy Baker, of Johns Hopkins University, pointed to the case of India, the country that had the single largest malaria eradication programme, and where malaria morbidity and mortality fell dramatically in the post-Second World War decades. Even though eradication was not achieved, malaria incidence was reduced from an estimated 100 million cases a year, and one million deaths in 1951, to less than 1,000 deaths a year 50 years later (in a population double the size of what it had been before). WHO today gives a higher figure of 15,000 malaria deaths a year (while other experts would put the figure even higher). Nevertheless, the drop in malaria deaths, Baker argues, 'underscores the value of the malaria program'.[8]

Meanwhile, of the estimated 300–500 million infections and one million deaths that still occur each year worldwide from malaria, 90 per cent occur in Sub-Saharan Africa, an area of the world that was essentially left out of the malaria eradication effort and is today the chief focus of international health aid. Does the contrast between India and Africa suggest what a single-disease malaria eradication programme could achieve, even if the programme never met the absolutist goals it had originally set itself? Is the time right for another try?

The answer given recently by Bill and Melinda Gates to this question is yes. In October of 2007, they startled their audience at an annual forum on malaria by announcing their intention to shift the focus of their anti-malaria work from the goal of control, to malaria eradication. They made it clear that in referring to eradication, they were using the term in its technical, absolutist sense. Since the Bill and Melinda Gates Foundation is by far the largest philanthropy working in global health today, with an annual spending budget that is bigger than that of the WHO itself, the Gates have an unprecedented power to shape the international health agenda, and so when they speak, they are listened to. 'Did they really say . . . eradication?', was the surprised reaction among many malaria experts present at the meeting, who took the view, according to reporters, that malaria eradication, 'though a noble goal, is simply unachievable'. The Director-General of WHO, Dr Margaret Chan, however, leapt to her feet to applaud the Gates's bold initiative.[9]

So is eradication a useful end-point to set for malaria, or is it yet another example of hubris and over-confidence in scientific approaches to disease? Does defining an absolute goal, an ideal, help focus efforts in the health field and sharply reduce the burden of a specific disease? Or does such a project lead almost inevitably to disappointment? What place should eradication have in the new era of globalization and global health?

My aim in this book is to answer some of these questions. When we speak of eradication campaigns, we are speaking of a characteristic form of public health intervention that has put its stamp on public health in the international arena. Historically, the adoption of eradication of disease as a goal has reflected enormous confidence in medical science and technical interventions, in the possibilities of international cooperation, and in public health know-how. At the same time, the sheer difficulty of achieving the absolutist goal makes eradication's pursuit as a key strategy in international health highly problematic.

My goal, then, is to identify the characteristic features of an influential model of public health, and to evaluate eradication's histories for what we might call their 'useful ambiguities'.

An Arch-eradicationist: Dr Fred L. Soper

Today, certain criteria have been established for deciding which diseases are potentially suitable for eradication. For instance, at a Dahlem Workshop held in Berlin in 1997 (twenty years after the last case of naturally occurring smallpox was identified), the criteria were divided into three – the biological, the economic and the political. The biological factors include the question of whether a non-human host or 'reservoir' of the disease exists (if so, eradication is extremely difficult, or even impossible, depending on the nature of the animal hosts); whether the disease is easily diagnosed; and whether an efficient method of intervention exists to stop transmission. Economic criteria relate to the assessment of the financial burdens the disease imposes on populations, and on cost-benefit analyses of eradication versus continued control. Political criteria relate to such things as the political salience of the disease, and the political will to achieve eradication.[10]

When we look at eradication historically, however, over the course of its twentieth century history, the selection of diseases looks much more 'messy', with decisions being shaped less by carefully weighed desiderata than by circumstantial events, often on the basis of incomplete knowledge of the disease in question, and under the influence of powerful metaphors of disease invasion. Little united the diseases medically and biologically; in addition, some of the diseases selected for the most intense efforts at eradication would simply not be candidates today on purely biological grounds (for example, yellow fever, because it has an animal reservoir of the virus, making it impossible to eradicate short of deliberately eradicating many animal species as well, which is virtually impossible and environmentally unacceptable). Eradication's histories are in fact many. They include the history of empire; the history of medical science and its technologies; the history of changing definitions of the 'public' in the 'public health'; the history of international public health agencies, and their ideologies and leadership; the history of the Cold War; the history of the shift from 'international health' to 'global health' and many others.

Aspects of these histories have been covered by many historians; there are also accounts of various parts of the story of eradication. The work of the Reed Board in Havana on yellow fever has been a particular favourite. The work of the Rockefeller Foundation's eradication campaigns in the 1920s and '30s is increasingly studied.[11] Hookworm has emerged in the historical literature more recently (but yaws almost not at all).[12] Malaria has been the subject of several excellent histories in recent years, with different aspects being emphasized according to the interest of the writer, providing, for example, a broad overview of the ecological and social history of malaria, as in Packard's recent and compelling book, or close examination of the post-war eradication campaign in a single country, as in Cueto's excellent study of malaria eradication in Mexico.[13]

No book, however, has attempted to tell the story of eradication as an idea *per se*, from its beginning in the early twentieth century to its present day incarnation in current eradication campaigns.[14] This is what my book aims to do.

In telling this story, I have used the life and career of an arch-eradicationist, Dr Fred Lowe Soper (1893–1977), as a constant reference point and as a means to give the book its chronological structure and narrative arc. In effect, I have tried to view the unfolding of eradication as a philosophy through his eyes, while at the same time keeping a critical distance from his point of view.

Soper was an American public health official whose life spanned the twentieth century.[15] He was a leading proponent of disease eradication in its absolute sense, and a man associated with some of the key eradication campaigns of the modern era. His life exemplified the new style of public health that emerged in this period – the international expert who, confident in his knowledge, moves from country to country, and from disease to disease, in quest of a world free from infection. Given to action, Soper seized on the possibilities opened up by developments in bacteriology, parasitology and the vector theory of disease that had emerged in the early twentieth century, and took to heart the view of the Rockefeller Foundation that the purpose of public health was the practical application of existing knowledge.

Born in 1893, one of eight children in a Midwest family, Fred L. Soper graduated in medicine from the Benjamin Rush School of Medicine in Chicago in 1918 before being almost immediately recruited to join the international health work of the Rockefeller Foundation (RF). Despite the almost boundless faith that the foundation had in American expertise and know-how, Soper in fact knew little about the problems and diseases facing poor populations. In fact, pretty much all he knew of tropical medicine he acquired in a three-week course in parasitology held at the School of Public Health and Hygiene at the Johns Hopkins University in Baltimore, before the RF sent him in 1920 to Brazil and then Paraguay, for years of disease control work in the field.

Rapidly becoming fluent in Spanish, and later in Portuguese, he gained years of detailed field experience in a number of tropical diseases; learned to exercise his authority over pathogens, insects and people; acquired confidence in his own judgement; and was given considerable scope to use it, in taking charge and administering large and complicated public health programmes. For several years he directed Brazil's entire yellow fever eradication programme.

Tall, with an almost military bearing, and at times a rather formal manner, Soper was charismatic, determined and meticulous. He made many enemies in the course of his career because of his dogmatic insistence on his own viewpoint; Dr Alan Gregg, another young RF doctor who overlapped with Soper in Brazil in the early years, described him as a 'very rough and tumble Kansan' who was 'too domineering to suit my fancy'.[16] But Soper also made many friends in Latin America, especially in Brazil where he spent so many years; he had a good sense of humour, and his self-certainty and energetic personality attracted as well as put off many people. He was physically tireless, capable of riding rickety cars, old buses, mules or horses for days to reach distant places in the rural hinterland in the pursuit of epidemiological data; of camping out in rough conditions; and of pushing himself to get to the bottom of public health puzzles.

He was an exacting leader, as demanding of others as of himself; he was once described as 'perhaps the most successful field general the Rockefeller Foundation ever had'.[17] Dr Marcolino Candau, the second Director General of WHO and a colleague from Soper's Brazil days, recalled at Soper's retirement dinner Soper's 'slave-driving leadership'.[18] In Brazil, he was known as 'the commander'.[19]

From a lifetime of work in international public health carried out in Latin America, North Africa, the Mediterranean and eventually even the Far East, Soper emerged as a man absolutely possessed by what he believed was a radical, even a revolutionary, idea – the idea of the possibility of the complete eradication of disease.[20] Developing his ideas from successes and failures in the field, Soper championed complete eradication as a panacea for the world's public health problems. In his own lifetime, he saw the reputation of eradication as a goal in international public health recover from a nadir in the late 1920s, to rise to a high-point of acceptance in the post-war period. This rise in popularity of the concept was widely attributed to Soper because, according to one commentator, it was Soper who 'showed that the eradication concept was feasible'.[21] Soper was the arch-eradicationist of the twentieth century, a man whom the historian of public health, John Duffy, characterizes as a 'secular medical missionary' who was convinced of the righteousness of the cause of eradication and who 'brooked no interference'.[22] The well-known British malariologist, Dr L. Bruce-Chwatt, was more generous, calling Soper 'one of the grand seigneurs of international public health'.[23]

Soper became a proponent of eradication in the 1930s and '40s when, as head of some of the Rockefeller Foundation's most important public health campaigns in Latin America, he became convinced that he had developed the technical methods needed to achieve the complete eradication of yellow fever and malaria by eradicating their mosquito vectors (this was even before DDT was on the scene). Following the Second World War, during which he worked on typhus and malaria in Africa and Italy on secondment to the US Army, and was one of the first to test the power of the new insecticide, DDT, in disease control, Soper took his eradicationist philosophy to the Pan American Health Organization (PAHO), which he directed from 1947–59, and which under his leadership greatly expanded its budget, personnel and activities, especially in launching eradication campaigns against yaws, yellow fever, malaria and smallpox.

In 1949, PAHO was made the WHO's Regional Office in the Americas (the only such regional office at that time).[24] Because of this link between PAHO and WHO, Soper was influential in the decision made by WHO in 1955 to launch the Malaria Eradication Programme (MEP). Latin America ended up being one of the regions where malaria eradication was most consistently pursued. Soper also put the energies of PAHO behind smallpox eradication efforts in the Americas, and later behind the WHO global Smallpox Eradication Programme, announced in 1959. After his retirement he travelled widely, lecturing on the goals and methods of eradication. PAHO maintained its leadership role in promoting eradication efforts, launching, for instance, the effort to eliminate polio in the Western Hemisphere in 1985, a campaign that who endorsed at the worldwide level a few years later.

Soper's reputation suffered when the MEP faltered in the late 1960s, when it was realized that complete eradication was probably unachievable, and the programme was scaled back to one of control. He died in 1977, before smallpox eradication was finally achieved, but with his faith in the idea still intact. Many years before, on a visit to New Delhi to assess the support for eradication campaigns, Soper was quizzed about eradication. 'You've never heard me say that eradication is easy', he said. His interlocutor rejoined, 'I've heard people say it is impossible'.[25]

But the eventual success with smallpox, and the prospect of future successes against other infectious diseases, suggest that Soper's life is ripe for reconsideration. He is in many respects a 'forgotten figure' in public health, unknown outside international public health circles (and even within these circles memories are short). For instance, in the RF's triumphalist book, *Yellow Fever*, published in 1951 and celebrating the RF's development of the yellow fever vaccine, Soper's preventive work occupies a rather minor place, despite the years he spent in the field. This was because the book was written in celebration of the final conquest of yellow fever, which the foundation viewed as a result of the successful identification of the yellow fever virus and the discovery of a yellow fever vaccine, in 1927 and 1937 respectively; this 'virus-centred' history of the RF's yellow fever, as Löwy calls it, leaves little space for Soper (not even a photo).[26] By the time the book appeared, the RF was moving away from practical public health work, and had abandoned the goal of eradicating the *Aedes aegypti* mosquito, to which Soper was completely committed.[27]

More recently, however, Malcolm Gladwell, in a *New Yorker* article, eulogized Soper as a type of public health expert that has almost disappeared – heroic, capable of almost super-human and single-minded (if at times also bloody-minded) dedication and effort, blessed with tremendous self-belief and with an almost fanatical faith in the humanitarian significance and scientific feasibility of the eradication of disease.[28]

Whether Soper is to be eulogized or criticized is matter of judgement and I will make mine clear. This book is not, however, a biography of Soper, but a biography of a concept, or idea, or style of conducting public health in the twentieth century. For my purposes, Soper has the merit of being a larger-than-life character, with many strengths as well as weaknesses. He left a massive archive, and his accounts of eradication and of the many public health campaigns he conducted, in Latin America, North Africa and Europe, make his life and work a rich resource for the historian. As a chief architect of the idea of eradication, Soper occupies the centre stage throughout this history of eradication.

But thc book is also more than an account of Soper's career. Many other figures who participated in the eradication story in public health, as friendly or critical colleagues of Soper's, are given their due. The book also looks beyond Soper's life, to examine the history of eradication and competing models of 'health and development' after his death, after smallpox eradication and into the present moment, as post-smallpox eradication campaigns inch their way to potential closure, and new diseases are put forward as candidates for eradication.

Eradication and 'Eradicationism'

Soper's zeal for eradication also serves another purpose in this book, in that it draws attention to the absolutism that both defines, and limits, modern notions of disease eradication.

To Soper eradication did not mean some vague or general reduction in disease incidence or prevalence; eradication to him was an all-or-nothing view of disease, a vision of the perfectibility of the human condition. Half-measures would not do. 'Once committed to eradication, all [disease] that continues to occur above zero has to be explained', he said.[29] The essence of eradication was the 'struggle to zero'.[30] Malcolm Gladwell calls him admirable because he was indeed an absolutist in his determination to exterminate diseases from the face of the earth.

To Soper, to accept eradication as a goal in public health implied a fundamental shift in psychology or in attitude toward disease, especially at the point when a disease targeted for eradication has almost disappeared; this is when most people tend to lose interest in continuing on to complete the job of eradication, and instead shift their interest and energies to other pressing public health tasks. To Soper, though, mere reduction to *near* invisibility of a disease in a population would not do; it was only at this point that the serious work of eradication actually began. Eradication had to be absolute.

With Fred L. Soper, in fact, we are dealing not just with eradication, but with 'eradicationism' – a belief system, a faith or a utopian dream of a disease-free world. As Jeffery has said, 'Eradicationism is an absolute term that demands a certain degree of perfection'.[31] The trouble with perfection is that it is hard to achieve; the world is not perfect, human beings are not perfect. More prosaically one could say that eradicationism is countered by the realities of evolutionary adaptation and ecology, and by the ever-shifting balance we achieve between human beings and disease organisms; it is countered by the facts of human history.

Though the philosophy of eradication had its critics from the start, sustained opposition became evident among the new environmentalists in the 1960s, when eradicationism was at its height. The new romance of the environment, the new ecology of the environmentalists, was fundamentally at odds with the 'war against nature' that is inherent to the eradicationist philosophy. The biologist and ecologist, René Dubos, in 1965 criticized eradication campaigns on these grounds, predicting that 'eradication programs will eventually become a curiosity item on library shelves, just as have all social utopias'.[32]

Dubos was proven wrong, as the success of smallpox eradication showed. In one form or another, disease eradication programmes are probably here to stay in international public health. They have powerful advocates, and are a goal-setting method of tackling health in poor countries, methods whose benefits and costs will continue to be debated and assessed. But in a larger sense, Dubos was without a doubt right to suggest that, for much of its history, eradicationism has been in tension with other modes of public health. This raises critical questions about eradication as a model in public health, and its adaptability, or otherwise, to fresh currents in public health thought.

In my judgement, merely to criticize eradication efforts as such seems wrong – a form of resignation to, or acceptance of, diseases in poor countries that would not be tolerated in rich ones. Removal of smallpox, or malaria, surely must be seen as a good in itself; it does not have to be evaluated only in relation to whether it increases economic productivity.

Yet the critics of eradication also have their point. Technically based eradication campaigns are not enough. Local ecologies, social conditions, political institutions, economic factors – all need to be taken into account, and this makes the task of completing an eradication campaign extremely difficult. Basic health infrastructures are found to be essential. Hostilities between the two 'camps' – pro- and anti-eradicationist – have often been intense and are historically understandable, but are now overdone. Today, we can find examples of eradication campaigns that, while specific in their focus on single diseases and dedicated to pursuing the goal of zero incidence, manage at the same time to correspond in their style of organization more closely to the ideals of preventive medicine and basic health care.

Eradication and basic health care need not be conflicting logics, and we should be able to imagine, politically, the integration of the two, so as to form mutually reinforcing policies.

1 Eradication and Public Health

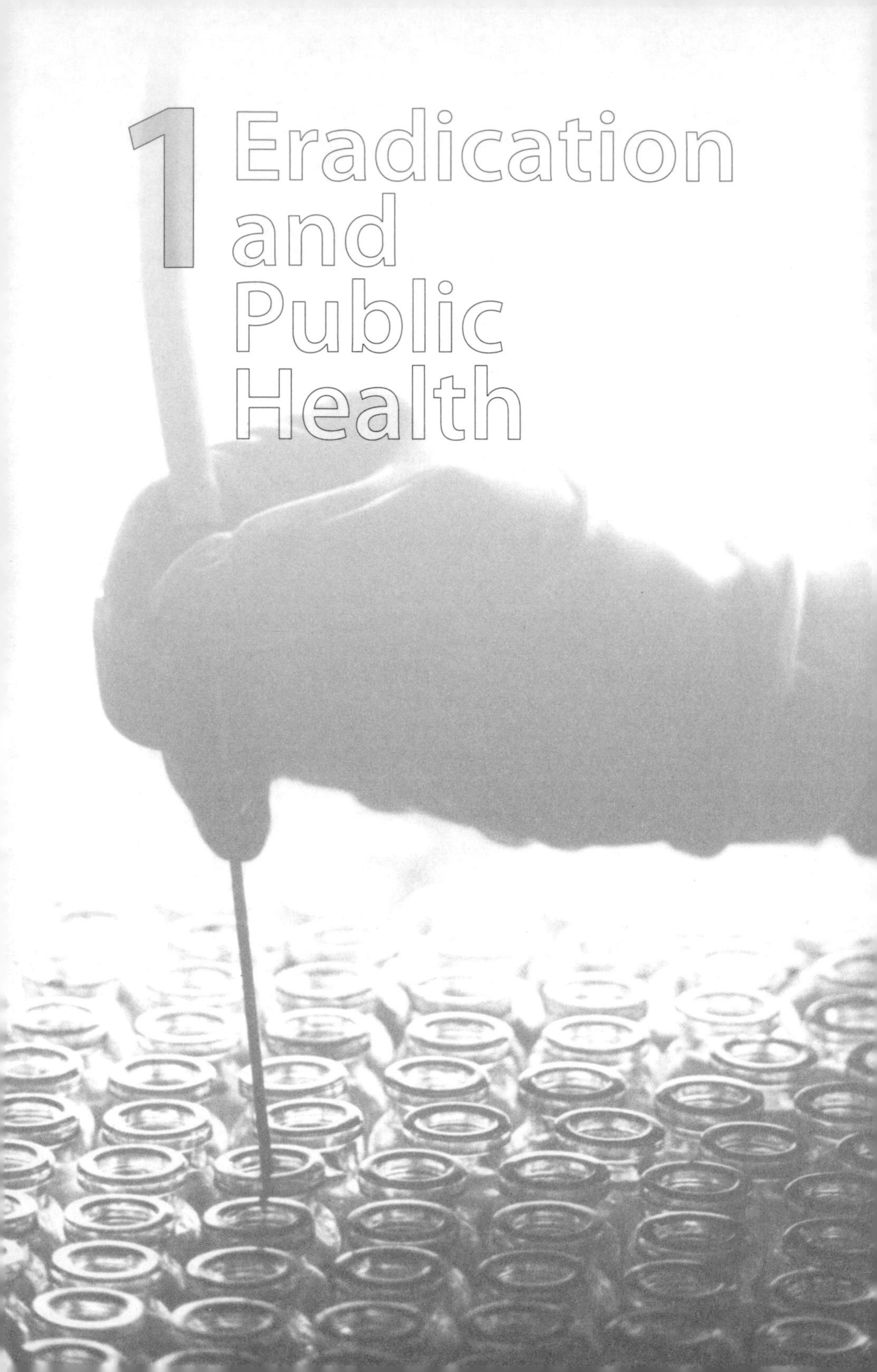

Two revolutions frame the discussion in this first chapter.

The first is the microbiological revolution that took place between roughly 1870 and the 1930s, a revolution that changed the way doctors thought about the causes of disease and the methods that might be used to control them. The second is the revolution in mortality and morbidity that has occurred on an almost global scale since the late nineteenth century.[1] The question is: What is the connection between the two?

Taking a broad overview of the second revolution, we see that there has been a more than doubling of average life expectancy in the world, from roughly 30 years' life expectancy at birth around 1830, to 67 years today, with some of the richest countries reaching life expectancies of over 80. These improvements in health began first in the industrializing, largely capitalist countries of Western Europe in the second half of the nineteenth century. Since 1950 the greatest gains in life expectancy have occurred in developing countries (starting as they did from much lower levels in life expectancy and higher levels of disease and mortality rates than those found in the developed countries). Such trends are not irreversible, as we know from Sub-Saharan Africa today where, by the year 2000, the devastating impact of the epidemic of HIV/AIDS, and the return of infectious diseases once believed to have been controlled, such as malaria and tuberculosis, combined with acute poverty and deteriorating political and economic conditions, have reduced overall life expectancy at birth to 47 years.[2] Nevertheless, in most areas of the world the gains in life expectancy have been remarkable. In his recent global survey of what he describes as the 'retreat of death and the democratization of survival into old age', James C. Riley goes as far as to call the mortality revolution, or 'health transitions' as they are referred to, as 'the crowning achievement of the modern era, surpassing wealth, military power, and political stability in import'.[3]

The question is: what explains such fundamental transformations in health and longevity? Specifically, what part have public health interventions, especially those based on the medical sciences of bacteriology, parasitology and the vector theory of disease transmission, played in bringing about such improvements? How have eradication campaigns contributed to, or otherwise affected, the health transitions?

I hope that by opening with these two revolutions, in medicine and health, this book can make a contribution to what is obviously a major debate of our day – the debate about the sources or causes of health and ill-health in human populations.

Disease Eradication and the Epistemological Revolution in Medicine and Public Health

Some historians consider the use of the word 'revolution' to describe the developments in bacteriology as somewhat of a misnomer. This is because the innovations in medical theory introduced by the new germ theory associated with scientists such as Louis Pasteur and Robert Koch, starting in the 1860s and '70s, were absorbed by different medical communities and different medical specialties only slowly and unevenly. There were also many continuities linking the pre-bacteriological and the post-bacteriological eras, especially in the area of practical public health policies, such as the isolation of the sick, quarantines, disinfection and fumigation.[4]

Nevertheless, conceptually, the new microbiological sciences signalled a revolution by shifting fundamentally the understanding of disease causation from what Stephen Kunitz calls a 'multiple weakly sufficient' model to a 'necessary' causal model.[5] Before the development of bacteriology, sanitarians had thought of infectious diseases as arising from multiple noxious sources, called 'miasmas' or 'effluvia', which were thought to emanate from the places in which people lived. These miasmas were conceptualized not as living organisms that reproduced themselves, but as invisible poisons of some kind, arising out of decaying matter, dirt and damp and swampy earth. They were multiple and weakly causal in the sense that the predicted effect – disease – only sometimes followed from the conditions. The goal of the sanitarians was to clean up man-made habitats (removing rubbish, cleaning up water supplies) and natural environments (by draining swampy lands), thereby reducing the miasmas and with them disease. Broad-based efforts to clean up the environment in these ways had the effect of reducing water and sewage-borne microorganisms that caused disease, even though their role in disease transmission was not understood at the time.

With the development of bacteriology and parasitology, the sanitarian model of disease was replaced over time by a narrower concept of disease causation, focused on the microorganisms themselves as the necessary agents in disease. The 1880s and '90s saw a flurry of discoveries of the microscopic living agents of numerous infectious diseases – including leprosy, tuberculosis, cholera, anthrax, typhoid and diphtheria. The discovery of microorganisms of disease led in turn to their experimental manipulation (by means of heat, or chemical treatment) to produce preventive vaccines (most famously, Pasteur's rabies vaccine in 1885, the first vaccine to be discovered since Jenner's smallpox vaccine in 1796), and also protective sera that could reduce the negative effects of infection after the fact (for example, the anti-diphtheria serum, introduced in 1882).

'Koch's postulates', named after Germany's leading bacteriologist, encapsulated the epistemological shift involved in microbiology. In a famous paper in 1882, Robert Koch identified the tubercle bacillus for the first time. More than this, Koch developed new staining methods to make microscopic bacteria visible, and a culture medium for the propagation of bacteria. By inoculating susceptible animals with bacteria, he proceeded to reproduce the symptoms of the disease in the animals and then recover from them the same tubercle bacterium, cultivating it once more in pure culture, thus proving that the bacillus was the fundamental 'cause' of the disease.

By setting out the necessary conditions for proof of a germ cause of a disease, Koch's postulates in effect located the disease in the pathogen itself.[6] Before the tubercle bacillus was identified, what we now call tuberculosis included many different conditions and terms, such as phthisis and scrofula; identifying the disease meant relying on very varied descriptions of clinical symptoms or pathological investigations. After 1882, a new unitary disease known as 'tuberculosis' emerged, based on the presence of the tubercle bacillus. Many other diseases were similarly renamed in recognition of the new epistemology. For example, 'elephantiasis', a disease that took its name from the characteristic elephant-like swellings of the limbs and genitalia found among people living in the tropics, was re-named 'filariasis' after the tiny filarial worms that were first identified in the 1870s as the cause of the infection.

A very important extension of microbiology came from the unravelling of the role of parasites in disease, such as the protozoa of malaria or the trypanosomes in African sleeping sickness. In addition, experimental work demonstrated the unexpected role played by insects in disease transmission, a finding of special significance to the emergence of disease eradication. Malaria transmission to human beings by the bite of female mosquitoes belonging to the anopheline genus was worked out by the British army doctor, Ronald Ross, and the Italian malariologist, Grassi, between 1897 and 1898. This was followed in 1900 by the Reed Commission's proof by experimental human inoculations that the bite of the female mosquito belonging to the *Aedes aegypti* genus (then known as *Stegomyia fasciata*) conveyed yellow fever to man.[7] These discoveries led almost immediately to the suggestion that getting rid of the insects would get rid of the diseases.

Very quickly, in fact, physicians and public health officials seized on the new germ and vector theory for the possibilities it offered in making what they saw as effective and economical attacks on diseases, by tailoring interventions to interrupt the weak point in the chain of causal transmission – whether by drugs, chemical attacks on breeding places of insects or other means. It was rather easy, in the circumstances, to dismiss as old-fashioned, and even irrelevant, the broad efforts to clean up sewage and provide clean drinking water that reformers and sanitarians had once engaged in. Dr Walter Reed's and Dr William C. Gorgas's conclusion that dirt had nothing to do with yellow fever transmission (but mosquitoes did) was very influential in this regard. Charles Chapin, the leader of the 'new public health' in the state of Rhode Island in the United States, cited the Havana story, arguing that Reed's and Gorgas's work 'drove the last nail in the coffin of the filth theory of disease'.[8]

It would be a mistake to think, however, that everyone agreed about the policy choices that followed from the new bacteriological and parasitological model – that disease control methods from now on followed a single script based on the logic of the new epistemology. The new microbiology opened up not one, but a variety, of policy choices, which tended to reflect not just medical judgement, but also the social values, ideological outlooks and political positions of the people involved. Malaria, for instance, could be said by the early 1900s to be caused by four different kinds of plasmodia (the single-celled microorganisms belonging to the protozoa and known as vivax, falciparum, ovale and malariae), which produce the four different kinds of malarial fevers known in human beings (falciparum malaria being the most deadly). Malaria can also be said to be caused by the 30 to 40 different species of anopheline mosquitoes, the females of which actually convey the plasmodia of malaria to human beings through their bites.

But malaria is also caused, or determined by, larger (or deeper) social, ecological and geographical factors such as particular geographical locations which, by virtue of their characteristic climate, terrain and overall ecology, encourage the breeding of particularly 'efficient' or deadly malaria-transmitting mosquitoes (for example, the *Anopheles gambiae* species in found in many parts of Africa); malaria is caused by poverty, because poverty, among its many effects, means people live in poor houses that lack the kind of windows that lend themselves to proper screening against biting mosquitoes. Poverty also stops people from getting to health clinics (if they exist) and from obtaining life-saving anti-malaria drugs, or paying for them; or from purchasing insecticide-saturated bed nets. Poverty causes malnutrition and reduced immunity to disease.

These different causes are all relevant to understanding malaria. We could add others. Development projects often alter patterns of human settlement by opening up new labour markets, which in turn bring non-immune, highly susceptible, people into malarial regions, often with disastrous results, such as malaria epidemics. Development projects themselves may alter local ecologies, which may in turn encourage (rather than suppress) anopheline mosquito breeding, thus increasing the risk of malaria to human populations. These geographical and ecological factors all play a part in determining whether and where people are likely to suffer from the disease of malaria.

Public health policy choices about how to proceed in order to reduce disease incidence are therefore not a given, but a matter of judgement about the most vulnerable points in a disease's transmission, the difficulty of carrying out a particular intervention, and an assessment of how long-term the impact of particular kinds of interventions may be. Groups of public health activists who share the bacteriological/parasitological understanding of disease may nonetheless disagree about what to do. In the first three decades of the twentieth century, for instance, Italian malariologists, many of whom had contributed to the development of the mosquito theory of malaria transmission, nonetheless continued to think of malaria less as a 'mosquito' disease than as a 'social disease' rooted in multiple factors of poverty. They focused their control efforts on protecting human beings with quinine and improving their living conditions. Rockefeller Foundation malariologists, on the other hand, tended to follow Ronald Ross in seeing malaria as fundamentally a mosquito disease and concentrated their interventions on finding new methods of controlling or eliminating mosquitoes or their larvae. My point here is that the public health policies derived from a particular scientific theory are variable, and tend to reflect the political contexts and ideological and other working assumptions of the groups involved. Science does not operate in a value-free or neutral environment, but is given meaning, and creates new meanings, in settings that are specifically social, economic and political as well as intellectual.[9]

Historically, however, we tend to find that the microbiological revolution was associated with more narrowly focused methods of disease control than in the previous era of public health. Attention was increasingly brought to bear on the proximate causes of infection, such as pathogens and vectors, while by-passing, if not actually ignoring, the deeper, and more intractable, social, economic and political factors that together with biological ones are responsible for ill-health. This approach has had a very long-lasting influence on the practice of medicine and public health, from the early twentieth century to the present.

In particular it defined the approach of most eradication campaigns, which were specifically designed as time-bound, technical and expert interventions to eliminate diseases across the world, one by one, without engaging with the social and economic determinants of ill-health. The words 'eradicate' and 'eradication' began to be used in their more strict and absolute sense in the first decade of the twentieth century, as discoveries in the new public health took off, with parasites and even hitherto completely unknown human diseases being discovered by the new experimental medicine.[10] In 1909, Rockefeller money financed a Sanitary Commission for the Eradication of Hookworm Disease; this was followed in 1915 by its Yellow Fever Commission, which set out for Latin America to investigate the possibility of eradicating yellow fever from the entire Western Hemisphere. The next year, in 1916, the American statistician Frederick L. Hoffman presented a 'Plea and a Plan for the Eradication of Malaria Throughout the Western Hemisphere'. Further discoveries in medicine and technology in the Second World War, such as penicillin, chloroquine and DDT, extended the reach of science-based public health, and led in the second half of the twentieth century to some of the most extensive eradication campaigns ever seen.

The basic model at work in all of these different campaigns was that of etiological universalism; wherever the disease in question was found, it was presumed to have the same cause and be open to elimination by the same methods, regardless of differences in the class, economic and geographical situations of the human populations involved. It was in this sense that eradication became international.

The Mortality Revolution and Public Health

Eradication campaigns have always had their defenders and their detractors, with their popularity understandably declining when an eradication campaign falters, and rising when the goal appears to be within reach. Underlying these swings in attitude are questions of feasibility, effect and alternatives. Is eradication feasible, given the technical, economic and political demands it makes on societies and international aid? What effect does removing a specific disease from a population have, beyond the very important one of simply removing a single and burdensome infection from populations? Is eradication the kind of public health intervention that contributes to overall health improvements, or does it tend to override or close out alternative paths to human well being?

In effect, these questions boil down to the issue of what the relationship is between public health interventions and secular improvements in human health. Those involved in public health naturally enough work with the assumption that their actions matter a great deal; and indeed, one has only to think of the success in reducing HIV/AIDS in Brazil, through public health activism and the free distribution of retroviral drugs, and compare this outcome with, say, HIV/AIDS in South Africa, to appreciate their point.[11]

Yet paradoxically, perhaps, the dominant paradigm in public health says otherwise. This paradigm, often referred to in public health circles as the 'McKeown thesis', after the British historical epidemiologist Thomas McKeown, whose popular and accessible books were published in the 1970s, still sets the terms of the debate today. McKeown maintained that the mortality revolution that occurred between roughly 1860 and the 1930s in Britain owed little if anything to medicine or targeted public health interventions, and almost everything to economic growth and rising standards of living, especially improved nutrition. Generalizing from the specific case of Britain, a universal and optimistic economic thesis has developed that the rising tide of economic growth raises all human beings in health.

One reason for the enduring appeal of this economic thesis is that in many ways it feels intuitively right. The recognition of the correlation between poverty and the ill-health was what had spurred the nineteenth-century sanitarians to action in France and England in the first place. Looking at the present world picture, we know that poor countries generally have poorer health than rich ones; and poor individuals, classes or ethnic minorities within rich countries have worse health than rich ones.

Nevertheless, there is more to be said about the economic theory of health.

McKeown began to write on health transitions at a time (in the 1960s) when he and others like him were increasingly critical of the biomedical and curative emphasis in health within Britain's National Health Service (NHS), which he believed was at the expense of broader economic and social approaches.[12] Using the first and historic mortality revolution in England as his central case study, McKeown emphasized its coincidence in time with the first industrial revolution and stressed the positive effect that economic growth had had on health. From a low overall level of life expectancy of around 30 years in the 1830s, mortality figures in England and Wales began to improve in the 1870s, as the more positive effects of industrialization were generalized and the toll taken by infectious diseases declined. Nevertheless, improvements came very slowly, with many variations across classes and regions within Britain. By 1900, life expectancy at birth had risen to an average of about 46 years (with lower figures for manufacturing cities like Manchester [36] and London [44]).[13] By 1950, the figure had risen to about 70 years. Looking back on this mortality revolution, McKeown concluded that none of the improvements could be attributed to the tools of curative biomedicine, such as drugs like penicillin, for the simple reason they were not available before the 1940s. By a process of exclusion, McKeown then went much further, to eliminate in addition the contributions of the sanitarians to the health improvements, concluding that improvements in per capita income, which translated into improved overall nutrition, were the major cause, or prime motor, of the mortality revolution.[14]

However compelling this economic thesis seems, many historians have now come to feel that McKeown's wholesale dismissal of public health interventions in bringing about improvements in health is a step too far, and indeed historically and conceptually misleading.[15]

After all, an equally compelling historical coincidence is that between the mortality revolution in England and the sanitary movement itself. Numerous historians, such as Simon Szreter and Anne Hardy, and social theorists such as Stephen Kunitz, have joined the fray, and in doing so turned a sceptical eye on the economic determinist theory of health. They argue, on the basis of detailed epidemiological and historical studies, that McKeown got many of the details of health history wrong (in overestimating the decline of tuberculosis) and neglected or downplayed many significant public health interventions that ameliorated the health of populations. Their conclusion is that, though economic factors are clearly important to health, the effects of economic growth are often negative in their impact on populations, and connected not to improved health but rather to what Szreter calls the four 'Ds' – Disruption, Deprivation, Disease and Death. Szreter and Moody's examination of the data on the impact of the industrial revolution in Britain in the decades between 1780 and 1850 shows that there were increases, not decreases, in mortality in the 1830s, thus confirming Hobsbawm's pessimistic view of the initial impact of industrialization on the UK population. Not until the 1870s and '80s did urban mortality begin to really decline.[16] In these nineteenth-century circumstances, Szreter argues, government actions, and especially local government actions, were extremely significant in transforming, through piecemeal reforms, the potential of economic wealth into actual health in populations.[17]

These actions were not the automatic result of the accumulation of economic wealth; on the contrary, manufacturers often resisted the costs of making outlays of capital to improve sanitation.[18] Rather they were the outcome of many different trends. The sanitation movement had many sources; it included diverse groups of reformers, including engineers, lawyers, doctors and some politicians. In reaction to the poor and overcrowded housing created by often unregulated industrial and economic 'development', to the polluted water supplies caused by manufacturing processes, and the equally polluted air in manufacturing towns like Manchester, and motivated by a mix of factors, from fear of epidemics in crowded cities, to humanitarian concerns for the lot of the those least able to protect themselves, sanitarians and others pushed to introduce sanitary and public health legislation. Hygienists and sanitarians on the whole put aside the problem of social inequality their investigations revealed, to focus on more 'manageable' reforms, such as the appointment of municipal Medical Officers of Health to monitor and deal with infectious diseases, municipally funded investments in water companies, the provision of effective sewage systems, and the extension of smallpox vaccination. Other important legislation was passed to improve housing, to ensure the supply of clean milk, to set up a system of inspection of food, to regulate filth and to establish special services for tuberculosis, venereal diseases and infant welfare.

Szreter also refers to more political developments, for example, the ability of groups such as trade unions to organize and represent themselves. The point is that, looking at the first examples of health transitions in Europe, Szreter finds there was nothing automatic in the equation between economic growth and health; ecological disturbances caused by industrialization were connected to periods of human health setbacks and increased mortality rates before the 1850s, setbacks which belie any steady association between economic growth and improved health. In his recent book, *Health and Wealth: Studies in History and Policy*, Szreter expands the scope of his analysis to take in globalization and twentieth-century health transitions in developing countries, identifying many instances, such as the growth of megacity urban slums, where the full force of disruption, deprivation, ecological disturbance and disease are felt, and where deliberate public health and political actions have mitigated some of these effects.[19]

Stephen Kunitz, in his *The Health of Populations*, takes a broad and comparative view of the various explanations given for variations in health and health inequalities in different countries across the world, and also concludes by emphasizing the importance of deliberate social interventions. He argues that the larger context of the population is more significant to health outcomes than economic growth *per se*, especially the actions of governments, as it is governments that determine to a large extent the contexts in which populations live. It is their ability and readiness to protect – or not to protect – populations that is important. In this regard, he says, 'political culture and institutions have a profound effect that may well be more significant than the standard of living as measured by income per capita'.[20]

The studies, contra the McKeown economic thesis, draw attention to the political contexts and the variety of interventions that have led historically to improved health in populations, rather than a single, universal path. James Riley, for example, in his book *Rising Life Expectancy: A Global History* (2001), finds that, in achieving their health transitions from high mortality and morbidity and low life expectancy at birth, to low mortality and morbidity and high life expectancy, most countries have pursued one or more of six basic strategies: public health, medical care, income redistribution, improved nutrition, changes in household behaviour and increased education. For example, in its compressed or rapid health transition in the 1930s and '40s, Japan did not invest heavily in systems of sewage disposal characteristic of the British health transition at the end of the nineteenth century, yet the country nonetheless saw rapid improvements in life expectancy and declines in morbidity and mortality because of actions it took in other areas of sanitation and social intervention.[21]

Eradication and Health Transitions

Understandably, perhaps, given the coincidence in time between eradication campaigns and health transitions in the post-Second World War decades, eradicationists have at times taken credit for contributing to sweeping improvements in health.

These improvements were most striking in developing or post-colonial societies, starting as they did from much lower levels of health than Europe. According to figures on Latin America provided by Marcos Cueto, for instance, in Mexico the mortality rate declined from 21.8 deaths per 1,000 people in 1940–44, to 8.9/1,000 in 1965–70. Other countries showed similar gains – even poorer countries, like Guatemala, where the mortality rate fell from 28.5/1,000 to 15/1,000 in the same period. By 1965–70, life expectancy reached an average of 61.2 years in the entire region, with some countries reaching higher figures, such as Costa Rica (64 years), Argentina (68) and Uruguay (69).[22]

India provides another example of a post-Second World War (and in this case, post-independence) health transition. The national death rate had been about 32/1,000 in the 1940s, but by the 1960s it had dropped to 21/1,000. Life expectancy improved, from around 33 years in 1947 (roughly what it had been in England in 1830), increasing steadily through the decades into the start of the twenty-first century, by which time it had almost doubled to about 62.[23]

These health improvements coincided with the intensification of commitment to health in the post-war era. Many mass health programmes targeting specific diseases, without aiming for complete eradication, were carried out. Between 1948 and 1960, for instance, WHO vaccinated almost 100 million people in Asia with the BCG vaccine against tuberculosis.[24] The mass application of penicillin against yaws was another project in many poor countries. Among eradication campaigns, malaria was the most significant, since the disease was largely rural and considered a great impediment to agriculture and food production. According to Tim Dyson, for example, India in the 1940s had seen tens of millions of cases of malaria and perhaps hundreds of thousands of malaria deaths every year. The national malaria programme, launched in 1953 after Indian independence, had by 1965 reduced the malaria burden to only 100,000 active cases and perhaps no deaths.[25]

Since malaria and several other eradication efforts did not eventually meet their goal of absolute zero, they have tended to be dismissed as failures; but if thought of as mass disease reduction campaigns, alongside other mass health campaigns, then they can be seen to have achieved a great deal.

As Sunil Amrith points out, many commentators at the time drew direct causal links between the observed mortality declines and mass health campaigns. In a recent survey of the evidence on India's health transition, Leela Visaria draws the same conclusion. 'There is little doubt', she writes, 'that the reduction in malaria was a major factor behind the decline in the national crude death rate' between 1940s and the mid-1960s.[26] We can probably assume that, in other places too, the concentrated reductions in malaria brought about by eradication campaigns helped to reduce mortality and morbidity more generally. We know from pilot studies in Africa, for example, that when malaria incidence in children is reduced, overall morbidity from other diseases is also reduced.[27] We can also say that in many places the eradication campaigns represented the first introduction rural populations had to Western medicine and public health work – to drugs, immunization and insecticides.

Along these same lines, it is perhaps reasonable to assume that post-Second World War health transitions owed more to medical technologies than the health transitions did in nineteenth-century Europe, when drugs such as penicillin and chloroquine, insecticides such as DDT and immunizations against measles, polio, diphtheria, mumps and yellow fever did not exist. In Sub-Saharan Africa, for example, improvements in life expectancy appear to have depended quite strongly on biomedicine, compared to the UK's much earlier health transition, in which clean piped water, adequate sewage systems, new housing and labour laws all played a major part.[28]

Some commentators go further, arguing that mass health campaigns of this sort could bring about health transitions without waiting for economic development.[29] The line of causation, on this view, runs from the massive reduction (or eradication) of a particular disease, to economic growth, instead of the other way around. Among leading economists today who have taken up the cause of international health, Jeffrey Sachs is perhaps the most prominent in making this case (though not the case for eradication itself). John Luke Gallup and Sachs have calculated that intensely malarial countries have on average 1.3 per cent less growth in GDP per person per year than non-malarial countries. They have therefore concluded that lowering malaria prevalence, by making massive investments in a range of anti-malaria activities, from drugs to insecticide-saturated bed-nets, would greatly aid in stimulating economic growth.[30]

It is, however, extremely hard to disaggregate the contributions made by eradication to improvements in health from other social, political and economic changes going on simultaneously (improvements in income and food production).[31] As already noted, studies of the late nineteenth-century health transitions in Europe indicate that multiple factors were involved, and this seems to be the case with the health transitions in developing countries after the Second World War as well. In 1945–71 in post-independence India, for example, Visaria shows that the national government took an active role in promoting health, with programmes aimed at reducing cholera, plague, leprosy and tuberculosis, in addition to making large commitments to malaria and smallpox eradication. But the government simultaneously made considerable improvements in transport and food distribution, and imposed price controls on food, which prevented the famines that had so often followed the failure of the monsoons in the pre-independence period. The connections between the various factors in improvements in health, and the directions of influence, were obviously very complex, making up, however, at least for a critical period of time, a 'virtuous circle' of interactions.[32]

This is in keeping with the findings of Szreter and other historical demographers and social scientists that, as already shown, and in contradiction to the McKeown or economic thesis that the increase in per capita income is the prime mover in bringing about improvements in health, human agency is of fundamental importance in transforming the *potential* of economic growth into the *actual* health of populations. In making the case for the significance of human agency and specific social interventions, historical demographers have included, along with basic sanitation, such factors as access to education, the right to vote, and other supports which have a bearing on citizens' health. This is not to deny the significance of economic wealth in providing a basic platform of well being to populations; it is, however, to widen the definition of social and political interventions beyond what is traditionally included in public health and to emphasize the role of deliberate political choices.[33]

The work of the extremely influential Australian demographer, John C. Caldwell, on economically poor but nonetheless 'high performing' countries in health, such as Costa Rica and Sri Lanka, or the state of Kerala in India, is especially pertinent in this regard; he emphasizes the mix of factors involved in achieving low rates of mortality and high life expectancy despite low per capita incomes. The factors he highlights are a substantial degree of female autonomy (and a concern for maternal and infant health); a commitment to education; a high investment in health services; an open political system and a history of egalitarianism. Investments in health services he found to be extremely important, but with success depending not on new and expensive technologies but on the density, efficiency and availability of services (for example, health worker visits to pregnant women at the time of birth and immunization campaigns). Political and social commitments were equally significant (in providing food subsidies and a basic platform of nutrition for all those who needed it).[34]

Caldwell takes these findings as a critique of the McKeown economic thesis of health. His conclusions about the importance of relative social equality in poor but well-performing countries (in relation to health outcomes) are supported by studies of the relationship between health, social equality and inequality in rich countries as well. For instance, the British researcher, Richard Wilkinson, who is very well known for his studies of social inequalities in health, shows that in wealthy countries, like the UK or the USA, overall per capita income is much less significant to health than the size of the gap between rich and poor individuals and groups within a society. The argument is that unequal societies are unhealthy societies.[35]

Caldwell does not address the impact of eradication campaigns *per se* on the health transitions he examines. Trying to measure the independent contribution is, perhaps, to miss the point; it is the dynamic interaction *between* social, political, economic and public health activities and interventions that brings about population health.

We can though, I think, single out eradication campaigns as being historically at times among the weaker of the determinants, despite their scale and the resources they deployed. For, although they often resulted in sharp declines in the incidence of the diseases targeted, the campaigns were usually set up as autonomous operations organized independently of the basic health services of the country; they relied on specific, technical, usually biomedical interventions that were not always flexible enough to adapt to unexpected variations in the ecological and other conditions encountered; and they set such a high standard of success, namely absolute zero, that it was hard to sustain the political will or the financial resources the campaigns needed over the long haul, especially when countries had many other competing health needs. The result was in many cases the abandonment of the effort, and the eventual return of the diseases that had been reduced to near-zero by the campaigns. As the external sources of money dried up and foreign advisory staff left the country, little was left by way of a legacy in basic health infrastructure (though in many places the disease incidence was much lower than it had been before the commencement of the eradication effort, and remained lower for a considerable length of time, even decades).

The limitation of eradication as a style of conducting public health internationally was recognized by WHO after the failure to eradicate malaria globally in the late 1960s. New ideas about health care in the 1970s, and a renewed emphasis on social medicine, also came to the forefront in WHO circles, leading to a movement to make the development of Primary Health Care (PHC) rather than eradication campaigns the chief focus of WHO's efforts to improve international health. By this time many people had come to question the massive international commitment to vertically organized, 'expert' public health campaigns focused on specific diseases, one after the other. Especially in poor countries, where individuals usually suffered from many infections at once and not just the targeted disease, an eradication campaign seemed short-sighted and narrow. People lacked adequate public health infrastructures and access to general preventive and curative care, and it was not clear why such fundamentals of health care should take a secondary place to 'one-disease', top-down and often foreign-directed disease campaigns that absorbed so much of the resources available for health care in the targeted countries.

People asked whether alternative approaches to public health were being foreclosed by an over-reliance on the complete eradication of a disease as the dominant approach in international public health; whether mobilizing the huge resources – financial, technical, human – that were called for in eradication campaigns was the best or most effective use of human and financial capital. On the other side of the debate, there were, and are, those who argue that foregoing the removal of specific diseases in the name of another goal – putting in place a system of Primary Health Care, for example – which is also extremely difficult to achieve, is not a solution either.

This is not a debate that will come to an end soon. Today the world is experiencing what some people see as the most profound public health challenge of the last 50 years. The appearance of new infections, such as HIV/AIDS, and the less devastating but potentially very worrying swine flu, SARS and avian flu; the resurgence of diseases once thought controlled, such as malaria and tuberculosis; and actual declines in life expectancy in the poorest countries in the world, hit by political collapse and even failed states (meaning the collapse of a usable state in a country), environmental changes, including devastating droughts or floods, and the economic disruptions brought about by globalization – all raise questions about what is to be done to relieve the intolerable burdens on the poorest and most vulnerable populations in the world. The United Nations' Millennium Development Goals (MDGs), announced in 2000, and spelling out broad targets aimed at reducing poverty and reversing the spread of diseases such as HIV/AIDS and malaria by the year 2015, are no doubt worthy, but remain an under-funded wish-list and do not and cannot tackle the underlying social and economic policies that create the very inequalities the MDGs are meant to redress.[36]

In this context we find a complicated mix of approaches in international or 'global' health, as it is now called (the significance or otherwise of this shift in terminology is something I discuss in chapter Seven). Eradication campaigns appear to be here to stay; WHO-supported global eradication campaigns against polio and Guinea Worm Disease are ongoing, as well as regional eradication or 'elimination' programmes, such as those against leprosy and Chagas disease.[37] Yaws is a possible candidate for eradication in the future, since an eradication campaign would complete what had been started in the

1950s, using the same basic method (mass use of penicillin) but would start from a much lower level of incidence than existed before. Measles is another.

Many people would probably argue that there is little chance that eradication (or even serious reduction) of a highly infectious disease like measles can be achieved without the development of basic or Primary Health Care services. But they would probably also argue that the Primary Health Care approach by itself is not enough. Special, targeted, immunization and other mass health campaigns will be needed as well.[38] Thus the gap between eradication and Primary Health Care may be closing, and the heated debates between the pro- and the anti-eradicationists are perhaps being re-configured. As I hope to show, we may be starting to see some examples of eradication efforts that overcome the limitations of the 'first generation' eradication campaigns and incorporate some of the features of basic health services, while nonetheless remaining focused on the removal of specific diseases.

2 Imperial Origins

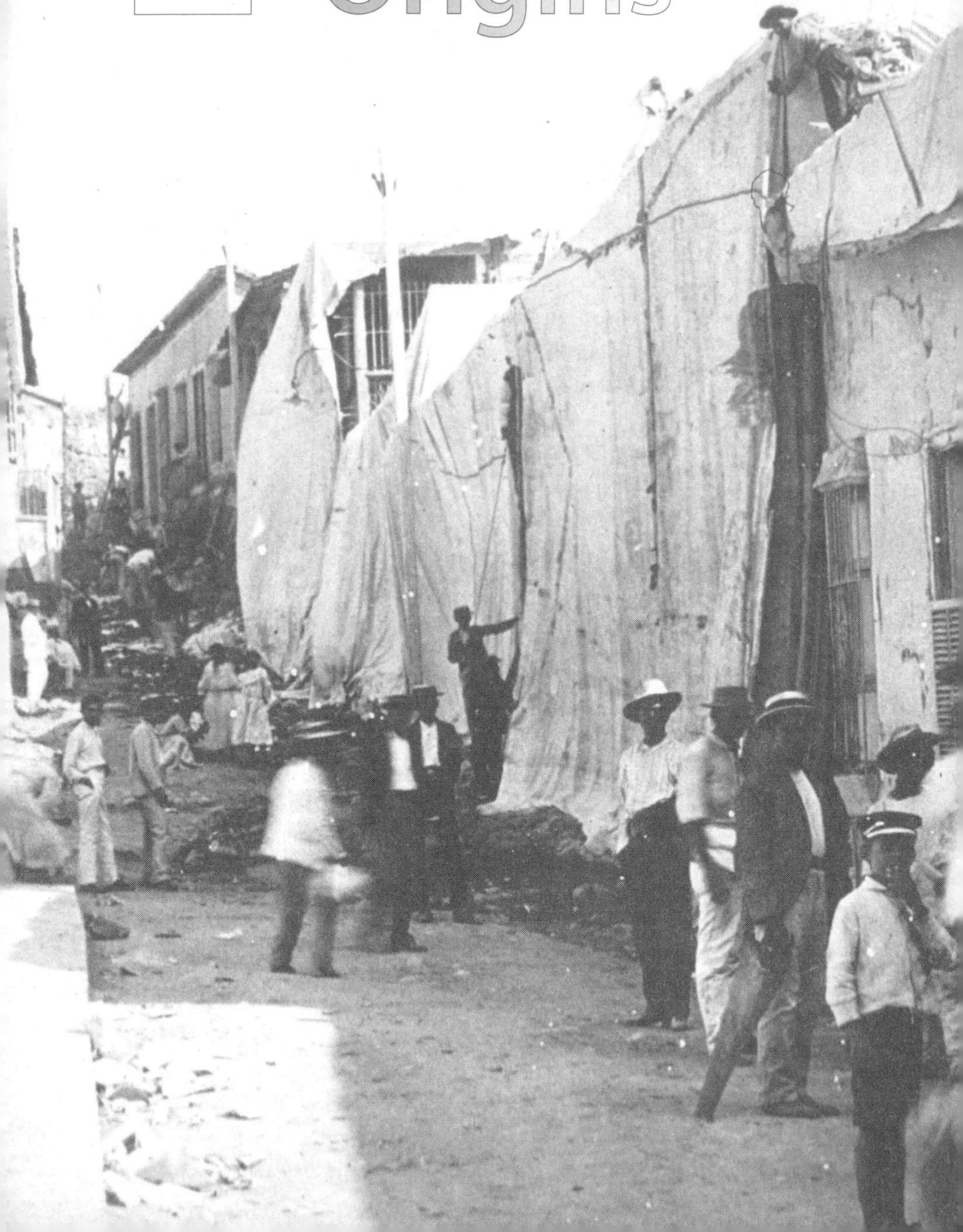

The history of eradication might be said to have started with one of the best-known discoveries of the 'new public health' – the experimental proof by US physicians in Havana in 1900 that yellow fever is transmitted by mosquitoes. Since yellow fever, unlike malaria, had no drug to treat patients once they were infected (and still does not); since it was not a chronic infection, which people learned to live with, but an often epidemic infection with high fatality rates; and because its pathogenic cause was unknown, getting rid of mosquitoes was recognized immediately as the logical method of eliminating the disease. The fact that the discovery of mosquito transmission was made while the US army was an occupying force in Cuba was another cause for the prompt move from research to application.

The rapid success of the campaign conducted against mosquitoes in Havana, led by William C. Gorgas in 1901, was followed very soon afterwards by similar anti-mosquito campaigns in other towns in Cuba, in the Panama Canal Zone, and cities such as New Orleans, and Rio de Janeiro in Brazil. So effective were the new methods that by 1911 Gorgas was already looking forward 'to a time when yellow fever will have entirely disappeared as a disease to which man is subject'.[1] In 1915, the Rockefeller Foundation recruited Gorgas to its newly founded International Health Division (IHD), and endorsed the goal of yellow fever eradication in the Americas.[2] Work on the project started in earnest at the end of the First World War.

Dr Fred Lowe Soper's path crossed Gorgas's in 1920 as this work took off. Soper, who had just finished his medical degree and been recruited to work for the IHD, had been sent to attend a three-week course in tropical hygiene at the Johns Hopkins University's School of Hygiene and Public Health in Baltimore, where Gorgas was giving some lectures. Exuding great confidence, Gorgas 'made everything so simple and straightforward', reported Soper, 'that it appeared yellow fever was on the way out and that we neophytes had come on the scene too late to have part in its glorious eradication [sic]'.[3]

How wrong Gorgas would prove to be, on all counts! Soper, the neophyte indeed, would come to play a crucial role in the yellow fever story; and yellow fever would never be eradicated. Nevertheless, yellow fever is a vital thread linking the eradication story from its origins in the early twentieth century, to the post-Second World War apotheosis in global eradication campaigns. Yellow fever was one of the first diseases to be proposed for eradication and the disease gave rise to the longest sustained effort in eradication's history; the early eradication campaigns left a lasting imprint on the eradicationist philosophy despite the fact that the yellow fever eradication effort in the end proved to be, in Soper's words, 'the most magnificent failure in public health history'.[4]

The encounter between Gorgas and Soper in 1920, brief though it was, connected two of the key figures in eradication and sets the themes of this chapter. These themes are the politics of yellow fever; the imperial origins of the eradication idea; the experimental basis of eradication and the concomitant confidence that the bio-medical knowledge and techniques necessary to achieve eradication were known and were well proven – an unwarranted confidence, as it turned out, but one that marked nearly every eradication campaign; and finally the role of Gorgas himself, in providing a new model of public health work in the international arena. This was a model that proved able travel – it was later adopted, with modifications, for diseases quite unlike yellow fever, and in situations quite unlike those of colonial occupation and martial law. After the Second World War, developing countries found their own reasons to collaborate with the World Health Organization (WHO) and take up eradication in what Amrith characterizes as a process of 'de-colonizing international health'.[5]

Though Soper did not meet Gorgas again (Gorgas died in London a few months later, on 4 July 1920, where he had stopped on route to West Africa to investigate yellow fever there), Soper was the truest heir of Gorgas's legacy in public health, as we shall see.

The Politics of Disease

Why yellow fever? Why did this disease become so central to the eradication story, setting the parameters for subsequent eradication campaigns against diseases very dissimilar to it, biologically and socially?

Historically, the importance a particular disease has to a particular society at a particular moment is rarely a straightforward function of health indicators, such as the number of people infected in a given population, or the mortality or morbidity the disease inflicts as a percentage of the overall disease burden. If the latter factors dictated social concern, then respiratory diseases such as pneumonia, or diarrhoeal infections, would have received by far the lion's share of public health efforts in the nineteenth and twentieth centuries – but they did not. Nor do the economic costs, or even the availability of an effective intervention, necessarily result in concerted efforts at disease control. Instead, we find that the alarm expressed, the attention given, and the action against a disease is determined by what I call the 'politics of disease', by which I mean its connection to larger political and symbolic issues of the day, as well as other class and economic priorities. In this regard, a disease can seize the public imagination to a degree that is out of proportion to the burden it imposes, relative to other infections.[6]

Yellow fever in the United States is an especially telling example of this. Yellow fever is largely confined, historically and today, to two geographical regions of the world, the Americas and West Africa. It was not by any means the most significant disease in the Americas by the late nineteenth century, as measured by mortality or morbidity. But the disease's dramatic epidemic character, its often high fatality rate and the disruption that epidemics and quarantines caused at a time of growing trade and immigration, combined to give yellow fever a national prominence that other diseases did not have.

First appearing in the United States in the seventeenth century along with the slave trade from Africa, by the late eighteenth century yellow fever had established itself as an endemic infection along the eastern seaboard; periodic and often ferocious epidemics continued to erupt at intervals until the last quarter of the nineteenth century, causing panic, mass flight and high death rates.[7] For reasons that are not clear, the geography of yellow fever in the United States shifted southwards after the Civil War. Improved sanitary and living conditions in the northeastern cities may have been responsible, by unknowingly reducing the breeding sites of mosquitoes.[8] The extent of epidemics diminished – the last major epidemic occurred in 1878, when yellow fever swept across the Mississippi Valley, causing over 100,000 cases and at least 20,000 deaths.[9] However, smaller but nevertheless deadly outbreaks continued to erupt in Mississippi, Texas and Florida often enough to make yellow fever a continued concern of local, state and federal authorities.

Yellow fever was not only often deadly, but also mysterious. Nothing the authorities did seemed to halt its spread. Neither flight nor quarantines were effective in stopping the disease. Sanitarians associated it with the grime, dirt and the dirty habits of townspeople, particularly poor and 'backward' populations. Yet this association failed as an explanation of the disease's transmission; during an epidemic, one person in a family might fall ill, while another seemingly subjected to the same conditions and influences escaped infection altogether. At times yellow fever seemed to invade a community or place from outside, for example through ports where ships and people from overseas arrived, or along transport routes, such as railways carrying apparently contaminated goods into towns; at other times the disease seemed completely local and internal in origin, springing up apparently spontaneously from the local soil.

Symptomatically, too, the disease was unpredictable; some people suffered little more than mild headaches, fever and nausea, symptoms that were not easily differentiated from those of other diseases, such as malaria (which is why retrospective judgements about infection and death rates are unreliable). But in about 15–20 per cent of the cases the patient would enter a highly toxic phase of the illness, with ghastly symptoms – extremely high temperatures, severe jaundice (hence its name, 'yellow' fever), bleeding from the mouth and gums and sometimes black vomit ('vómito negro' in Spanish), indicating internal haemorrhaging. Sudden death awaited many of those entering this toxic phase – mortality rates of 10–20 per cent of those with toxic symptoms, and sometimes as much as 90 per cent, were not uncommon.

The fact that yellow fever struck newcomers with particular ferocity was one of the disease's most characteristic and fearsome features, especially as the United States increasingly acquired the character of an international trading and immigrant country. How immunity was acquired was not known, but long residence in a warm climate seemed to 'season' or acclimatize people and make them resistant (unknown to observers at the time, such individuals had almost certainly survived a mild case of yellow fever, usually in childhood, which had then conferred life-long immunity upon them). The black population was assumed to be inherently or racially immune. This assumption was contradicted repeatedly by events on the ground, but to many southern doctors it was an article of faith, held to through thick and thin; it is a telling example of how disease interpretations were shaped by political racism.[10]

Because yellow fever targeted newcomers, immigration 'fed' the disease. As Margaret Humphries shows in her excellent study, *Yellow Fever and the South* (1992), so important was yellow fever judged to be as a public health menace to the United States as a whole, with its large immigrant population, that what was largely a regional and southern problem had an unprecedented influence on national public health institutions. The first national public health organization, the American Public Health Association, for instance, was founded in 1872 largely in response to yellow fever. The 1878 passage of a National Quarantine Act was similarly prompted by the threat of yellow fever epidemics; the act gave the US Marine Hospital Service (originally established to protect the health of seamen) the authority to declare a quarantine when necessary to stop the spread of the disease. In fact, between 1872 and 1910 the US Marine Hospital Service was funded and staffed with yellow fever very much in mind.[11]

The increase in shipping to United States in the last quarter of the nineteenth century put further pressure on the federal authorities to control yellow fever. By 1890, the number of ships arriving from foreign ports had risen to 20,000–22,000 per year, compared to the 10,000–12,000 ships a year that had made the passage in the 1850s. Ships also travelled faster, which meant that by the turn of the twentieth century a city like New Orleans lay 'within easy epidemiological reach of many African, Asian, European and Latin American ports'.[12] Starting in 1887, foreign consular officers were required to report cases of yellow fever abroad on a weekly basis to the US Marine Hospital Service. With increased shipping there came a huge increase in passengers, whose arrival prompted ever more elaborate health checks at their points of entry, and strict quarantines.

An important factor in the growing emphasis placed on ports and shipping in the US was the growing conviction that yellow fever, whatever its supposed germ or mode of transmission might prove to be, was not in fact native to the country, but was largely an import from other countries where it was endemic. Yellow fever occurred in warm climates, and did not overwinter easily in the frosty conditions that occurred in even many southern cities in the United States; it seemed it had to enter anew each year from the outside. To stop yellow fever in its tracks, older methods of burning sulphur compounds to ward off local miasmas, or applying disinfecting agents, therefore began to be supplemented by more rigorous systems of disinfection and quarantines at the points of entry into the United States. The port emphasis in yellow fever control further strengthened the hands of the US Marine Hospital Service and its federally contracted medical officers – an interesting example of the federalization of public health at a time when there was otherwise very strong southern resistance to federal authority.

Alternatively yellow fever might, if the methods were at hand, be stamped out at its origin points, like Cuba, only 145 km (90 miles) off the coast of Florida. America's intervention in the Spanish–American War came, then, at an interesting conjuncture: the growing importance of experimental methods in medicine, and the growing conviction that the solution to yellow fever lay outside the US. The 1898 war put Cuba in US hands, allowing the US public health authorities, under conditions of martial law, to impose stringent measures on the island, with far-reaching consequences for Cuban independence and for public health.

The United States as an Imperial Power

The entry of the United States in 1898 into what was a 30-year-long struggle by Cuban insurgents to throw off the yoke of Spanish colonial rule marked the emergence of the US as an imperial power. As Louis A. Pérez, Jr says: 'The intervention transformed a Cuban war of liberation into a US war of conquest.'[13]

Compared to the British, French, Belgian and German powers, which by 1900 had divided up much of the world between them, with 90 per cent of Africa and over 50 per cent of Asia in their hands, the United States viewed itself as a reluctant imperial power.[14] To this day, Americans define the origins of their nation in terms of its anti-imperial struggle against Britain; they are uneasy at being called imperialist, and like to think that they differ from Europeans in this regard. They often claim that American imperial influence is indirect, based on an empire of free trade, of ideas and cultural influence, and not the conquest of peoples and the occupation of foreign lands. They argue that, historically, the country has been 'limited in its appetite for territorial expansion overseas'; it 'prefers the idea that foreigners will Americanize themselves without the need for formal rule'.[15]

Much of US history contradicts this view of US imperialism.[16] As the pace of imperial possession by the European colonial powers accelerated at the end of the nineteenth century, so the US also began to shift towards a more aggressive imperialism beyond its own shores, notably in Central America and the Caribbean. After 1898, US–Latin American relations would be marked by a history of repeated military invasions by the US of Latin American countries to the near south, and by extensive economic and cultural influence throughout the entire Latin American continent.[17]

The new era of US imperialism began when a ship, the USS *Maine*, which was anchored in the bay of Havana as if in preparation for an invasion of the island, blew up on 15 February 1898, with considerable loss of US life. The American bully-press quickly blamed the Spanish colonial government for the explosion (though such involvement has never been proved), and the event gave the American government the excuse it needed to intervene in the last stage of what had been until then a prolonged anti-imperial struggle for independence by the Cubans against Spain. The rapid defeat of the Spanish military forces in Cuba led to US military control of the island by January 1899, the acquisition of a permanent military base at Guantánamo Bay, and the eventual imposition of the infamous Platt Amendment as the terms of US withdrawal from the island in 1902; the latter secured for the United States the right to further interventions and veto powers over the island. At the same time, Puerto Rico came under US control. Another military annexation in 1903 in what became Panama gave the US possession of a 16-km-wide (10-mile-wide) strip of territory through the heart of the country. Through this strip the US built the Panama Canal; the canal opened to shipping in 1914, and remained under US control until 1979.[18] The quick surrender of the Spanish led the US further afield to the annexation of the Spanish Philippines, where a bloody and prolonged struggle took place between the Filipinos and US forces, with the US responsible for many atrocities. The Philippines would not become independent until 1946.

Yet even with these acquisitions of territory overseas, the US rejected the imperialist label and liked to claim that its interventions were essentially benign and in the best interests of others. This peculiar mix of philanthropy and power that is characteristic of US imperialism was captured very well by Simone de Beauvoir, in her fascinating and astute book of travels in the US entitled *America Day by Day* (1947): 'In the eyes of the average American, imperialism takes on the guise of charity. Their arrogance lies not in their love of power. It is the love of imposing on others that which is good. The miracle is that the key to paradise should be in their hands.'[19]

One of these keys was believed to be modern medicine and sanitation. The newly acquired colonies had long been seen as epicentres of disease; indeed, among the motives for imperial involvement or occupation was that it gave the US the chance, or, the argument went, even the right, to sanitize sources of infection threatening to invade mainland USA. The Spanish–American war energized the emerging speciality of tropical medicine in the US, and notably in relation to a disease that was not already the preserve of European physicians. Yellow fever had once been part of the epidemiological landscape of southern Europe (striking as far north as the French Atlantic port of St Nazaire in 1861, and Swansea, in Wales, in 1865), but by the late nineteenth century was restricted to the Americas and West Africa.[20] US success in discovering the mode of transmission of yellow fever in 1900 put US tropical medical research on an equal footing with Europe for almost the first time. Thereafter, the US kept yellow fever research as a kind of imperial scientific possession.

Havana, Yellow Fever and the Reed Commission

Historically, perhaps no medical investigation has been more written about or more celebrated in US history books than the work of the Reed Board on yellow fever in Havana. The events surrounding the solution of a long-standing puzzle about yellow fever transmission, in the space of a few months in 1900, have given rise to numerous hagiographies of the principal parties involved and to heroic accounts of the risky inoculations undertaken. Many of these accounts are short on accuracy, make almost no reference to the medical failures surrounding the US military occupation, and ignore the Cuban context in which the events took place.

It is not my purpose here to retell the story of the inoculation experiments (which I have done before).[21] My goal here is to focus on the question of how military occupation affected the discovery process and the conclusions about disease control that were drawn. My argument is that the investigations were cut short by the requirements of military occupation, with the result that eradication was based on inadequate knowledge of the disease.

To start with, we have to recognize that even though the Spanish army, exhausted by yellow fever among other things, surrendered quickly, the war was a near medical fiasco for the United States.[22] This early fiasco goes some way to explain the sometimes exaggerated praise that has historically been heaped on the Reed Board's experiments. It was in such marked contrast to what had gone before that it seemed to make up for what had otherwise been a very sorry showing indeed of supposed American medical know-how and efficiency. 'Thank God', wrote Dr Walter Reed, the head of the Yellow Fever Commission, 'that the Medical Department of the US Army, which got such a black eye during the Spanish–American War, has during the past year accomplished work that will always remain to its eternal credit'.[23]

Unlike Britain, the United States had no Colonial Office or its equivalent to direct its new colonial affairs; its imperialism was essentially a military matter, and its public health in Cuba, Panama and the Philippines was largely in the hands of army doctors. When the US invaded Cuba in 1898, its peace-time army was small, and the invasion force had to be brought up to strength by recruiting thousands of untrained volunteers (among them the future President of the USA, Theodore Roosevelt, and his 'Rough Riders'). Medically, the army was equally under-staffed and under-prepared; many doctors had to be brought in hastily under contract to the military to make up an adequate medical corps.[24] According to Cirollo's recent and careful account, 345 US soldiers were killed in combat during the war, but about 2,500 died of disease. Two thirds of the deaths occurred not in Cuba itself but in US-based camps where volunteers were assembled.[25]

So serious were the reports by newspapers of the medical incompetence of the US Army, and the chaotic disease conditions in army camps, that they provoked an outcry, which in turn led to the appointment of a commission to examine the charges, and eventually to the setting up of three different medical commissions of enquiry, of which the Yellow Fever Commission is the best-known.[26] From the start, yellow fever in some of the army camps and in surrounding small towns threatened the occupation force and dented the US's reputation for scientific expertise and administrative competence. Until late 1899, the city of Havana itself remained relatively free of yellow fever, owing largely to the fact that the port itself was blockaded by the Americans, thus preventing the entry of non-immune people, especially Spanish immigrants. The main effort was to clean up the capital. Years of war had left the city in a chaotic state, littered with the debris of war – not just mounds of rubbish, dead animals and decaying matter but also beggars, orphans and the generally impoverished. In the city of Havana, the Chief Sanitary Officer, Major William C. Gorgas, a competent, southern-born medical officer, began a systematic clean-up, including house fumigations and disinfection of the streets, in some places on a daily basis. Bars, saloons and cafes were closed. As a result, the overall death rate in the capital city fell steadily. No expense was spared; some 300 men were employed daily in environmental cleanups.

But in July 1899 cases of yellow fever were again on the rise on the island. In August 1899 the port of Havana itself was finally re-opened to commerce, and by the end of the year some 12,000 immigrants had entered the city, 60 per cent of whom settled in the capital itself. By December 1900, yellow fever was epidemic in Havana once again. Altogether in 1900 there were 1,400 cases.[27] Gorgas found he was powerless to check the march of the disease; cleaning the city was obviously not enough.

By this time the four members of the US Army's Yellow Fever Commission, usually referred to as the Reed Board, set up in May of 1900, were already in Cuba. Dr Walter Reed, who taught bacteriology at the recently established US Army Medical School in Washington, led the Board. The second member, the British-born Canadian, Dr James Carroll, served in Washington as Reed's assistant. The third, Dr Jesse Lazear, an American doctor working at Johns Hopkins University, had studied yellow fever, and also worked in Italy and knew something about medical entomology, while Dr Aristides Agramonte, the fourth member of the team, was a Cuban-born, American-trained pathologist. None could be considered real experts on yellow fever. However, Dr Henry R. Carter, with whom the Reed Board was very fortunate to be in close contact, was a highly experienced quarantine officer with the US Marine Hospital Service who had studied yellow fever epidemics closely; his epidemiological investigation of yellow fever in Mississippi in 1898 had established the very important fact that a roughly two-week or greater interval of time separated the appearance of the first cases of yellow fever during an epidemic, from the appearance of the next or secondary cases. Carter called this interval one of 'extrinsic incubation', and in a paper published in 1900 proposed that it indicated that, whatever the 'germ' of yellow fever might turn out to be, it had to undergo some kind of change in the environment before it could infect another human being.[28] Carter had been posted to Havana and had put his paper in the hands of the Reed Board on their arrival.

It was some time before this information could be digested and made central to yellow fever epidemiology. The members of the Reed Board, who set up their experiments at Camp Columbia, an army base some miles from Havana, instead spent several weeks testing various hypotheses about the possible bacterial origins of yellow fever, work which proved fruitless (the causative organism is a virus which would not be isolated until 1927).

What led the Reed Board to turn their attention eventually to the 'mosquito' hypothesis of yellow fever transmission is not clear; the evidence leaves a gap at some critical junctures. What is known is that the idea of a role for insects in spreading disease was 'in the air' at the time; in particular, there was the model of filariasis, but also malaria, whose transmission by anopheline mosquitoes had been proven experimentally by Ronald Ross and Battista Grassi in 1897–1898.[29] By analogy, several other diseases were hypothesized to involve intermediary insect vectors. One of these was yellow fever. There was, moreover, a quite specific mosquito hypothesis of yellow fever transmission at hand that had been put forward by the Cuban physician, Dr Carlos Finlay, as early as 1881. Trained in the United States, as were so many Cuban doctors at the time, Finlay had carried out human inoculation experiments in order to transmit yellow fever to non-immune individuals by the bite of infected mosquitoes.[30] Finlay's inoculation experiments were, unfortunately, not persuasive.[31] He was nevertheless resident in Havana at the time of the Reed Commission's work, having volunteered his services to the US authorities; and once the Americans decided to test the mosquito hypothesis, it was Finlay who was able to identify the most likely mosquito species involved, the *Stegomyia fasciata* mosquito (later called the *Aedes aegypti*), from among the more than 600 mosquito species found in Cuba (it was very different in type from the anopheline mosquitoes responsible for malaria transmission); and it was he who provided the female mosquitoes (which alone fed on human blood), and their eggs, for use in the inoculation experiments. Without Finlay's specific theory of transmission to hand, it is hardly possible that the Reed Commission would have been successful so quickly.

In fact, the Reed Commission made many mistakes in their initial mosquito inoculation experiments; the first human tests, carried out in August of 1900, proved nothing, as no one bitten by a supposedly infected mosquito came down with yellow fever.[32] The significance of Carter's conclusion that, after an *Aedes aegypti* mosquito had been infected by feeding on a yellow fever patient, it could not infect another human being for a period of ten to twelve days, had clearly not been grasped. The critical second round of inoculations was undertaken in late August and early September, while Reed was away in the United States; the inoculation tests, led by Lazear, involved the deliberate biting of himself, Carroll and a volunteer army private by mosquitoes that had been made to feed previously on yellow fever patients. All three got yellow fever; the private and Carroll recovered (though Carroll became extremely ill). But Lazear did not, dying of yellow fever on 25 September 1900.[33]

Lazear's death was a turning point. A telegram to Reed brought him back to Havana and led to immediate action. The three cases of yellow fever infection strongly suggested that the mosquito theory was right, but the inoculations had been undertaken in such a way that Reed realized they could not be counted as definitive experimental proof of the theory. Lazear and Carroll had not followed strict experimental protocols during the work; Carroll, for example, had not been isolated from non-experimental sources of infection either before or after being bitten, so another mosquito, or even direct contact with a patient, might have caused his infection; and Lazear's deadly infection was the result of an imprecisely documented bite.[34]

Nevertheless, on his return to Cuba in October, Reed realized from studying Lazear's notes that Carroll and Lazear had both been bitten by mosquitoes that had fed on yellow fever patients twelve and sixteen days previously, so that the results of their yellow fever infections were congruent with Carter's epidemiological conclusions about a period of extrinsic incubation. On the strength of this realization, Reed decided to make a public statement, largely to claim priority for the discovery. On 23 October, at the meetings of the American Public Health Association held in Indianapolis, Reed made the historic announcement that yellow fever was indeed transmitted by the bite of the female *Aedes aegypti* mosquito. The paper was published shortly afterwards, under the authorship of all four members of the Reed Board.[35]

On his return to Cuba, Reed authorized a further series of human inoculation experiments, starting in October, which were carried out with rigorous supervision of experimental protocols at the specially constructed Camp Lazear, situated outside the city, using army and civilian volunteers.[36] Altogether, the new set of human experiments produced sixteen cases of yellow fever that were indisputably the result of the bite of infected mosquitoes and occurred after the necessary twelve to fourteen days of incubation of the infective material in the mosquito; miraculously, no one died, and the results appeared in a second historic paper.[37]

A separate set of inoculation experiments, carried out by the Cuban doctor, Juan Guiteras, was not so fortunate; deliberately inoculating blood infected with yellow fever into the skin of non-immune volunteers, in order to see if it were possible to provoke mild cases deliberately, and so create immunity (by a kind of vaccination, much as Finlay had done), Guiteras infected eight people, three of whom died.[38]

This was too much, even in an age which, viewed from our present-day perspective, was only too casual in conducting human experiments. All further inoculation experiments by the Reed Board were terminated, on the grounds of the great risk of death they posed to all those involved.

As a result, though the breakthrough in knowledge was very considerable, many things about yellow fever remained unknown for a very long time; several erroneous assumptions were made, and for a number of reasons, including the success Gorgas had initially had in applying the new mosquito theory in controlling yellow fever, no further investigations, either epidemiological or experimental, were carried out for many years thereafter.

The period of experimentation had in fact been remarkably short, only a few months, and essentially ended with the proof of yellow fever transmission by the *Aedes aegypti* mosquito. The members of the Reed Board were unable to isolate experimentally the infective organism of yellow fever itself, though they were able to establish that it was sub-microscopic in size – so small, in fact, that it could pass through a very fine porcelain filter.[39] It was therefore much smaller than a bacterium. They were also unable to infect animals experimentally, something which would have allowed them to carry on experiments without the risk to human life. The reasons for this failure are not evident. It was widely believed that animals were not hosts for yellow fever, since during epidemics they were not seen to fall ill or die. Reed in fact took the decision to proceed with dangerous human experiments because of the absence of an experimental animal with which to work; if the Board had not been so pressed to come up with answers, perhaps more time would have been taken to pursue the matter. Early in the twentieth century, Sir Patrick Manson and other British doctors raised the possibility, based on their knowledge of yellow fever in West Africa, that forest animals, especially monkeys, formed natural hosts or reservoirs of yellow fever, but this was not followed up at the time.[40] Not until much later, in the late 1920s, in a new phase of experimental research sponsored by the Rockefeller Foundation, were scientists able to infect monkeys experimentally, and identify the yellow fever virus, thus making possible an animal model and eventually, in 1937, the production of a workable yellow fever vaccine; these events are recounted in chapter Three of this book.

In the absence of a cultivable pathogen or an animal model, and therefore of a potential vaccine, and with no known medical therapy available for the treatment of yellow fever victims, attention understandably focussed on the *Aedes aegypti* mosquito itself, which provided a potentially vulnerable target in the transmission chain. Here again, however, a conclusion was drawn that proved over the long term to be premature, namely that only one single *Aedes* mosquito species was involved in yellow fever transmission.[41] Only a few other mosquito species were tested at the time, with negative results.[42] The major role played by the *Aedes aegypti* species in transmitting yellow fever in urban settings was in fact correctly ascertained, but it did not give the whole picture of how yellow fever is sustained as a virus in the wild. The assumption may have been a result of the Reed Commission's reliance on Dr Juan Carlos Finlay for his very astute identification of the *Aedes aegypti* species, from among the hundreds of other mosquito species he had studied, as the likely candidate as principal vector. The fact that Finlay was dealing with yellow fever in Havana, and that he, like the Reed Board members and Dr Henry R. Carter, believed yellow fever to be a fundamentally urban disease, may also explain why it took so long to recognize the existence of what is now called 'jungle' or 'sylvatic' yellow fever, with its different mosquito vectors and epidemiological profile (the jungle form of yellow fever transmission is anyway not found in the United States).

Yet even at the time, there were those who raised the possibility of a role for other vector species. Dr Henry Carter himself, for instance, commenting on how few experiments had been made with other mosquitoes, pointed out that, 'from analogy, not always a safe guide, we would suspect that some other species of this genus, or maybe subfamily, would convey yellow fever, and none of any other subfamily would'.[43] He noted, quite rightly, that this was not just of academic interest, but of practical importance, since methods used to control one kind of mosquito might not work with another species with a different habitat and behaviour.

The consequence of the truncated investigation of yellow fever was an incomplete epidemiological model of yellow fever whose shortcomings did not become evident for more than three decades.[44] As a rough and ready guide to yellow fever control, the knowledge proved workable and assured a US dominance of the yellow fever problem for several decades. In the longer run, the incomplete epidemiological model proved to be yellow fever eradication's undoing.

The Practical Campaign

The yellow fever story was characterized by a remarkably rapid translation of the mosquito theory into practice – a quite different outcome than with malaria, as we shall see later. One reason for the rapid resort to a campaign based exclusively on anti-mosquito methods was the quasi-wartime conditions and occupied status of Cuba. Another was the rapid confirmation that anti-mosquito programmes worked.

The Reed Board's work opened up two new control strategies. The first was to prevent the mosquitoes from biting anyone infected with yellow fever; this meant identifying, and then isolating behind mosquito screens, all those sick with yellow fever. The second was to destroy the mosquitoes themselves, either in their adult form as they came into houses to bite, or in their larval form in pockets of water.[45]

For the latter purpose, various chemicals and fumigation techniques were used. For many years, crude oil mixed with paraffin was applied to surface water as a chemical larvicide; various other chemicals, such as sulphur-based compounds, or powder composed of pyrethrum (a product of the chrysanthemum plant and a known insecticide) were also burned inside houses to kill adult mosquitoes (though pyrethrum tended to stun rather than kill the insects). The new methods of mosquito control were unfamiliar, of course, to the Havana residents. They had already been subjected to strict public health measures before mosquitoes became the target; anti-mosquito work now subjected them to new kinds of public health surveillance.[46] Public health officials had to remove, or cover, or chemically treat and otherwise get rid of, any and all possible sources of breeding sites in and around people's houses. Drinking tanks had to be sealed, or their water surface covered with a thin layer of oil (to suffocate any larvae), and spigots attached (in later campaigns, special larvae-eating fish would sometimes be introduced into the water tanks); elaborate house fumigations often left behind films of dust or caused smoke damage.

Major William C. Gorgas was not a research scientist, but a military man with a job to do. He was not at all involved with the work of the Reed Commission, and at first was not convinced that the mosquito was the sole source of yellow fever transmission. Nor did he think it possible to get rid of all the mosquitoes; nevertheless, as an army officer he followed orders.[47] Told in early 1901 by the military Governor General of Cuba, Dr Leonard Wood, to concentrate the anti-yellow fever sanitation efforts almost exclusively on the new mosquito theory, Gorgas set to work in Havana in February, eventually shifting two thirds of his Sanitary Department's crews from cleaning streets to house-to-house oiling tasks. The results came remarkably fast. The summer months were historically the months of epidemic yellow fever; but the outbreaks that occurred were few and had few deaths. When cases in August (six in all) were identified, Gorgas got authority to put inspectors on all railroads entering Havana from potentially infected places outside the city. Any non-immune individual trying to enter the city was reported, and then put into quarantine for a week. Only a few cases and deaths were recorded in Havana in August and September. The last cases (and no deaths) were recorded in early October; after that there were none, nor did yellow fever return in the next yellow fever season in 1902. 'I submit', wrote Gorgas, 'that this is evidence of the practical demonstration of the mosquito theory'.[48] A disease that had attacked Havana with regularity for over a century or more seemed to have been conquered.

As a practical matter, the campaign against yellow fever was run as a military operation, and conducted under martial law, which allowed hierarchical command over personnel and the rapid harnessing of the resources needed – not a model easy to copy in ordinary civilian circumstances.[49] Attention was paid first to identifying and isolating all yellow fever patients; these individuals were sealed off from contact with non-immune people, and from further mosquito bites (which would have resulted in re-infecting the insects), by bed netting, either in rooms in their own homes, or in an isolation hospital.[50] Their houses, and those of their immediate neighbours, were then also sealed and fumigated by burning sulphur-based chemicals or pyrethrum powder, to kill or stun any adult mosquitoes on the premises. This meant papering over cracks in the house walls and windows (quite a challenge in the dilapidated structures most people lived in), and burning chemicals inside houses without burning them down; and following the burning, un-sealing the rooms and sweeping up all the dead or stunned mosquitoes and removing them. Factories and warehouses were fumigated with sulphur or tobacco smoke; cafes and bars where people congregated were shut.

To get rid of mosquito breeding places, Gorgas mapped the city in detail, marking the position of every house or premise. The Sanitation Department had already divided the city into sanitary districts for the purpose of cleaning streets; now the city was re-divided into mosquito inspection districts, each district comprising the number of houses that an inspector could inspect in a designated period of time, at regular intervals of a day or week, with the same inspector attached to the same district throughout the campaign. Each inspector appointed to the special anti-yellow fever service was accompanied by a squad of oilers, who poured oil onto puddles of water; the inspector also carried with him printed-up forms devised for the campaign, on which he entered information about the condition of the water closets, cess pools and sinks on each of the premises visited and the rates of mosquito infestation. These reports were turned in every night to a centralized office of the sanitary department, and were consolidated day by day, so that a running inventory of the larval and other conditions of the entire housing stock of the city was compiled. Old bottles, discarded cans, any container-like rubbish found lying about in yards and gardens that might attract breeding mosquitoes were inventoried and removed. House gutters were cleaned and straightened to prevent water build-up; screens were put in windows wherever possible, according to the conditions of the houses. In principle, every house was re-inspected once a month to see that the regulations were being obeyed and that householders were maintaining vigilance against the mosquitoes.

The US authorities paid for much of this work; but continued vigilance against open water sources in houses that could serve as breeding places for larvae was made the responsibility of individual householders. To enforce compliance, the Mayor of Havana issued an ordinance fining each householder ten dollars if the premises were found to have larvae present during subsequent inspections, with the fines being collected by the Cuban courts.[51] As many as 1,000 such cases would sometimes be brought to the courts in a single month.

By March of 1901, Gorgas's inspectors had identified in Havana about 26,000 different water deposits infected with mosquito larvae, most of them of the *Aedes aegypti* variety. Many of these water sources were simply destroyed. By January of 1902, after ten months of mosquito work, inspections showed that within the city limits the number of infected water sources had fallen to less 300.[52] House infection by larvae had as a result fallen from an estimated 100 per cent in early 1901, to 0.6 per cent in March 1902. As noted already, long before this yellow fever had been extinguished in Havana; no cases of yellow fever were detected after the end of October 1901.[53]

In 1902, the US occupation forces left Cuba, placing public health under the direction of the now aging, but much fêted, Dr Juan Carlos Finlay. This was not quite the end of yellow fever on the island, however. It remained a constant concern of the US authorities, who did not trust the Cubans to keep up the surveillance necessary to stop further transmission unless pressured by the United States. Yellow fever did in fact return to the island, first in 1904, and again in 1905; this (and political instability) led the US to re-occupy the island in 1906 for a further three years. Extending the anti-mosquito measures to every town in the island, by late 1908 yellow fever was extinguished once again, this time to stay out of the island for decades. In 1909, the US finally left Cuba, having instructed the Cuban authorities on their 'colonial responsibility' to keep the United States safe from re-invasion by the yellow fever virus.[54]

Making the Tropics Safe for the White Man

The new anti-mosquito methods were quickly tried elsewhere – in the United States itself, in Brazil, in Mexico and of course in Panama. The feeling was that a method had been found to stop yellow fever in its tracks in a kind of surgical intervention, without the need to carry out general sanitary improvements or address underlying issues, such as poverty and general lack of sanitation.

In 1905, New Orleans, like Havana, was infected by yellow fever. This time, the local authorities made a direct appeal to President Theodore Roosevelt for federal help; the US Marine Hospital Service sent twenty medical officers to join forces with local public health officials who, with the support of funds raised voluntarily by local citizens, applied the anti-mosquito methods developed in Havana. The epidemic was terminated, but not before 3,402 people caught the disease, and 452 died (one in seven).[55] The British physician, Sir Rubert Boyce, who was keenly interested in yellow fever in West Africa, was sent by the Liverpool School of Tropical Medicine to New Orleans to observe the anti-mosquito campaign. He described in admiring terms the efficiency and almost military style of the operation.[56]

The elimination of yellow fever in Brazil's capital, Rio de Janeiro, between 1903 and 1906 was important in spreading the anti-mosquito model and its public health methods further, because Brazil was considered one of the true homes of yellow fever in the Americas; sharing its borders with all but two countries in South America, Brazil's endemic yellow fever was viewed as a potential threat to the entire New World. The country also had a political goal which provided an incentive to its public health programme; it was bent on 'whitening' its largely black population by attracting white immigrants from Europe. But since newcomers were known to be especially susceptible to yellow fever, the national vision of a European civilization in the tropics was jeopardized by the repeated epidemics of the disease. Yellow fever, in short, had a political profile in Brazil comparable to that in the United States.

In 1903, the French-trained, modernizing Brazilian bacteriologist and Director of Public Health, Dr Oswaldo Cruz, launched a campaign against the plague, smallpox and yellow fever. In tackling yellow fever, Cruz employed Gorgas's methods of house fumigation, the isolation of yellow fever patients and destroying mosquitoes and their breeding sites. Another feature of the sanitary campaign was a tight, centralized command over the city's population which, while falling short of martial law, nonetheless involved draconian measures. At the time, the city had a population of over 600,000 people (twice that of Havana), with a high percentage of non-immune, foreign residents. With the backing of the President, Cruz pursued the goal of sanitation relentlessly, relying on special tribunals to enforce compliance with anti-mosquito requirements. Within three years, Cruz succeeded in ridding Rio de Janeiro of yellow fever; the city remained free of yellow fever until 1928.[57]

Of all the demonstrations of the effectiveness of the new anti-mosquito methods, however, that in Panama was the most significant to the eradication idea, since the opening up of a sea connection between west and east opened up at the same time potentially new and rapid means of disease communication, perhaps even the spread of yellow fever to the Far East, where mosquitoes were plentiful but yellow fever was absent. The building of the Panama Canal Zone was, of course, a massive engineering undertaking that was constantly in the news, and one whose ultimate success depended on the ability of the United States to control the spread of disease among its largely imported workers.[58] Success in sanitation, led by Gorgas, widened his reputation in circles far beyond the United States; and it gave support to his opinion, shared by colonial officers in Britain and the other European colonial powers, that the application of the new tropical medicine would make the tropics safe for the white man.

The US took possession of the Panama Canal Zone on 8 May 1904, under the overall authority of the US Secretary of War.[59] The building of the canal was concentrated in a highly artificial geographic space, a quasi-militarized slice of another country, Panama, the slice being just over 64 km (40 miles) long and about 16 km (ten miles) wide. In the next ten years, this artificial space was to be transformed into a gigantic sea passage for shipping. Much of the population working in the Zone was artificial too, in that at the height of the construction it contained huge numbers of people brought in from countries other than Panama; at its peak, the workforce included over 20,000 men imported from Barbados, who were ruled over by equally imported white engineers and officials brought in mainly from the United States.[60]

The US knew that thousand of workers had died of disease during the failed French effort, led by de Lesseps, to build a canal through Panama in the 1880s and '90s. Yet despite this history, the membership of the Panama Canal Commission appointed to administer the canal's construction did not include a senior medical expert (Gorgas, now elevated to the rank of Colonel, was recommended by the American Medical Association for such a position, but was turned down). Appointed Chief Sanitary Officer in Panama, Gorgas soon found the situation less satisfactory than it had been in Cuba, as far as his authority to impose public health measures was concerned; the budget designated initially for sanitation was also completely inadequate, and the anti-mosquito work of Havana either not known to the Panama Canal Commission or ignored by it. Lacking funds, material and personnel, Gorgas found himself unable to stop a yellow fever epidemic that erupted in March of 1905, as the first non-immune workers brought in to carry out the back-breaking work of blasting a canal through the isthmus arrived in Panama.

The result of the epidemic was panic; many US officials promptly left Panama for home and, for a time, work on the Canal came to a virtual halt.

Gorgas himself came close to being dismissed by the Canal Commission as incompetent. President Roosevelt, who was heavily invested politically in the gigantic undertaking that the construction of the canal represented, overruled his dismissal. He was also mindful of the costs of disease, both from the past experience of the French failure to complete the canal, and from the fact he had witnessed at first hand the impact of disease on the US war effort in Cuba.

Finally getting the backing he needed, Gorgas managed to stop the yellow fever outbreak within a few months; the disease would not re-appear in the Panama Canal Zone until 1954.[61] Once again taking the mosquito theory as the key to yellow fever control, and following the lessons learned in Havana, Gorgas began by tackling the two towns of Colon and Panama City, which were situated at the northeastern Atlantic end and the southwestern Pacific end, respectively, of the projected route of the canal. They were both towns where yellow fever had been repeatedly epidemic in the past, and where now many non-immune northeastern workmen, officials and workers from the Caribbean lived. Gorgas introduced the isolation and fumigation strategies he had employed in Havana, using 136 kg (300 lb) of sulphur and 54 kg (120 lb) of pyrethrum – the entire year's supply for all of the northeast, according to Litsios, and all that Gorgas could find on the market.[62] The towns struck visitors as horribly run-down, straggling, dirty and without any basic sanitation. But Gorgas's focus was on yellow fever only. As in Havana, towns were mapped and divided into anti-mosquito districts, each with its own inspector in charge of the fumigation and mosquito-killing teams, and all the premises were searched for larvae-breeding containers of water, which were emptied, sealed or oiled as the case required. Many houses for white workers were screened. A new law was introduced, making it a misdemeanour punishable with fines to have mosquitoes in the larval stage on the premises. By early 1906, the number of those dying from yellow fever was in decline, and in September, 1906, Gorgas was able to announce that the yellow fever epidemic had ended.

Malaria control was equally important to the success of the Panama Canal project. While not as dramatic a disease, malaria was much more widely distributed than yellow fever, being found throughout the entire length of the Zone where work was being carried out; at any one time, it left a high percentage of the work force chronically ill, hospitalized and unable to work. Quinine could be used as an effective preventative and therapy, and Gorgas made it widely and freely available, but at the high doses necessary to control malaria, quinine could have nasty side effects, and many people resisted taking it.

Anti-mosquito work was therefore a chief focus; this method had been promoted and tried by Sir Ronald Ross in Sierra Leone in West Africa, and by the British authorities in Northwest India, but with very mixed results (as we shall see in chapter Five). Malaria was ecologically complex and sustained reductions depended on understanding the habits and habitats of the different species of malaria mosquitoes, as well as their interaction with human-made environments – a long-term process.

This was not, however, Gorgas's way. His method was an all-out assault on the insect vectors. According to Gordon Harrison's account, the attack on the mosquitoes along the 76-km-long (47-mile-long) railway lines from Panama City to Colon involved an area of some 160 sq. km (100 sq. miles) and some 80,000 people scattered in some 30 villages or work camps.[63] Dividing the area into 25 sanitary districts, Gorgas sent out teams of labourers, each under the direction of a sanitary inspector, to distribute paraffin oil on breeding sites and to carry out extensive ditch digging and ditch filling; they also cleared brush and cut back grasses to within 183 metres (200 yards) of towns and villages, techniques aimed at exposing the terrain to sunlight and/or reducing water collections to reduce anopheline breeding.[64] The problem was that the work of construction of the Panama Canal, achieved by blasting through rock, and digging out and removing tons of soil, constantly multiplied the potential breeding places of the anopheline mosquitoes that conveyed malaria. It was a story of the repeated creation of malaria-breeding environments, and then the attempt at their elimination by ditching, mowing and massive oiling. Essentially, malaria was controlled by a tremendous environmental assault of paraffin oil, some 189,270 litres (50,000 gallons) a month, and hang the costs to the environment, and financially. Malaria did not disappear from the Canal Zone, as yellow fever did, but it did fall steadily as a percentage of the cases admitted to hospital, and as a percentage of the overall death rate.[65] In three years Gorgas had reduced malaria incidence by half.

To people at the time, the sanitation achieved under Gorgas was a model of effectiveness and a major step in imperial development.[66] The mosquito theory of yellow fever and malaria transmission, and experimental medicine more generally, were seen to have broad implications for colonialism. Until the late nineteenth century, it was believed that the white race could never be fully acclimatized in tropical climates, where it risked the constant threat of physical and moral degeneration brought about by the heat, disease and the moral laxity of uncivilized cultures. The development of the new tropical medicine, however, meant that European control over the tropical environment might now be much improved through specific interventions. Gorgas went so far as to suggest that, with both yellow fever and malaria eliminated, 'life in the tropics for the Anglo-Saxon will be more healthful than in the temperate zone'; within a few years, he believed, tropical countries – which offered, he thought, a much greater return on man's labour than did temperate zones – would be settled by white men so that the 'centers of wealth, civilization and population will be in the tropics'.[67] Sir Malcolm Watson, the British expert on malaria, made the same point; through sanitation, the tropics would become 'if not the permanent home for the white race, at least a part of the world in which the white man may live with little more danger to health than in his own country'.[68]

In fact, of course, what was achieved in Panama was quite limited. At huge expense and effort, a small slice of an otherwise foreign country had been made free of yellow fever, and partly free of malaria, the diseases considered most relevant to building the canal, while the majority of diseases remained untouched, and the general public health conditions beyond the Panama Canal Zone remained outside the scope of US action. Even within the small area of the Canal Zone itself, some benefited much more from the new public health than others. The disparities in health between whites and blacks were striking. Segregation of black workers from white workers was enforced, as was the rule in the United States at the time, with different rates of pay being established for each group, different kinds of housing provided (only the white workers had access to purpose-built housing with screened windows), and consequently different outcomes in health. The US authorities maintained strict control over the entry of people into and out of the work areas, rejecting those considered unfit, or nuisances, or unnecessary to the canal effort.[69]

Nevertheless, the British malariologist, Sir Malcolm Watson, on visiting the Panama Canal Zone in 1915, called it 'the Mecca of the modern Sanitarian'.[70]

Military Metaphors and Models of Disease Eradication

A characteristic feature of the new public health was the use of military metaphors and military language to describe disease control measures – 'campaigns' were conducted against 'enemies', meaning the pathogens and insect vectors, against which people had to do 'battle' or make an 'assault', using chemical and other 'weapons' such as mosquito 'brigades', so that 'victory' could be achieved.

Such military metaphors were not an invention of anti-yellow fever campaigns; they had a longer genealogy, acquiring currency in the 1860s and '70s when verbs such as 'invade', 'defeat', 'overwhelm' and 'combat' were used by Louis Pasteur and Robert Koch in their discussions of bacteriology. Vaccines were described as 'weapons against disease'. Such metaphors provided 'a central vision of the "wrong" that a disease presented to a community, and therefore the framework of "intervention" needed for making it "right".'[71] Examples like these are easily multiplied. Sir Ronald Ross, for example, declared that 'Sanitation is a Form of War'.[72] A more recent example comes from an analysis of the failure of the global malaria eradication campaign led by WHO, which is attributed to an 'underestimation of the enemy and over-confidence in the available weaponry'.[73]

As I have argued elsewhere, there is a strong tendency in science for metaphors to become naturalized, so that they are used not as figures of speech, but are taken instead to be true descriptions of the world as it actually is.[74] Given this tendency to reduce metaphor to reality, one is not surprised to find that military metaphors easily get connected to the idea that disease eradiation itself requires military-like strategies: 'One obvious result from this, on a grand scale, is the feeling that solutions and cures must also follow the military line: disease can be "defeated" only by massive mobilizations, involving more money, more personnel, more research, more effort of every kind. This quantitative argument arises directly, even logically, from the ideology of "battle".'[75] The lines of influence go both ways; the historian, David Arnold, remarks that the involvement of the military in medical interventions is one of the striking features of the imperial period, but that no less important was the tendency to think of medical investigations in military terms.[76] These kinds of analogies are historically constructed; they may be contrasted with an alternative set of medical metaphors that developed much later in the twentieth century, in which an analogy was drawn between disease and the environmentalist concept of 'the web of life', pointing to the idea of the co-existence of pathogens and humans. The implications of this latter set of metaphors of nature and disease for public health interventions were understood very differently from those arising from military metaphors, as we shall see.[77] For one thing, they were taken to exclude the idea of a surgical strike against disease, such as eradication represented.

Along a more historically specific line of analysis, Edmund Russell argues for an intimate metaphoric and actual connection between war, public health language and the use of chemicals to destroy pests. Ideologically, he suggests, pest control created a set of values that warriors used to argue for combating and even annihilating hidden enemies, whether parasites or humans; scientifically and technically, 'pest control and chemical warfare each created knowledge and tools the other used to increase the scale on which it pursued its goals'.[78]

A New Model of Public Health?

Russell does not refer to the US campaigns against yellow fever in Havana and Panama, but they would seem to be paradigmatic examples of his thesis. In Havana and the Panama Canal Zone, an American military or quasi-military model of imperial public health was actualized in which the chemical elimination of pests and disease was central. It was a model that was admired and emulated. Given the importance of this model, it is worth highlighting some of its characteristic features, particularly in regard to how key aspects of the model represented a departure from previous public health practices. What Gorgas did in an eight-month period in Havana under military command, after all, 'set the pattern of attempts to control yellow fever for the next thirty years'.[79]

As a first characteristic of the new model I would list its biomedical character. The focus on dirt, miasmas and overcrowding of human beings, which had traditionally been associated with the eruption of epidemic fevers, was replaced with a focus on microscopic organisms and biting insects as the true causes of ill health. This was not a social view of disease. As already mentioned, Gorgas noted with satisfaction that in Havana he had got rid of yellow fever without tackling any of the traditional problems of public health, and had in fact shifted two thirds of his men from cleaning houses to mosquito brigades. Putting in piped water to replace water storage receptacles, or replacing hovels with adequate housing, which would allow window and door screens to be put in place, was not considered part of the new public health (even though, in retrospect, it appears that better housing and screens were factors in the disappearance of yellow fever in the United States in the twentieth century). In the United States the waning of the reformist, social agenda in public health was especially marked; the professionalization of public health was connected to the embrace of bacteriology, a focus on individuals at risk of disease rather than on populations at large, and on technically expert interventions.[80]

A second feature of the model was its single-disease focus and the organization of the control methods as a 'campaign' set up independently of, or outside, existing public health services. In Havana, the single-disease focus and the separation of the yellow fever service from the rest of public health was justified by the US authorities in terms of its military efficiency and urgency. The US was an occupying force, had to act quickly, was not there to stay over the long haul, and did not take on responsibility for the general health of the Cuban population. Its focus was on stabilizing its own political and military presence. The resident Cubans were often indifferent, if not hostile, to the yellow fever control efforts, either because they were already immune to the disease from infections in childhood, or because they lived outside the designated geographic area of interest to the US authorities. The Cubans were largely poor, and reeling from years of death and disease caused by their struggles against the Spanish (struggles which had resulted in one of the highest *per capita* death rates of any war of independence); to them, tuberculosis, respiratory infections, high levels of infant mortality, and lack of adequate food were at the forefront of their problems, not yellow fever.

Away from an actual war situation, the rationale given for organizing yellow fever as a freestanding, autonomous service outside the normal public health routines was its technical and administrative requirements, namely the need to train usually low-level and uneducated personnel in the techniques of mosquito killing, and to supervise them separately. It was additionally argued that only by keeping the service as a special unit could it be insulated from political pressures. The specialized service was to be run like a unit of the army, with teams or squads of mosquito killers working under strict hierarchical discipline, as though they were indeed army brigades. This idea of an autonomous service, dedicated to eradicating a single disease, and lying outside routine public health, was very dear to Fred L. Soper's heart, as we shall see.

Though the model has something to recommend it in certain circumstances (a sudden eruption of a highly contagious disease like SARS may call for a highly targeted, swift and semi-independent public health effort), generally speaking dealing with diseases, even epidemic diseases, in separate organizations risks fragmenting public health and reducing its effectiveness. People, especially people in poor countries, do not necessarily get ill with one disease at a time; someone with HIV/AIDS is likely to suffer periodic bouts of malaria while also suffering from galloping tuberculosis. A holistic and integrated approach to health is required.

A third feature of the 'Gorgasian' campaign model of public health was its detailed mapping and record-keeping. Maps had of course been used before in epidemiological work, while the keeping of bio-statistics, such as the register of the causes of deaths in a population, or records of compulsory disease notification, were very important features of the European sanitary revolutions of the nineteenth century. But the eradication campaign was now planned, mapped and recorded with a new precision; record-keeping not only tracked how the campaign was going, but in effect defined it.

Gorgas had begun his yellow fever campaigns by drawing up detailed maps of the places to be targeted, showing the location of all the houses on all the streets. The map was kept in a central office, so that all the data sent in by inspectors could be evaluated at one place in a comprehensive manner.

The work of the inspectors, and of the teams of oilers or mosquito-killers, was also precisely planned; the number of houses an inspector had to inspect in a day or a week, the route he should follow, and how the inspection was to be carried out, were worked out in advance and precisely adhered to.[81] An inspector had to expect his own work to be inspected in turn, with deviations from routine, or failures to carry out tasks, being punished by fines, or even dismissal from the service. Later, inspectors would be given a uniform to wear, to make clear their identity and authority (sometimes they also carried a bell with which to announce their arrival). In Brazil, where the same system was used, the teams of mosquito-killers were given the military name of 'brigades', Ronald Ross's suggested term.[82]

All of these activities were regulated by a system of record keeping on specially designed forms, with inspectors filling out on a daily basis the details of the houses visited, the work carried out, the numbers of sources of mosquito larvae found, and the numbers of premises found violating the regulations. Many years later Fred L. Soper developed Gorgas's system of record-keeping in even greater detail in the eradication campaigns he ran; he invented and had printed numerous report cards for all the different aspects of the campaign and the inspectors' work; and he compiled them into a massive volume, a kind of 'Bible of Eradication', which conveniently, in the case of malaria, he was able to put (in an English version) into the hands of the Egyptian authorities in 1943, when they mounted a campaign against mosquitoes following a massive malaria epidemic.[83]

The fourth characteristic of the new public health campaign model was its top-down, authoritarian character, growing initially out of its military origins but reflecting a tendency in public health more generally to want to impose on people regulations the experts believed would protect the population at large. Such regulations, and resistance to them, is a constant theme in modern public health. Reflecting on his initial failure to control yellow fever in Panama, Gorgas concluded the reason was that sanitation in Panama was not in fact under direct military rule, as it had been in Havana. In thinking about a model organization for yellow fever work, Gorgas listed the requirements as first, adequate resources; second, complete authority over the public; and third, special ordinances or legislation to enforce compliance, in this order.[84] Guiteras, who in 1903 had been sent to deal with an outbreak of yellow fever in Laredo, Texas, using the new anti-mosquito methods, had found it a challenge because he had no authority over the population living in the Mexican side of the city; he agreed with Gorgas that to stop an epidemic it would be wise to impose martial law.[85] Sir Rubert Boyce concurred; he maintained that relying on what he called propaganda, meaning by this the use of publicity, notices and announcements during an epidemic to persuade people to obey public health measures, was useless; only special laws to enforce them would do.[86]

On the other hand, as one commentator noted, quite rightly, the severe methods employed in Panama 'could probably not be enforced at all in a democratic community in ordinary times'.[87] Law has in fact always been an instrument of public health (for example, in laws against nuisances such as rubbish, or the laws making vaccination obligatory). Public health is a field of social intervention in which, to an inescapable degree, the rights of the individual are at times pitted against the rights of the community as a whole. It is the community at large that makes up the public for whom public health is ostensibly carried out (even when the 'public' in public health excludes many categories of people, as it often has in the past). Given the tension between individuals' rights to liberty of action, and the community's need for health, the acceptance by individuals of the inconvenience, and at times actual risks, of public health measures (for example, the risk of side effects from vaccination) depends on a certain convergence of values between individuals and public health authorities about the greater good that cooperation or compliance will bring them. Individuals have to believe that knowledge is on the side of the authorities, and be prepared to give up their rights (for example, a right to refuse to be vaccinated) because they perceive the good of the community as in some sense congruent with their own.

Education, full citizenship, participation and political equality are the historical routes to achieving the cooperation between individuals and the authorities that is necessary to make public health work; public health fiascos have many causes, but non-compliance tends to occur when the public do not in fact share the values of the authorities, or have lost confidence in their expertise – witness the refusal of many parents in the UK to submit their children to the MMR vaccination, a vaccine made of three live, attenuated viruses against measles, mumps and rubella (German measles), because of their fear that the vaccine may have unacknowledged side effects such as autism, and because they no longer trust the advice given to them by doctors.[88] In all these regards, the resort to martial law represents a very blunt instrument of public health – an emergency measure, at best. Yet again and again, those responsible for eradication efforts have referred to the need for mandatory laws, for compulsion, or even martial law. When Soper was put in charge of the entire federal anti-yellow fever service in Brazil in the 1930s, the first thing he demanded from the government was special legal mandates to enforce compliance with the rules and regulations of his campaign. He was used to working in a semi-authoritarian or authoritarian political framework, where citizens had few rights, and in this sense also was Gorgas's direct heir.[89]

Finally, we need to draw attention to the role of chemicals in eradication campaigns. Again, nothing new here in principle; chemicals had been used for public health purposes before. Lime and other corrosive substances had been dumped into pits as disinfectants; chemical insecticides had been used against agricultural pests. What was new in the eradication campaigns was the scale of chemical use. The twentieth century was a century of chemical innovation and of the massive employment of chemicals in agriculture and public health. In the early twentieth century, paraffin and oil were the main chemicals used to destroy larvae in the environment; at the peak of the anti-mosquito work in Panama, in the town of Colon alone, 100,584 sq. metres (330,000 sq. ft) of surface terrain was oiled; according to Abernathy, 567,812 litres (150,000 gallons) of oil were used each year over all the canal zone.[90] In the 1920s, an arsenic-based chemical called 'Paris Green' began to replace oil as an efficient larvicide, giving rise to the term 'greening' used by the Rockefeller Foundation personnel who promoted it and used it in anti-malarial work (this greening had, of course, nothing to do with the 'green' issues of the environmentalists today).

Sir Ronald Ross had remarked in 1902 that he had long wished for an ideal poison for mosquito larvae: 'What a boon it would be', he wrote, 'if we could keep the surface of a whole town free from larvae simply by scattering a cheap powder over it, once every six months or so. It is very possible such a substance exists, but unfortunately we have not yet discovered it.'[91] A prescient remark! After the Second World War, DDT would fit the bill. It became the all-purpose, wonder insecticide, being cheap and long-lasting. It was often sprayed in spumes over large areas of the environment from air planes, largely in order to destroy agricultural pests, but also against the vectors of human diseases. The environmental consequences of such massive reliance on powerful chemicals did not become a political issue until the 1960s. The environmental movement resulted in a new attitude towards chemical pollution and its long-term effects on environmental and human health. The outcome was not just an eventual ban on the use of DDT as an agricultural pesticide, but also its virtual withdrawal from health campaigns against diseases like malaria.

The correctness or otherwise of this decision is still being debated within public health circles, and will be returned to at the end of this book; but the ban on DDT and similar insecticides represents a basic challenge to the style of public health campaigns that had originated in the Americas in the early twentieth century, under the circumstances described in this chapter.[92] It would be modified in subsequent eradication campaigns, but certain features remained as a legacy from the Gorgasian era: it was a top-down health strategy organized around a single disease. It was often costly, not cheap as its advocates claimed; it was in its own way intrusive; it was independent of other activities in public health. But for a long time it worked.

The International and the Global

The 1905 New Orleans yellow fever epidemic was the last to occur in mainland America. Why yellow fever disappeared thereafter from North America is not known; it was certainly not due to the systematic destruction of the *Aedes aegypti* mosquitoes and their larvae, as had occurred in Cuba. Humphries speculates that the virus itself might have undergone a mutation (different strains of the yellow fever virus, with different virulence, being known to exist) but this is only speculation; perhaps the increased use of piped water and sewage, improved housing with screens and the growing use of insecticides, held it at bay.[93] Whatever the cause, yellow fever's disappearance in the United States consolidated the idea that, henceforth, the essence of the problem lay overseas; the task was to extirpate the remaining seed beds of yellow fever elsewhere, in order to protect the US at home. The impulse in preventive medicine is always to prevent the invasion of harm from the outside; this was the origin of the first quarantines in the fourteenth century, and the same principle underlay various efforts, none of them very successful, to set up a system of quarantines between states in Europe in the nineteenth century, in order to protect them against the invasion of cholera and other communicable diseases. In the early twentieth century, steps were taken to institutionalize a system of notification of disease among participating countries. An early example was the Pan American Union, established in 1902 by US initiative largely with yellow fever in mind.

The opening of the Panama Canal in 1914 crystallized worries about the internationalization of disease. Gorgas and other public health officials learned that colonial officials in India and elsewhere were fearful that the Canal would open up a new route by which yellow fever could be transmitted from the Americas to the Far East, where the *Aedes aegypti* mosquitoes were widely distributed but where hitherto yellow fever had never penetrated. Colonel S. P. James, of the Indian Medical Service, had investigated the problem of the potential spread of yellow fever to India, and had called for permanent quarantine stations to be maintained in Panama, Hong Kong or Singapore, at the expense of the European colonies in the East; he also recommended that the Indian government make a systematic attack on mosquitoes.[94]

Might it not be better, however, to aim to extirpate yellow fever completely from its endemic homes, first in the Americas where yellow fever eradication had already been tried, and then in West Africa, before increased contacts between west and east (by the new air transport, as well as by sea) spread it even further? Was complete eradication a possibility?

Colonel Gorgas, for one, thought so; he believed that the anti-mosquito work in Havana proved 'the practicability of eliminating in the Tropics the two diseases malaria and yellow fever'.[95] Similarly, Dr James Carroll, one of the original members of the Reed Commission, claimed in 1905 that 'It is now certain that before the lapse of many years, the disease, yellow fever, will have become extinct. The length of time necessary for complete eradication will depend on the readiness of our southern neighbours to accept the mosquito theory in toto, and to institute for their infected seaports, vigorous and energetic measures based upon it.' He added 'Another epidemic of yellow fever should never be seen in the US.'[96]

The term 'eradication', derived from the Latin and meaning 'to tear out by the roots', had often been used to describe the aims of public health, but it had been used loosely, to mean the control of a disease, or its general reduction. Now a more precise and absolute idea was being introduced. We see this, for example, in a 1911 lecture given by Dr Henry R. Carter, who had contributed the concept of extrinsic incubation so critical to the mosquito theory of yellow fever; the aim of yellow fever sanitation, he said, was to 'eliminate yellow fever where it exists'. And he added: 'I say eliminate, not control. The latter is allowable for malaria, but I think that for yellow fever the sanitarian should be satisfied with nothing short of elimination. It is easy.'[97] To the idea that the techniques were available and easy, there was added a high-mindedness about the duty, even the obligation, to take action against yellow fever. Dr James Carroll maintained that so simple was it now to stop yellow fever that any outbreak could only be the result of the 'culpability of some irresponsible person'.[98] Something that had hitherto been viewed as immensely difficult, the elimination of yellow fever, was now being presented as within reach, and even morally imperative.

But though the proponents of eradication insisted that yellow fever eradication could be achieved easily, even cheaply, the truth was the opposite. Panama told the true story. In one year alone, in the single town of Colon, some 100,584 sq. metres (330,000 sq. ft) of the city's surface was oiled, 60,960 linear metres (200,000 ft) of ditches were cut, of which 6,096 metres (20,000 ft) were stoned and cemented, and 19,202,400 sq. metres (21,000,000 sq. yards) of grass were cleared. 'Never had a crusade been carried out with such completeness', said Ronald Ross, 'for never has a chief sanitary officer had so free a hand'. This remark referred to what Gorgas had achieved with malaria, as much as with yellow fever; nevertheless, taken together, the overall expenses of the operations were enormous. Gorgas's sanitation department spent $2 million per annum, estimated at one tenth of the total annual cost of the canal work, to achieve what was, as we have seen, a result that was limited in its geographical extent.[99] This did not make Panama an easy example to follow. Where were these kinds of resources to be found in, for instance, the British colonies, where Dr Ronald Ross, Nobel laureate in medicine, found himself unable to persuade the colonial authorities in West Africa to fund even a single anti-mosquito brigade for malaria control?

The Rockefeller Foundation Takes Up the Challenge

The answer lay, in the first instance, not with individual governments, but arguably the most significant philanthropic agency to work on health between the two world wars, the International Health Division of the Rockefeller Foundation (RF), inaugurated in 1913. By the time Soper met Gorgas in 1920, the RF had already been involved with disease eradication for some years. In the case of yellow fever, to which the RF devoted the largest percentage of its resources in its overseas work in the Americas, there was a direct line of influence running from Havana and Panama to the RF, the RF's International Health Division (IHD) having recruited Gorgas, Carter, Guiteras and other veterans of Panama, in a full-time or an advisory capacity, because of their experience with yellow fever and their belief in its eradicability.

When the young, newly married doctor, Fred L. Soper, presented himself in Washington in late 1919 for an interview with Mr Wycliffe Rose, then the head of the IHD, he arrived at just the right moment for a new kind of career overseas. It is not evident what decided Soper to choose a life that meant spending years abroad, working in tough conditions, on diseases in poor countries; it was not a humanitarian gesture. Soper says he was attracted by Wycliffe Rose's view that the special function of the IHD 'was to help bridge the gap between existing medical knowledge and its practical application'. Rose mentioned to Soper the IHD's work on hookworm and 'a campaign for the eradication of yellow fever which he thought would take from five to 10 years for completion'. Soper, as we shall see, was not a research scientist, but a man given to action and command, and he accepted the offer from Rose and prepared to be sent immediately to Brazil. 'Thus I began a career in international health', says Soper, 'a field which scarcely existed prior to 1915 except for the work of colonial officials, military officers, or occasional missionaries.'[100]

The RF opened the next stage in the story of disease eradication, sharpening the concept, applying it to diseases other than yellow fever and helping define, as it did so, the meaning of the 'international' in international public health.

3 Paradoxes: The Rockefeller Era

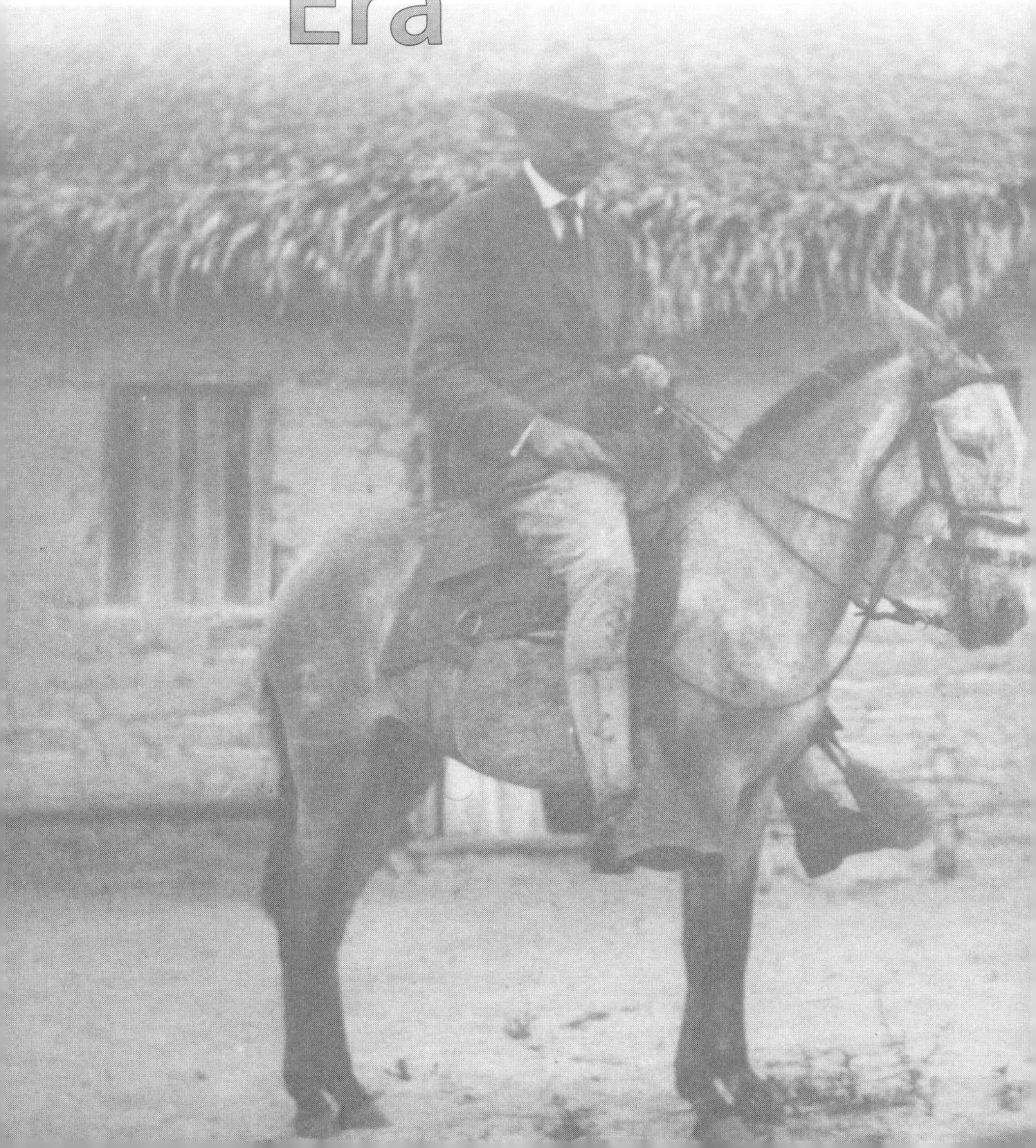

By 1927 Dr Fred Lowe Soper had been one of the 'Rockefeller medicine men' for seven years.[1] He had spent the time working on hookworm disease, first in Brazil and then in Paraguay, and was not yet the formidable medical baron of the organization he would later be. He was about to be transferred to Rio de Janeiro, then the capital of Brazil, where he was to take over the task of running one of the Rockefeller Foundation's (RF) regional offices.[2]

At this point, the RF's International Health Division (IHD) had been conducting eradication campaigns against yellow fever in the northeast of Brazil, where yellow fever was endemic, since 1923.[3] It was certain its methods were working, and expected to stay on in the country for only a few more years. Steps were even being taken to close most of the RF's mosquito eradication stations, and to hand back responsibility for any remaining yellow fever work to the Brazilians.[4] So confident was the RF about the imminent disappearance of yellow fever in the country that in January 1928, Dr Michael E. Connor, who was directing the RF's yellow fever operations in Brazil at the time, announced that, if no further yellow fever cases appeared in the country in the next three months, he would consider the disease finally eradicated from the entire Western hemisphere.[5]

But by May this confidence was utterly dashed; yellow fever re-appeared in epidemic form. At first, just a few cases were registered, in the north, then in Rio de Janeiro. Soon the capital city, which had been free of the disease for twenty years following the anti-mosquito campaign early in the twentieth century, was in the middle of a full-blown epidemic.[6] In addition, cases of yellow fever were identified in 40 other towns in the state of Rio de Janeiro. It took months of frantic efforts, the hiring of 10,000 public health workers, and the expenditure of some $10,000,000 over the next two and half years to finally free the capital of the disease.[7] Over the next three years, cases of yellow fever also appeared in many other towns, in the interior of Brazil, and in port cities from Buenos Aires to Belém at the mouth of the Amazon. In 1929, Recife, in the northeast, had new cases despite five years of continuous anti-*Aedes* work.

This epidemic overlapped in time with a burst of RF-funded laboratory and epidemiological discoveries that in the space of only a few years would reveal that much of what the RF had thought about yellow fever had been simply wrong. More – the RF slowly came to understand that *yellow fever was not the kind of disease that could ever be eradicated from the face of the earth,* owing to the belated realisation that the virus of yellow fever was harboured by animals, mainly monkeys, which could not themselves be eradicated short of the massive slaughter of many forest species. This biological fact, the existence of animal reservoirs of microorganisms that are pathogenic to humans, has become one of the fundamental limiting principles of the eradication concept. The discovery ended for the RF the romance of yellow fever eradication; eventually, it also spelled an end to the RF-era of large-scale, practical public health programmes.

By an accident of timing, Soper was in Rio de Janeiro to witness yellow fever's re-appearance. Knowing almost nothing about yellow fever ('I never had killed a mosquito in my life', he boasted), he was drawn into yellow fever work.[8] By the early 1930s he was running Brazil's National Yellow Fever Service. But paradoxically, as the RF gave up its ambitions for eradication, Soper converted to the cause, pursuing it as the goal and purpose of his lifetime in international health. Over the years, indeed, he became eradication's most forceful proponent.

The purpose of this chapter is to try to resolve this and other paradoxes in the history of eradication in the pre-Second World War, and Rockefeller, era. Without Soper's conviction about eradication, which his experiences in the Second World War only strengthened, and which he then took into new organizations, notably the World Health Organization (WHO), eradication might not have been taken up as enthusiastically as it was by the international community after the war, to become a global public health effort.

The Rockefeller Creed and Eradication

The RF originated as a philanthropic organization focused on medicine and health in the early years of the twentieth century, when the immensely wealthy John D. Rockefeller Sr sought to redeem his unsavoury reputation as a robber baron, by becoming a baron of charity.[9] In 1901 he founded the Rockefeller Institute for Medical Research (later called the Rockefeller University). In fairly short order thereafter, Rockefeller money funded a Sanitary Commission for the Eradication of Hookworm (in 1909); the Rockefeller Foundation (established in 1913); and the International Health Division (the IHD, also begun in 1913), which was responsible for health work overseas. By the time the IHD closed its operations in 1951 its field staff had worked in public health in 80 countries, including Canada, the United States, 25 countries in Europe, fifteen in the Caribbean, every country in Latin America and several countries in Africa and the Middle East.

The Foundation based its public health activities on what came to be known as the 'Rockefeller Creed'. Enunciated by Fred Gates, the first head of the Rockefeller Foundation, the creed, says the historian Farley, 'has become a cliché but still warrants quoting': 'Disease is the supreme ill of human life, and it is the main source of almost all other ills – poverty, crime, ignorance, vice, inefficiency, hereditary taints and many other evils.'[10] In a reversal of the idea that the direction of causation runs generally from poverty to disease, disease was assumed to lead to poverty. Historically this idea – that disease makes people poor, and that by removing a disease we remove the chief barrier to economic productivity – has been deeply embedded in public health. Louis Pasteur, for example, famously remarked that 'whatever the poverty, never will it breed disease' – a 'brazen statement', comments the historian, Anne-Marie Moulin, but one which 'signified the mood of the new hygiene'.[11] Disease being considered easier to eliminate than poverty, the goal of the Rockefeller Foundation was to remove disease and thereby all the ills enumerated in the Creed.

To achieve this end, the RF believed that what was needed was a new and permanent organization 'capable of acting on new scientific discoveries'. With a strong biomedical orientation, the RF clearly favoured the application of technical know-how over broader social approaches to ill health. The RF's 'philanthropic universalism', in Weindling's words, implied that scientifically based knowledge was universal in its application; the same methods could be applied in the same way in very different political and social settings, even in places where the most basic health infrastructure was absent.[12] This technical approach, suggests Darwin H. Stapleton, fitted in well with the RF's desire to avoid political involvement, and with the general bias in American culture, dating back to colonial times, but especially evident in the Progressive era, towards finding technical approaches to social problems. The technical approach had the advantage of yielding immediately quantifiable results that could then be used to justify the large expenditure of funds. Data on the number of houses screened, pipes laid, larvae sources found, and blood samples taken could flow back from the field to the RF headquarters for statistical analysis and budgetary assessments.[13] Every field officer working for the Foundation in public health was required to keep a daily diary of activities, which was circulated among the other field officers; strict financial accounting was also demanded. Woe betide those who overspent their allowances![14]

Two other aspects of the RF philosophy need noting. First was the RF's principle of working only with governments (and not with other private, non-governmental organizations). This reflected the RF's desire to make a permanent impact on health services; it wanted to make formal agreements with national or local governments, which would then serve as partners in health projects, with a system of shared work and distribution of costs such that, by the end of an agreed-upon period of time, the financial and administrative responsibilities of projects would pass from the RF to the governments themselves. Second, in keeping with these approaches, the RF thought of itself as a tutelary organization, demonstrating to public health and government officials how to apply scientific knowledge, but not itself running public health departments. The number of people working for the RF directly at any one time was never very large; over the entire course of the RF's yellow fever work in numerous countries in the Americas and West Africa, the total number of salaried RF officers amounted to only 76 people. Most of the people working on the RF-sponsored yellow fever projects were in fact doctors and field workers from the various host countries.[15]

Retrospectively, the limitations of the RF approach are evident – a distance from, at times even a disdain for, clinical knowledge or local medical practices and an over-confidence in expert knowledge. On the plus side was this same confidence, the ability to put money where the RF saw fit, and to be bold. The RF in this respect had a great deal more freedom of action than the WHO probably has today.

Among many historical analyses of the RF, the recent account by John Farley is especially valuable in giving an overview of the IHD's public health work overseas.[16] Farley's critique of the RF is not that the RF was a part of a capitalist plot to dominate the poor countries of the world (as Farley shows, more RF money was spent on Canada, the United States and Europe than on poor, developing countries over the course of the IHD's history, nor did its public health efforts follow specific US government capital or imperial interests), but that its approach to public health was reductionist, as well as surprisingly naive in its faith in its quantitative measures of success. In Farley's analysis, as in the newer histories of the RF more generally, the neo-imperialist context of the Foundation's work is not ignored, but taken as a given – the starting point for an analysis of the complex arrangements, and the push-and-pull features, of a well-endowed public health organization that worked over the course of the inter-war years, cooperatively and by invitation, with governments as diverse as revolutionary Mexico, progressive Costa Rica, authoritarian Brazil and fascist Italy. The historian, Steven Palmer, in his account the RF hookworm campaigns in the Caribbean and Central America that launched the RF in global health, starting in 1914, is especially convincing about the initial adaptability of the field methods the IHD field officers used, as they learned how to collaborate with local officials and come to terms with the realities of local customs and cultures.[17] Later, as in the case of Soper's work for the IHD in the 1930s, the IHD acquired the more familiar characteristics of the top-down and autonomous mode of operations generally ascribed to the RF; but the international division of the RF always worked with a broad range of governments, even fascist ones, as already noted. The RF also gave considerable financial and technical support to the League of Nations' Health Organization, the other important international organization of the inter-war years (set up in 1923).[18]

The RF prized its political neutrality. In fact its best field officers, like Fred L. Soper, were shrewd assessors of the political situations in which they operated, and were given considerable leeway to use their political skills to promote the Foundation's goals.

Getting to Work: From Hookworm to Yellow Fever

The RF's first efforts in public health overseas were directed against hookworm disease. This chronic and debilitating disease is one of the most common infections of poor people today, infecting some 576 million people in developing countries (in sharp contrast to the disease's absence in the developed world).[19] Considered one of the most significant 'Neglected Tropical Diseases' (NTDs), hookworm's roots in poverty and the lack of sanitation could not be more striking.

But in an earlier era, between roughly 1900 and the mid-1920s, hookworm had a high profile; it was the target of many health campaigns, and was a key disease in the emergence of 'international health'. Hookworm was first identified in the late nineteenth century by scientists working in areas of agricultural and industrial capitalist expansion, where mining, plantation agriculture and labour migration brought large numbers of people to work in conditions of grinding poverty and minimal sanitation.[20] The hookworms were identified as microscopic organisms, the largest specimens of which can *just* be seen with the naked eye. The worms, either *Ancylostoma duodenale* or *Necator americanus*, the latter found in the Americas, as its name indicates, are parasitic organisms called nematodes that, once in the digestive system of human beings, attach themselves to the gut with their hooks (mouth parts), and proceed to disrupt the digestive processes, causing symptoms of anaemia, lethargy, disorders of appetite, emaciation and sometimes mental retardation; in very severe cases it can be fatal. The worms and eggs are excreted from the body during defecation and in poor sanitary situations, where there is no piped water or latrines, they pollute the soil. The eggs develop into larvae in the moist and humid soil; from there they enter the human body, usually through people's bare feet, working their way eventually into the digestive tract, where the whole cycle starts again.

In the early twentieth century, hookworm disease was very common throughout the hot, southern states of the United States, where it was believed to be responsible for the 'backwardness' and lack of productivity of the rural population. The disease attracted the attention of the RF because it was seen as amenable to diagnosis and scientific prevention. Whether the RF really aimed for complete eradication is not entirely clear, though Soper claimed it did. Certainly, the 'Rockefeller Sanitary Commission for the Eradication of Hookworm', which was set up in 1909 to conduct anti-hookworm campaigns in the South, used the word 'eradication' in its name. The Commission may have taken its inspiration from the achievements in Cuba and Panama with the eradication of yellow fever – a very different disease. The Director, Wycliffe Rose, in describing the aim of the Sanitary Commission, said 'eradication must . . . be made a world campaign – not for altruistic motives merely but because no one country can be safe until all have been cleared of this pest'.[21] This gave a succinct definition of eradication: in its strict sense, it had to encompass the entire world. The more immediate goal, though, seems to have been to demonstrate the presence of hookworm disease in a location and to show how local populations and public health officials could take steps themselves to eradicate a disease, by following the RF's scientific methods.

Operating in eleven US states between 1910 and 1914, the work of the Sanitary Commission was based on mobile dispensaries that tested people for hookworm infections and offered treatment with drugs. Since testing for worm infections required faecal samples from the population, the programme touched on delicate, indeed taboo topics, and required, therefore, great efforts at public education in hygiene. It is worth noting that, though the lack of shoes, the lack of sanitation, especially latrines, and the lack of food (malnourished individuals being affected by the worm burden much more severely than well nourished ones), were known to be the prime determinants of hookworm disease, the RF concentrated its own work on surveillance, testing and effecting a 'cure' by dosing people with a strong vermifuge, thymol, followed by a purgative such as Epsom salts, which moderated the unpleasant (and at times dangerous) side effects of the thymol. The expectation was that two or three, or even four, treatments would rid an individual of worms for good. During the First World War, another drug, oil of chenopodium, was often used instead of thymol. By 1914 more than one million people had been examined in the southern states of the US for the presence of worms in their stools, of which over 440,000 were infected.[22]

In 1913, the International Health Commission (later the International Health Board, and later again the International Health Division) was formed, and in 1914 it took the hookworm programme overseas. The first efforts outside of North America were organized in six small countries in the British Caribbean and in Central America.[23] Dr Hector H. Howard, the physician chosen to first test the RF's methods abroad, in British Guiana, said in the manual he drew up after returning from the British colony, 'There is not a missing link in our knowledge of the Ankylostome [hookworm]'.[24] But Howard also conceded 'that while the complete eradication of [hookworm] in a given territory is theoretically possible, practically it can only be approximated'.[25] In fact, the US experience already showed that re-infection rates, following treatments or 'cures', were very high.

In British Guiana the RF developed what came to be known as the 'intensive' (or 'American') method; by this was meant a more comprehensive mapping of the population to be treated and larger and more rapid dosing of people so as to effect a cure.[26] A team of people, involving nurses, microscopists and a doctor, would carry out a careful survey of the designated population, identifying and registering on special, standardized forms, every person as to their age, sex, race and location; the population would then be asked to supply stool samples, which would be collected and analysed in a laboratory by microscopy to confirm infection by worms. Those found to be infected were then treated systematically with drugs, until each individual was free of worms. The all-encompassing character of the hookworm campaign, the requirement to test and treat everybody in a population, gave it an inclusive stamp which Soper later liked to emphasize (calling it 'egalitarian'); the method of mapping an entire population, the data collecting and centralization of command also gave him a kind of blueprint for later work on yellow fever and other eradication campaigns. In fact the centralization of data seems to have been borrowed from the yellow fever campaigns in Cuba and Panama. The intensive method worked best in colonial situations, where to a certain extent it could be imposed on local populations. The RF field officers certainly thought the method worked well enough that more than 90 per cent of those infected received at least one drug treatment.

When Soper joined the IHD in 1920, to be sent abroad after a short introduction to parasitology to work on hookworm control, he knew nothing about the disease or, or for that matter, about the country he was going to (when asked by a RF staff member what he knew about Brazil, which Soper had ventured as one of the countries he would like to be assigned to, he could name only coffee and rubber; when pushed for something more, he added monkeys).[27] In this regard he was not untypical of the young doctors the IHD recruited to spend years working in foreign places 'on their own' (as was often said, though actually with a staff from the country concerned, some of them also doctors). Soper's contemporary, Dr Alan Gregg, who met Soper in Brazil at this time (and did not like his brash manner), commented in his reminiscences: 'the fact is that we didn't know how to do public health work', adding 'It was much more a guerrilla warfare on disease than a planned campaign.'[28] But Soper learned, and quickly.

When Soper arrived in Brazil in February 1920, the RF had been working on hookworm in various parts of the country for three years. Brazilian doctors and public health officials had already discovered the importance of hookworm infections for themselves before the First World War, through numerous medical expeditions and surveys in the rural hinterlands. In the state of São Paulo, the centre of coffee production, there was particular interest in dealing with hookworm, since the First World War was cutting off the supply of European immigrants; this led local officials to concentrate attention on reducing hookworm infections in the local labour force.[29] The RF added to these pre-existing efforts in Brazil, bringing its own ideas about how to address hookworm, together with its far greater resources. However, the huge size of the country, the deep poverty of its rural populations and the absence of even rudimentary health structures in the rural areas, meant that while the RF's dispensaries were often welcome, eradication was not in the cards.

Like the hookworm programmes conducted in the Caribbean, the IHD's methods in Brazil had to be adapted to the realities on the ground – to the fact of people refusing to take the medicine, to migrating away from their homes in search of work or to resisting entering their names on a registry (young men in rural areas feared that, in doing so, they were being conscripted into the army). The intensive method, the IHD's innovation, proved to be unsuited for use in rural Brazil, where populations were often scattered. Instead a system of mass treatment was used which bypassed both the pre- and the post-treatment testing of individuals. This was justified on the grounds that a quick survey of several hundred random stool specimens from each of a number of communities in the area showed that a high percentage of the population was infected with worms; it was decided to treat everyone in the community (with thymol or oil of chenopodium), regardless of the degree of infection, or even whether a person was infected at all. It was a system of blanket coverage. Exceptions were made for the very young, pregnant women, the very old and people known to have heart disease. Most of the treatments occurred without the supervision of a physician.

Soper found by experience in the northeast and in the south of Brazil that it was impossible to treat 100 per cent of the inhabitants in any given area; he said it was considered a good result if 70–80 per cent received one treatment, with progressively fewer people receiving a second or a third treatment. He also found it very difficult to introduce latrines, or where introduced, to persuade people to actually use them.[30]

In the autumn of 1922, Soper returned to the US for a year, during which he obtained a Certificate in Public Health at the Johns Hopkins School of Hygiene and Public Health, and acquired a further four months of field work experience in Alabama and Georgia, where he learned something about malaria and typhoid fever, as well as more about hookworm disease. He also learned at Johns Hopkins that there were serious doubts regarding the eradicability of hookworm disease.

He was then assigned to Paraguay, where he was put in charge of setting up a new hookworm programme. He was to spend the years 1923–7 based in Asunción. Though Soper was apparently quite a good linguist, eventually becoming fluent in Portuguese and Spanish, he and his wife, Julie, never managed to learn Guaraní, the lingua franca of Paraguay; as Soper acknowledged, this failure militated against their identification with the people. It didn't stop Soper, however, from becoming an expert and determined public health administrator, who got used to running his own show, and commanding both people and parasites.

From the years working on hookworm Soper learned how to conduct a survey of a population, map a district's houses and locations, keep and manage personnel and put in place a system of inspection of work done as well as checking those inspections – all features of his later eradication methods.[31] In Paraguay, hookworm operated as an autonomous programme (independent, that is, from other sanitation work or institutions); Soper hired and fired his personnel, kept careful financial accounts and was his own boss – a model of operations he kept in mind henceforth.

During his years working on hookworm, Soper learned both to keep very careful records but also to trust no statistics unless he knew the manner in which they had been compiled. In his memoirs (1977) he tells the story of a woman in the northeast of Brazil who was registered in the books as having shoes (and therefore in principle protected from getting hookworm infection); but Soper discovered that she used her shoes only for attending church, carrying her shoes to the church door, putting them on for the service, and removing them afterwards.

Dr Lewis W. Hackett, who was to have a long career with the IHD, and at the time had oversight of the hookworm programmes in Brazil, said he thought hookworm a 'sound choice' for eradication, because it allowed for a much better 'entering wedge' for long-term health programmes than malaria or yellow fever, since the worm could be seen without a microscope, the disease held 'no mysteries', and huge areas of the world were infested with the worm.[32] In fact, it proved to be a poor choice of a disease to work on, given the RF's preference for technical solutions over social ones. According to most accounts, the IHD made little real dent in hookworm's incidence in countries overseas in the long term. The records the RF field officers kept showed an amazingly painstaking approach to identifying those infected and treating them, but Farley nevertheless calls the RF's assessments of their supposed success in reducing hookworm infestations 'forays into a mathematical never-never land', since however quantitative the data collected appeared to be, it was not of a kind to actually answer the questions asked.[33] First and foremost a disease of social misery, hookworm disease was probably incapable of being eliminated short of a real improvement in the standard of living of the rural poor among whom hookworm infections were rampant.[34] In his reminiscences of his time working on hookworm in Brazil, Gregg commented that the RF officers in the field knew that when people were properly fed, they were less likely to have worms, and added: 'We might have been able at a far greater cost to get rid of parasites in Brazil by feeding the population extremely well.' But this was something that the RF either did not feel in a position to do, or perhaps wish to do.[35]

At any rate, the RF approach by itself would not eradicate a disease so entangled in multiple determinants of a social and economic kind. Better housing and incomes, better diets, indoor sanitation, piped water and the widespread use of shoes were what was needed; the RF's chosen methods – registering a population of sometimes several hundred people at a time; testing them for worms (rates of 100 per cent infection were common); persuading people infected with worms to take medicine, with nasty side effects; measuring hookworm infection rates afterwards and encouraging (but not paying for) latrines – were not enough. The IHD knew that building latrines was crucial to preventing re-infection, but considered it the responsibility of individuals, all of them very poor, or the local authorities (equally without funds). As a result, latrine building was haphazard and completely inadequate for the job. Two years after a treated population was tested again, infection rates were found to be as high, or almost as high, as before – and the process of testing and treating had to start again.[36]

In the early 1920s, the RF arranged for a Dr W.W. Cort, of the Johns Hopkins School of Hygiene and Public Health, to conduct detailed epidemiological studies of hookworm in Trinidad, Puerto Rico and China; these studies showed that eradication could not be achieved in a reasonable length of time by the methods then being used.[37] In this regard hookworm was rather like tuberculosis; the IHD had campaigned against tuberculosis in France from 1917 to 1924, and when the campaign ended (with disappointing results) the IHD directors had decided never to get involved with a 'social disease' like TB again.[38] At the end of the decade, the IHD's hookworm campaigns were being quietly folded – without, Farley notes, any acknowledgement of failure.[39]

Soper was very surprised to learn he was to be phased out of hookworm work and Paraguay, and sent instead back to Brazil, to do administrative work. He had been working away on hookworm for years, even as the IHD had lost all practical interest.[40]

Instead Soper found himself getting involved in yellow fever, the next disease for eradication that the RF took up. The anti-mosquito techniques employed against vector-born diseases seemed to lend themselves to the RF's bio-medical, interventionist and accounting approach better than did hookworm disease. The possibility of eradicating yellow fever completely seemed realistic.

The RF's interest in yellow fever dated back to before the First World War. In 1913, Wycliffe Rose, the director of the IHD, travelled through Europe and Asia, where he learned that many colonial medical officers were worried, as we saw earlier, that the imminent opening of the Panama Canal to shipping the next year might lead to the spread of yellow fever to Asia, where there were plenty of the *Aedes aegypti* mosquitoes but no yellow fever.[41] Asian populations therefore had no immunity to yellow fever should it ever reach the region. Dr William C. Gorgas, the Chief Sanitary Officer of the Panama Canal Zone, agreed about the potential danger of the eastward spread of yellow fever, and in 1914 persuaded Rose and the IHD to take on the task of eradicating the remaining foci in the Americas.[42]

As we know, Gorgas was confident that the methods to eradicate yellow fever were at hand. What was needed was the means, and this the RF was willing to provide. The goal of complete eradication of yellow fever was announced by the RF in 1915 (and endorsed at the Second Pan American Scientific Congress, held in Washington in 1915–16).[43] The next year Gorgas joined the RF's Yellow Fever Commission, which included, among others, Dr Henry R. Carter and Dr Juan Guiteras (both veterans, like Gorgas, of Havana and Panama), and was sent on a six-month tour of Latin America to assess the yellow fever situation and advise the foundation on a comprehensive plan of action. The Commission concluded that, as Gorgas had maintained, there remained in the American continent only a few remaining endemic foci of yellow fever (for example, Ecuador, Peru, Mexico, Panama, Brazil), and that yellow fever could 'be eradicated from the face of the earth within a reasonable time and at reasonable cost'.[44] Eventually, yellow fever would receive the lion's share of the foundation's attention and money. From 1925 to the late 1930s, in fact, over 50 per cent of the RF's budget for overseas health was spent on this single disease.[45]

In her study of the RF in Africa, Heather Bell argues that the yellow fever problem was in effect an 'invention' of the RF and the international community – not in a literal sense, since yellow fever certainly existed in Latin America and West Africa (as it still does today), but in the sense that the RF gave it its high profile, and made it a global concern that trumped local health priorities. In both Latin America and Africa, 'the IHD directed resources at yellow fever out of all proportion to the disease's impact on local health. In both places, local resistance to the global goal – whether by the general population or a government – was regarded by the IHD and its allies as selfish and irresponsible.'[46]

Of course the impulse in public health has always been to prevent the invasion of harm from the outside, for example, by state-to-state agreements concerning mutual notification of diseases and by quarantines. As empire and trade expanded in the early twentieth century, several new organizations were founded to improve international cooperation in health, such as the Office d'Hygiène Internationale in 1907, based in Paris, and the Interamerican Sanitary Bureau (the predecessor to the Pan American Health Organization), established in 1902 on the US's initiative, with its headquarters in Washington. Its original purpose was precisely to stop the transmission of yellow fever between the American republics (especially from the Latin American countries into the United States). But the executive capacities of both organizations were limited (the League of Nations Health Office was more effective, but was not founded until 1923).

The RF carved out a place for itself in these years, when the mechanisms of international cooperation in health were less effective than they would become after the Second World War. Its distinctive contribution was to take its disease control methods overseas, for a mix of utilitarian and humanitarian reasons. Yellow fever was represented as a danger to the global community because new paths of communication were being opened up, especially air travel. The RF thought that the US could not rely on countries where the disease was endemic to deal with it effectively (despite the evidence that Brazil, for one, was in fact controlling yellow fever reasonably well, given the huge size of the country, its poverty, and its limited public health resources). As a well-endowed philanthropic organisation, the RF proposed to go to the sources of yellow fever abroad and tackle them there. The term 'international' in public health, as with the term 'global' in 'global health' today, stands for less than it seems to imply. In the case of the RF, its internationalism meant the pursuit of selected diseases across political and national boundaries, in the name of a greater good for the world community of nations. Eradication encapsulated this distinctly qualified notion of international public health; it was carried out 'for' the United States, as a form of what might be called 'defensive internationalism'.

The Start of Yellow Fever Eradication

Action on the yellow fever eradication plan was delayed by the entry of the US into the First World War in 1917 (during which Gorgas served as Surgeon-General of the US Army). It was not until the war's end, in 1918, that the RF was in a position to send a Yellow Fever Commission, composed of several field experts, to Guayaquil, in Ecuador, the first country selected in which to tackle yellow fever; the bustling port on the Pacific coast of Latin America was considered the most likely place from which yellow fever might spread to Asia.

The initial assessment of Guayaquil and yellow fever by the RF team in 1916 had focussed on the inadequate water supply in the city, which had led the residents to rely on open containers of water in their houses – perfect breeding places for 'stegs' (short for *Stegomyia*, as the *Aedes aegypti* mosquito was then called). The RF team proposed to delay tackling yellow fever until after a water supply was put in; or alternatively, suggested tackling yellow fever right away if the RF would pay to put in a water supply – an idea, Farley says, that Wycliffe Rose 'squashed'. The Yellow Fever Commission returned to Guayaquil in 1918, and again reported on the need for better water as well as improved street paving; but Rose insisted, once more, that these amenities were the responsibility of the city itself.[47]

This was a missed opportunity, an alternative to the RF's preferred technical fixes in public health, since in the long run it is likely that yellow fever disappeared in the United States because of improved piped water supplies (which reduces mosquito breeding in or near houses). But long-term social investments of this kind were not the RF's 'way'. Nonetheless, approaching yellow fever (which was epidemic in the city) entirely as a problem of mosquitoes, the RF's team had a quick success by following the Gorgas model; by imposing strict quarantines, isolating suspected patients, fumigating houses and identifying and destroying all foci of *Aedes aegypti* breeding, the team cleared the city of yellow fever in six months.

The Ecuadorian campaign was followed by others, in Mexico and Peru. In Peru, the campaign was very much a case of 'sanitation from above'.[48] The authoritarian government gave support to a short and ruthless campaign that 'never managed to have most of the public co-operate actively'.[49] In Mexico, the campaign was more cooperative, despite Mexican hostility to any interference by the US government and the difficulty the RF had in representing itself as quite independent of US authorities. But the sudden appearance of yellow fever in the port of Veracruz in 1920, and changed political circumstances, resulted in an invitation to the IHD to collaborate in controlling the epidemic. That year, the country had 505 cases of yellow fever (though this figure was no doubt an under-estimate); by 1921 the number had fallen to 115, and by 1922 to 14; in 1923, Mexico closed its anti-*Aegypti* control centres.[50]

West Africa now beckoned Gorgas, who set out on yet another RF-sponsored Yellow Fever Commission to investigate yellow fever in the only other geographical region of the world believed to be endemic to the disease. Visiting London in 1920 en route to Africa, Gorgas was much fêted; but while there, he fell ill and subsequently died, though not before being knighted in his hospital bed by King George V for his contributions to public health.

There remained in Latin America the country of Brazil, which was, in yellow fever terms, the 'prize' as far as the RF was concerned – the largest country in the southern continent, and the country that contained the most numerous endemic foci of the disease. As we have seen, Brazil had mounted an anti-mosquito campaign against yellow fever in the capital city within two years of Gorgas's success in Havana. The campaign in Rio was followed by campaigns in a few other Brazilian cities (for example, Belém in the Amazon in 1910). An extremely poor, largely black country – the last country in the western hemisphere to abolish slavery, in 1888; a country encompassing vast hinterlands that were almost unknown to the political elites living on the eastern seaboard; a country lacking democratic traditions, and lacking, too, even the most rudimentary of health infrastructures – Brazil's conquest of urban yellow fever in the capital of the country was a highlight in an otherwise neglected field of public welfare. Hoping to present the world with an image of a country free of an infection that targeted the very immigrants from Europe Brazil wanted to attract in order to 'whiten' its otherwise black population, the control of yellow fever had acquired a symbolic importance in the national imagination that perhaps no other disease had at the time.[51]

The RF first approached Brazil about collaborating in the country's anti-yellow fever efforts as early as 1920. That same year, Soper had his first introduction to yellow fever when he travelled with General R. C. Lyster (Gorgas's nephew) to spend several days in the northeastern state of Pernambuco, looking into Brazilian control efforts. Here Soper saw for the first time the living forms of the *Aedes aegypti* mosquito – the larvae, pupae and the adult insects – and was introduced to his first 'foco' (breeding site). The director of the state's health service had at the time fifteen doctors and 300 men working under him on anti-mosquito activities. Lyster and Soper were impressed with the detail and efficiency of the service, Lyster concluding that, if maintained in all of Brazil, yellow fever could indeed be eradicated.[52]

The RF representatives on this visit were rebuffed in their request to get involved in yellow fever work in the country; the Brazilian government was proud of its expertise in yellow fever control, and declined any outside assistance. In 1923, however, this changed when a new, more autocratic President took office, and the director of the National Department of Health, Dr Carlos Chagas (of Chagas disease fame) agreed to allow the RF to try out its methods in endemic areas in five states in the north of the country. This was conveniently far away and out of sight of the elite in the nation's cities in the south, and so protected the Brazilian government from the charge that it had handed over the country's yellow fever control to foreigners. To the IHD this agreement seemed of historic significance, allowing them to tackle what appeared to be the last holdout of the yellow fever virus in the Americas.

Within a few years of work, as we have seen, the RF was confident that yellow fever was on the verge of being eradicated in the country, a confidence that proved unwarranted when the epidemic of 1928–9 erupted in the capital city and surrounding areas.

Eradication and the Problem of Expert but Incomplete Knowledge

In retrospect, this unanticipated epidemic put in sharp relief a problem that has been a feature of almost every eradication campaign – the problem of expert but incomplete knowledge. Again and again, eradication campaigns have proven to be more complicated than expected; diseases in general tend to be more complex than experts predict; applying the same methods of disease control in different contexts often proves to be a mistake. The idea that one method fits all is a mistake.

Of course, scientific knowledge is always uncertain and medical and public health practices are always running up against the limits of what is known about the aetiology or nature of disease. But the problem of incomplete knowledge is compounded in an eradication campaign, since to a greater degree than in traditional sanitation, an eradication campaign tends to be narrowly focused; it is usually concentrated on a single disease at a time, and depends for success on a specific biomedical intervention; it often runs the risk of unravelling when it encounters unexpected challenges, is unable to adapt quickly to changed circumstances, and so fails to meet the absolutist goals it has set for itself.

With no disease were these lessons learned more painfully, perhaps, than with yellow fever. The RF scientists held several strong beliefs about the disease, all of which proved over time to be untrue. They believed that yellow fever was essentially an urban disease whose continued transmission required a large population of many thousand people. This reflected the US's main experience of yellow fever, where it had been almost entirely urban. The RF also thought that yellow fever was readily diagnosable, with clear clinical symptoms, such as high fevers, black vomit and high fatality rates; that yellow fever was transmitted by a single species of mosquito; and that it had no animal reservoir. And finally, by 1919, they believed they had in their possession a workable vaccine.

The trouble was, all of these beliefs were wrong.

The belief in the vaccine was perhaps the most egregious of the foundation's errors. It represents a bizarre saga involving the tenacious but, in the end, unwarranted faith the RF placed in the work of one of their researchers, the Japanese-born bacteriologist, Dr Hideyo Noguchi. The discovery of a preventive vaccine would obviously have contributed greatly to solving the yellow fever problem. A vaccine is often the holy grail of infectious disease research (think of the current search for a malaria vaccine); a vaccine was the crucial intervention allowing eventual smallpox eradication; and the production in 1937 of a genuinely effective yellow fever vaccine changed the RF's anti-yellow fever strategy, as we shall see. But for almost ten years, between 1919 and 1928, the RF backed a vaccine that was based on a series of errors and mistakes of understanding. The strong support the RF gave to Noguchi's work is especially striking (if very much understated in the foundation's official history, which managed to avoid a frank account of the events), because of the profile the foundation had as an institute defined by its commitment to the highest standards in scientific research.[53] The history of microbiology is replete with mistaken identifications of pathogens, and vaccines that did not work; but the striking thing about Noguchi's yellow fever vaccine is that some quite obvious and very basic follow-up investigations that should have been done at the time were not. It was not until doubts by scientists, many from outside the RF, forced a re-assessment in the mid-1920s, that the RF finally decided to investigate Noguchi's work.

A flamboyant, indeed eccentric, character, Noguchi was an established bacteriologist working at the Rockefeller Institute when he was asked to go with the RF's Yellow Fever Commission to investigate yellow fever in Guayaquil, Ecuador in 1918.[54] Getting to work immediately, collecting blood from yellow fever patients and then inoculating a number of animals, within less than two weeks of his arrival in July, Noguchi had concluded he had found the elusive pathogen of yellow fever – something no one else had been able to do since the work of the Reed Commission almost twenty years before. He identified it as a small bacterium known as a spirochete, which he named *Leptosira icteroides* (like, but he claimed, distinct from another spirochete called *Leptospira icterohaemorrhagia,* which was known to cause a different human infection called Weil's disease).[55] A furious period of experimentation resulted eventually in a series of fourteen papers between 1919 and 1921.[56] His final paper in the series described his method of prophylactic inoculation against yellow fever, using liquid cultures of the *Leptospira icteroides*. This method was tested on animals and humans in Ecuador during an epidemic. The Rockefeller Foundation proceeded to send Noguchi's vaccine out for use as a preventive, both for its own researchers, and for Latin American populations.[57]

The trouble was that his vaccine flew in the face of everything known about yellow fever up to that point. The causative organism, though unknown at the time, was not considered to be bacterial at all, but an organism that was much smaller – smaller, certainly, than a bacterial spirochete. Nor was the guinea pig, Noguchi's chosen experimental animal, considered receptive to, or suitable for, experimental inoculations of yellow fever. In fact, Noguchi inoculated a startling number of mammals and birds – startling, because all the researchers before had failed to inoculate any. There was also the problem of lack of corroboration of his findings by other researchers, especially by experienced medical scientists from Latin America. Critics asked why they could not find Noguchi's leptospira in yellow fever victims, why Noguchi did not try to inoculate more suitable or likely animals and why he did not spend more time clearly differentiating 'his' leptospira from the leptospira of Weil's disease.[58]

The story of Noguchi's yellow fever work is, as Clark puts it, 'long and confusing', involving visits to many countries in search of materials, such as Mexico and Brazil, and ending only with his death in Africa in 1928. Clark, who knew and liked Noguchi, attributes his mistakes to his careless and disorganized laboratory habits, his driving ambition to make a name for himself in science, and his undisciplined personality.[59] But Noguchi was also oddly persuasive, and this may explain the strong support some key RF figures gave to his work (notably, Simon Flexner, the Director of the Rockefeller Institute). Noguchi himself dismissed all those critics who could not duplicate his findings by claiming they lacked either his experimental dexterity or adequate laboratory facilities for dealing with what he said was an organism that was highly sensitive to contamination by other organisms. Dr Juan Guiteras published a refutation in 1921, pointing out that Noguchi had simply confused the spirochete of Weil's disease with that of yellow fever, but to no avail. In 1923, Dr Aristides Agramonte, the only surviving member of the original Reed Board, made an even more trenchant critique of both Noguchi's leptospira and his vaccine, whose use he said had endangered the people who relied on it. But Noguchi seemed to shrug off such attacks.[60]

Eventually, though, the criticisms became impossible to ignore. In 1925, the RF decided to send out scientists to West Africa, ostensibly to carry out investigations to see whether Latin American yellow fever was different from, or the same, as yellow fever in Africa. The real purpose of the Yellow Fever Commission, which set itself up in a laboratory in Lagos, Nigeria, was to re-examine Noguchi's work to see if it really stood up to rigorous experimental examination. Already in 1926, Max Theiler and A. C. Sellards, of Harvard University, had shown that Noguchi's spirochete was indistinguishable from the spirochete responsible for haemorrhagic jaundice.[61] All further efforts to find Noguchi's *Leptosira* in yellow fever patients had negative results. The scientists with the Yellow Fever Commission went on to show that yellow fever in the two continents was indeed identical; for the first time, they were able to infect rhesus monkeys with yellow fever, thus making possible an animal model. In 1927, the true causative organism of yellow fever was isolated, and identified as a small, filterable virus, as had been originally believed, and not a bacterial spirochete, as Noguchi had claimed.[62] Eventually, a particular strain of the yellow fever virus (known as the 'Asibi' strain after the African man from whom the first sample was taken) was identified, and sent to the RF's Yellow Fever Laboratory in New York City for further study; through many experimental stages, it became the basis of our modern yellow fever vaccine, the 17D vaccine in 1937 (Max Theiler received the Nobel prize in 1951 for his part in this work).

Thus the RF's claim to have produced an effective yellow fever vaccine was now correct, but it was obviously a quite different vaccine than Noguchi's. Noguchi, who had gone to look into yellow fever in West Africa himself, working as always, secretively, carelessly, and obsessively in a laboratory the RF set up for him in Accra, Ghana (and so independent of the Lagos-based RF scientists who were undoing his theory), died of yellow fever on 21 May 1928, still experimenting, and without ever repudiating his work.[63]

Commenting years later on the Noguchi episode, Soper remarked that 'The extent and duration of the Noguchi fiasco in yellow fever is really surprising. This mistake was not a single false observation . . . it was a series of false observations repeated in different geographical areas over several years.'[64] Hindsight no doubt makes judgement easy, and few disease campaigns have been conducted on the basis of perfect knowledge. Nonetheless, the yellow fever story was dogged by blindness and over-confidence.[65] It may be that the long and troubled history of Noguchi's yellow fever vaccine made Soper suspicious of substituting vaccination for the eradication of mosquitoes, even after the highly effective 17D vaccine had become available in the late 1930s and was administered to millions of people.

Re-Thinking Yellow Fever

Noguchi's death coincided almost exactly with the return of yellow fever to Rio de Janeiro, in an epidemic that tested the RF epidemiologically, and which heralded a period of several years of re-examination of other long-held beliefs about yellow fever.

The RF had inherited a model of yellow fever transmission from Gorgas and the Reed Board that, though an adequate general guide to yellow fever control in cities, was inadequate when it came to complete eradication. The core of the RF's yellow fever strategy, as it existed in the 1920s and into the early 1930s, was encapsulated in what was known in RF circles as the 'key-centre' theory of transmission. First articulated by Dr Henry Carter in 1911, the theory held that yellow fever was fundamentally an urban disease, because it was only in large centres of population that sufficient numbers of *Aedes aegypti* mosquitoes existed to transmit the virus, as well as sufficient numbers of non-immune humans entering the population, by birth or by migration, to keep the virus circulating and transmission sustained.

The epidemic in Rio de Janeiro in 1928–9 seemed at first to confirm this key-centre, urban model. It was thought that the city had been re-infected from the north and the epidemic was due to failure to eradicate the yellow fever mosquito in key urban centres. But the model was undermined when outbreaks of yellow fever occurred in very rural and often isolated places, where no urban mosquitoes were found. As early as 1907, a Colombian doctor, Roberto Franco, described yellow fever cases he had seen in forested or jungle areas remote from towns; another outbreak in 1916 in the same place was dismissed by Gorgas, because he found none of the expected urban *Aedes aegypti* mosquitoes present in the vicinity.[66] Many other Latin American physicians had in fact had doubts about the RF's model; they knew that yellow fever was often found in small and scattered villages in the interior. Some British colonial physicians, such as Sir Rubert Boyce, said the same about West Africa.[67] It was clear that much about the epidemiology of yellow fever was simply not known.[68]

The discovery of rural yellow fever challenged another of the RF's beliefs, namely, that the disease could be readily diagnosed. As North Americans, the RF doctors thought of yellow fever in terms of the often dramatic symptoms seen in victims who were newcomers; but physicians in Latin America knew yellow fever as an often 'silent' or mild disease, frequently infecting children, and causing headaches, malaise and a slight fever – symptoms easily overlooked in places without doctors, and anyway not easy to distinguish from those caused by other infections. Over the years, when faced with reports of such cases in rural areas, RF doctors tended to reject the diagnoses and identify them with some other condition. In his memoirs Soper drew attention to many such occasions, in 1923, for instance, the RF staff officer, Dr Joseph H. White, clashed repeatedly with Brazilian experts on the existence of yellow fever cases in small rural towns, refusing to recognize them as such because the clinical signs did not match his expectations. Dr M. E. Connor, the IHB field officer in charge of anti-yellow fever work in Brazil who so confidently predicted yellow fever's elimination in 1928, was another RF officer only too ready to dismiss local clinical knowledge.[69] 'Regrettably', wrote Soper, 'the Foundation workers were unable to appreciate the wealth of experience and keenness of observation of their Brazilian colleagues.'[70] Soper did not mention that he himself had initially taken a similarly sceptical attitude.

Both the clinical signs of yellow fever and the idea of a single vector were thus being undermined by clinical and epidemiological experience. By the early 1930s it was becoming evident that the overall picture of yellow fever was very different from what had been thought, and that vectors other than *Aedes aegypti* were involved. In 1932 Soper himself travelled to the southern state of Espiritu Santo to investigate an outbreak of yellow fever in the Valley of Canaan. It is clear that he could not make the epidemiological pattern of yellow fever he encountered fit the old expectations. Outbreaks like the one in Espiritu Santo established definitively the presence of yellow fever without the known *Aedes* vector; and within a few years, several non-*Aedes* species were implicated and a new epidemiological pattern was identified.[71] In 1934 Soper coined the term 'jungle yellow fever' to differentiate a non-*Aedes* cycle of rural yellow fever transmission from an urban *Aedes* cycle. Jungle fever's tardy recognition was due to the fact that the cases fell outside the urban, endemic areas recognized by the RF.[72]

It was because it was realized that yellow fever is indeed often silent or difficult to diagnose that laboratory tests became significant to the yellow fever story. There were doctors (for example, some of the British) who had said early on, on the basis of clinical and epidemiological knowledge of yellow fever in West Africa, that what was needed was a method of sero-diagnosis (some kind of blood test to confirm the presence of a disease that was sometimes easy to miss). Such a test was eventually developed by RF scientists once the yellow fever virus had been identified in 1927. This was the ingenious 'mouse protection test', which allowed scientists to identify immunity in individuals whose past history was not known, or who were not known to have had a bout of yellow fever.[73] The test, then, was a test of infection after the fact, allowing medical doctors to identify yellow fever areas in the apparent absence of clinical diagnoses of the disease. It was very useful, therefore, for mapping the geographical distribution of immunity in populations. Immunity surveys using the mouse protection test were carried out in the 1930s, in Africa and Latin America; the surveys found that indeed rural populations harboured yellow fever, even though no outbreaks of yellow fever cases had been recorded.[74] These numerous cases had gone undetected, either because no doctors were at hand to diagnose them, or because the symptoms were so mild they had passed unnoticed (or had occurred in children who suffered from many other childhood illnesses and fevers, such as malaria). The RF took a perverse pride in its work when, in 1940, a yellow fever epidemic, predicted on the basis of their immunity surveys, actually occurred in the Sudan, against the British colonial doctors' expectations. The epidemic resulted in 20,000 cases and 200 deaths between early 1940 and early 1941. According to Heather Bell, many of the experts involved took satisfaction when it happened, treating yellow fever not primarily as an illness but as affording proof of their theory. She quotes a local district commissioner remarking: 'For the specialist an epidemic like this, which has killed its thousands, is a glorious field day.'[75]

In the summer of 1932 Soper told the then head of the IHD, Frederick F. Russell, that the foundation no longer had the 'holy formula'.[76] By the late 1930s doctors were indeed beginning to piece together the elements of a fundamentally new picture of yellow fever, based on new epidemiological information and experimental data coming out of Rockefeller laboratories. This new picture indicated that the primary hosts of the yellow fever virus were not humans, but animals, mainly monkeys, living in the forests; these animals represented a *permanent reservoir of the virus*.[77] Human beings were only the secondary, or incidental, hosts. Jungle yellow fever (or 'sylvatic' yellow fever, as it is now called) refers to the cycle of yellow fever that occurs when non-*Aedes* mosquitoes, living in the jungle canopy, transmit the virus they have picked up by biting infected monkeys or other animals, to human beings working at the edge of the forest. Then the movement of infected people from forest areas to local villages and towns initiates the cycle of yellow fever based on the bites of the urban-breeding *Aedes aegypti* mosquito.[78]

The result of the compounding errors in the understanding of yellow fever had been that many outbreaks of yellow fever had been unanticipated and inexplicable for several years. After the epidemiology of jungle yellow fever was established, it was realized that, while urban yellow fever could be controlled, yellow fever eradication itself was impossible, short of destroying all the forest animals that harboured the yellow fever virus. There had to be a reckoning with the fact that, as Farley says, 'contrary to earlier beliefs yellow fever seemed to be a disease that would never disappear'.[79]

Soper Takes Charge: Authority and Mastery in Public Health

When Soper took over the direction of the RF's yellow fever project in 1930, most of these developments lay in the future. Looking at yellow fever from a practical point of view, he attributed the recent epidemic in Rio de Janeiro to the fact that the federal yellow fever service, which had been set up originally as an autonomous, single-disease service, with its own mosquito-brigades and bureaucratic regulations, had been merged into the general public health service. From this Soper derived his lifelong belief in single-disease organizations and personnel, preferably organizations and personnel over whom he himself had complete command.

And command them he did. Within three years of his return to Brazil in 1927, Soper found himself in charge of a nation-wide, federally organized, cooperative yellow fever service – running a Brazilian department, in effect, a remarkable turn in the career of a man who at the time knew nothing at all about yellow fever. The epidemic in Rio in 1928–9 had shone a very unwelcome spotlight on a disease of great symbolic significance to the country that most public health officials had believed to be on its way out. The brunt of the criticism in the press, and among the political class, fell less on the RF, which had been working far away in the northeastern states, than on the federal authorities in charge of sanitation in the capital city. The outcome was an opportunity for the RF to widen its role in the country. In 1929, the RF and the Brazilian government began to discuss a new agreement, which resulted shortly afterwards in the establishment of a joint Cooperative Yellow Fever Service (CYFS), which steadily expanded its area of authority until it eventually came to include the entire country.[80] By the terms of the agreement, the operating expenses were to be paid by the Brazilian government, amounting to 60 per cent of the total costs, and the other 40 per cent of the expenditures by the RF (excluding the salaries and allowances of the RF staff, who never numbered more than half a dozen at any one time). In the single calendar year 1930 the Brazilian government spent $2,500,000 as its contribution to the new cooperative yellow fever service alone.[81]

It was this cooperative service that Soper took over in June 1930. Having engineered the removal of his predecessor, Dr Connor, Soper took charge of a much-expanded programme, holding on to the position until 1942, when he left Brazil for public health service in the Second World War. It was a leadership role for which he was entirely suited, by temperament and skill.

Soper was not a laboratory man, but a public health administrator of genius. In the administration of a huge and taxing public health campaign Soper found his métier. Whereas to many RF field officers, the actual tasks of finding mosquito breeding sites, and spraying or chemically treating them, were viewed as a 'deadly routine not suitable for RF staff', they were exactly what interested Soper.[82] He loved the details, the commands, the organization and the accounting that a practical public health campaign depended on. He set to work to understand them, master them and refine them. To him, administration was, as he put it, 'the Essence of Eradication'.[83]

Soper's assumption of the direction of the RF-Brazilian Cooperative Yellow Fever Service in 1930 took place against a background of political events in Brazil that greatly helped him achieve his goals. The 'Revolution of 1930', as it is referred to in Brazilian history, represented a political revolt against the institutions of the Old Republic and its 'liberal', semi-democratic system (very limited though the voting rights were). It ushered in an era of strongman politics, under a President, Getúlio Vargas, who ruled Brazil in authoritarian, neo-corporatist fashion in his 'New State' (Estado Nôvo, established in 1937) until the end of the Second World War. Under Vargas, Congress and all political parties were abolished.

Considered one of the most influential Brazilian political figures of the twentieth century, Vargas was a canny politician but essentially a pragmatist rather than an ideologue.[84] Sometimes called the Mussolini of Brazil, for his mix of authoritarian and modernizing impulses, he lacked Mussolini's fascist trappings, such as a black-shirt militia. Brazil at the time was a country of some 30 million people who were desperately poor, largely illiterate and locked in dependence on local rural bosses, a dependence Vargas tried to break. Vargas was a centralizing force who used the power of the centre to incorporate, selectively, the industrial working class into the political system. Equally selectively, Vargas supported programmes aimed at solving social problems; the yellow fever programme was one of them, and another a massive anti-malaria campaign in the northeast in the late 1930s. Both diseases were important to Vargas because they affected negatively the international reputation of the country.

To Vargas, government was 'chiefly a question of administration', and so, in a country short of administrators and skilled workers, he invited many foreign experts to come to Brazil to advise on how to modernize.[85] He carefully balanced his leanings towards the United States with his leanings towards Nazi Germany, before committing the country belatedly, in 1944, to the side of the Allies in the Second World War.[86]

Vargas's commanding style suited Soper's methods in public health extremely well.[87] Arranging a meeting with Vargas within two months of the Revolution of 1930, Soper found support for his ideas about yellow fever, and was given the scope to innovate in administrative methods, to have complete authority over his personnel, and to get the legislative backing he needed to impose his public health methods. Soper found that Vargas, having already appointed military men as 'interventors' in place of elected governors in the states, had made effective rule from the centre much easier than it had been in the era of decentralized politics, at least in programmes that were run with determination, as Soper's was. In effect, between 1931 and 1942, Soper found himself the leader of a large national department of health focussed on a single disease.

The RF Abandons Yellow Fever Eradication, Soper Converts: Resolution of a Paradox

However, as Soper took over this greatly expanded national programme and developed new methods to control yellow fever, he found himself on a course of action that went far beyond what, by the mid-1930s, the RF wanted – a course that was in fact no longer compatible with the foundation's goals. This leads me to the central puzzle of Soper's yellow fever work: his embrace of disease eradication right at the moment that the RF realized that yellow fever could never be eradicated.

With typical hyperbole, Soper described the RF's yellow fever programme as 'the most magnificent failure in public health history'.[88] This failure derived from the discovery in the early 1930s of yellow fever's animal reservoir. This 'underlined one of the most important principles in the selection of human diseases as candidates for global eradication – this was impossible if there was an animal reservoir'.[89] By the mid- to late 1930s, the RF had accepted this fact; by 1937, they also had a new weapon, a vaccine.

Soper reasoned, however, against these conclusions, that if the disease of yellow fever could never be eradicated, then *at least the main urban vector of the disease, the well-known Aedes aegypti mosquito, could be*. Eradication, in this formulation was thus shifted from the disease itself, to an entire species of insect. True, jungle yellow fever would remain, but this cycle of disease was sporadic and confined to the rural borderlands with forests. Brazil was an increasingly urbanized country, and it was in the cities that the greatest number of deaths from yellow fever occurred. The new perspective Soper brought, then, was to turn an old goal, namely the reduction of the urban vector of yellow fever to a point at which transmission stopped, to a new absolute – to the complete elimination of a vector. In this way, urban yellow fever itself would be eliminated.[90]

The trouble, as Soper saw it, with aiming for mere *Aedes aegypti* control (that is, simply a reduction to low numbers of mosquitoes and/or their larvae), as previous yellow fever campaigns had done, was that the authorities invariably relaxed controls over mosquitoes when yellow fever itself seemed to disappear. The result was the eventual return of yellow fever, often in explosive epidemic form, after years of absence, as had occurred in Rio. Why not, argued Soper, get rid of the *Aedes aegypti* mosquito once and for all, from an entire port, or city, or a region, a country or even a continent – the crucial test of success being the ability to discontinue all control methods even in the presence of suitable breeding areas for the mosquito, without any recurrence of the disease?

Soper acknowledged that such an absolutist goal was hard to achieve; it required more money and effort up front, and more determination. But once achieved, there were huge savings to be had in terms of safety and costs; all controls could be relaxed, because the species is wiped off the face of the earth and cannot return to act as a vector again. Making urban areas safe in this way, control and surveillance would be focused eventually on rural areas where yellow fever was only sporadic. The majority of the population, located in cities and towns, would be free of yellow fever forever.

To work, however, this new concept of eradication had to be absolute. Any chance that *Aedes aeygpti* mosquitoes might be re-introduced from the outside, into an urban area that had been made free of them, would be potentially disastrous, as meanwhile a whole city would be filled with people who had never had yellow fever and so never acquired the immunity conferred through childhood infections. Of course, after 1937 a yellow fever vaccine was available (and Soper was responsible, as head of the yellow fever service, for supervising its production in Brazil, testing it, and finally giving it to several hundred thousand Brazilians). But because yellow fever was often a hidden disease, it could pass unnoticed into urban areas that, if still infected with *Aedes aegypti* mosquitoes, could have outbreaks of the infection before vaccinations could be introduced to halt its spread. For this reason, Soper always remained sceptical that yellow fever control could depend solely on vaccination.

When Soper began to talk about exterminating the *Aedes aegypti* species from all of Brazil, 'yellow fever experts from Rio to New York laughed at him. They declined to be Soperized.'[91] But to Soper, getting rid of the mosquito was everything.

Perfectionism at the End of the Line

The question was: could it be done? How was eradication of the *Aedes aegypti* mosquito to be achieved? The answer was – through meticulous and systematic methods of insect extermination, based on almost superhuman attention to detail and accuracy in inspection. Here was where Soper came into his own, elevating public health administration, as Litsios put it, to as 'exact a science as one can imagine possible'. Someone else characterized Soper's administrative method as one of 'perfectionism at the end of the line'.[92]

As Soper looked back over his time in Brazil in the 1930s, he reflected that there were three problems he had faced: the epidemiology of yellow fever was not fully known and the disease could spread sight unseen for months if not years; the *Aedes aegypti* mosquitoes could maintain themselves in hidden breeding places despite careful inspection; and it was difficult to maintain an efficient anti-mosquito service in the almost complete absence of cases of yellow fever disease. These problems were to be solved by discovering when and where silent endemic yellow fever existed; uncovering hidden mosquito breeding points; and ensuring absolute accuracy of reporting on such sites, even in the absence of yellow fever victims.

In essence, his model was that of Gorgas's quasi-military one, in its administrative style, its centralized leadership, its detailed prescription and management of inspectors, its attention to the generation of reliable records and the autonomy of the yellow fever service. In 1930, when he took over the Cooperative Yellow Fever Service (CYFS), Soper knew nothing about how yellow fever control methods worked; taking himself off to the northeast of the country, he spent several weeks following mosquito inspectors around, as they did their house-to-house searches for mosquitoes and larvae, oiled containers of water and repeatedly returned to make their inspections again. Losing 12 kg (27 lb) in the course of such work, Soper came to appreciate how hard it was, and also how easy it was to make mistakes. Gorgas had famously remarked that to control mosquitoes, one had to learn to think like a mosquito. Soper famously amended Gorgas, saying that to kill mosquitoes, one had to think like a mosquito inspector.[93] Rigidly controlled inspection of the inspectors therefore became the key to mosquito eradication under Soper.

Soper's employees had better pay than public health workers outside the yellow fever service, but more was expected of them; they reported directly to him and were independent of other public health officials; they had exacting work schedules which were worked out in detail, by means of a clock, establishing the exact routes the inspectors were to follow, and the times of day, the numbers of houses to be inspected and so on (25 per cent of the entire CYFS budget was spent on checking the checkers). Extremely careful accounting of all tasks done, and bookkeeping, was also demanded, Soper inventing numerous new tables and forms whereby the results of inspections were recorded and tabulated.[94] Inspectors could be dismissed for any unwarranted infringement of the rules (for example, if an inspector could not be found within 10 minutes near the correct location stated on his pre-assigned schedule).

This expectation of responsibility and duty led to one of the most repeated anecdotes about Soper's administrative style; on learning that one of his men had managed to avoid being killed in an accidental explosion at an arsenal because he had failed to go to work, when he showed up the next day Soper fired him for dereliction of duty.[95] Löwy has called the system of public health administration associated with Soper 'Taylorism of the *sertão*' (the name given to the parched lands of the northeast of Brazil but used to convey the 'hinterlands' or 'backlands' more generally).[96]

Two other innovations of the national yellow fever service concerned the issue of visibility: how to make visible the locations of yellow fever when the disease was often invisible or invisibly mild; and how to make visible the hidden breeding sites of the mosquitoes.

The first problem was resolved largely by the development of a 'viscerotomy' service. A viscerotome was a simple instrument invented in 1930 that allowed the rapid extraction of a sample of liver tissue from someone who had recently died of a fever or unknown infection; once extracted the sample would then be sent to a pathologist to see if it showed evidence of the characteristic signs of yellow fever infection. These signs had been described correctly by the Brazilian medical scientist Dr Henrique Rocha Lima in 1912, but the significance of his findings had been overlooked for years. Not until it was accepted that yellow fever was widely found in rural areas, and often passed unnoticed or undiagnosed, was it realized that autopsies could be effective means of identifying yellow fever infections after the fact.

Eventually, Soper put in place a system of gathering such autopsy data from all individuals who had died within eleven days of falling ill with an unknown fever. Between May 1930 and June 1933, some 28,000 liver exams were carried out; among these, 54 cases of yellow fever deaths were documented, 43 in places not known to have yellow fever at all.[97] By 1948, the viscerotomy system consisted of no fewer than 1,310 viscerotomy posts throughout Brazil, and a system for paying local individuals to extract the samples and send them on to Rio de Janeiro for analysis. By this time, a total of 385,728 liver specimens had been obtained from people who had died after illnesses of up to ten days in duration, with 1,487 cases of yellow fever being identified.[98]

Many people understandably objected, at times violently, to having the burials of their dead relatives interfered with by nosy officials intent on removing from the bodies specimens of tissue for autopsies (especially since their permission was not asked for in advance). In the early days of the service, at least five viscerotomists were killed, a fact that led the RF to order the service cancelled. This order Soper simply ignored, in the name of public health necessity – as he saw it.[99]

The second technique for making visible what was otherwise invisible was the introduction of special squads, or teams of inspectors, whose job was to hand-capture adult breeding mosquitoes found in people's houses. When Soper had followed the yellow fever inspectors around in 1930, step by step, house by house, water receptacle by water receptacle, he had discovered how hard it was to identify every place where *Aedes* mosquitoes could breed – in standing water in all sorts of receptacles near or in houses. In poor areas, these receptacles could be almost anything suitable, from abandoned tins, to old rubber tyres, to the many jars and containers people used to store water in their homes (no piped water being available in most areas of the country). Even the best inspector, the most careful, would find on returning to a house he had inspected a few days before, that mosquitoes were still flying around, indicating that somewhere, hidden from view, a female mosquito was laying eggs and producing new mosquitoes that could transmit yellow fever.

Taking a tip he acquired around 1930 from malaria specialists that the most sensitive indicator of hidden breeding sites of mosquitoes was the presence of even a few adult mosquitoes, Soper sent in special teams of 'mother squads' to detect any flying mosquitoes and trace their sources back to their hidden mosquito 'mothers'. With this technique, in 1932 Soper managed to achieve the first zero index of mosquito house infection. Failure to eradicate *Aedes aegypti* had been explained until then, said Soper, 'on the basis of the sanctity of the species, the law of diminishing returns, and the irreducible minimum'. But these explanations become, he said, 'untenable' in the face of hand capture techniques and meticulous administration.[100]

Finally, I come to the issue of what Soper called, with approval, 'coercive legislation'.[101] Vargas, who ruled by presidential decree from 1937 to 1945, was a firm believer in power of the centre, the need for a firm hand, and he was especially important in giving Soper the backing of the law. By May 1932, new legislation not only gave Soper a free hand in setting the terms of employment and the firing of employees; it also gave Soper and the CYFS the absolute right to impose sanitary policies as they saw fit – to inspect and investigate sources of mosquitoes in houses, and to make the families living in the houses responsible for keeping them mosquito-free following inspection. Soper described the legislation as 'purposely draconian'.[102] Compliance was enforced by means of monetary fines. It was one of the first times since Gorgas in Havana and the Panama Canal Zone that the authoritarian, sanitary bureaucracy had been worked out in such detail in a civilian situation.[103]

The legislative decrees passed in Brazil satisfied Soper's need for the coercive legislation to get public health work done. Soper looked like a military man and thought like a military man. He believed that the seriousness of the job of eradication demanded an autonomy of service and a principled, single-minded focus on the work, with autonomy especially in the bureaucratic routines, and freedom from interference, if the work was to get done.

Soper's Law

It was well-known that you did not have to get rid of the *Aedes aegypti* completely to interrupt yellow fever transmission; reduction to 5 per cent (meaning 5 per cent or less of the houses inspected were found to be infected with the *Aedes* mosquito) was sufficient, but of course this meant the mosquitoes remained and could re-populate cleared houses. Soper began to find, however, that under the rigorous system of inspections he introduced in 1930, without initially intending to he was actually reducing the incidence of mosquitoes to almost zero; by 1933 he found that the *Aedes* mosquito had disappeared completely from many coastal cities in the northeast of Brazil, and it was this that gave him the idea that actual eradication of the entire species of *Aedes aegypti* was possible. 'I wish I could say we carefully planned to eradicate aegypti and then did so', wrote Soper: 'In truth, this was a free ride, so to speak; some would call it serendipity. It was not planned, but came as a reward of careful administration and of lowering the visibility of aegypti breeding below the survival threshold.'[104] He maintained that it was easier in fact to chase after every mosquito, than after every yellow fever victim.

As Soper gained more and more confidence that his teams of mosquito killers were indeed able to wipe out the urban vector of yellow fever, he began to promote the concept of species eradication, and propose that the Brazilian government set up permanent nationwide services for *Aedes aegypti* mosquito eradication to achieve this aim.[105] As Soper put it, 'The discovery of the permanent reservoir of infection in the jungle in the absence of *Aedes aegypti* paradoxically forces the organization of permanent anti-aegypti measures throughout threatened regions.'[106] Soper recognized that with the collapse of the key-centre theory of yellow fever, the eradication concept had been thoroughly discredited compared to the optimism of the days when he heard Gorgas speak in 1920; but he was confident that his new idea about insect eradication would resuscitate its fortunes.[107]

From 1934, this was the theme Soper began to mention – the possibility of extending his techniques of species sanitation to the entire country; and then to other states; and finally, to the entire Americas.

To him this was a revolutionary concept. It signified much more than simply improving existing control efforts; it was a demand for new standards of efficiency in local health services, and coordination across regions and countries to cover the entire range of a particular vector under attack. It was a revolutionary concept because it was absolute and total. In many respects, all the new ideas about yellow fever, even jungle yellow fever, were merely incidental debating points when it came to species eradication; what was needed, Soper believed, was administrative competence and commitment – the push to be 100 per cent efficient. It needed certifiable results, based on organized operations, printed forms, mapping of towns, numbering of blocks of houses, measured itineraries, flags, responsibility on the part of every inspector, uniforms, records of every visit, bonuses for work done properly, the capacity to fire workers who did not carry out their tasks meticulously for dereliction of duty, legal backing for rules, independent checks of all the checking and so on. 'Aa [sic] eradication born of efficient administration of known techniques' is how a lecture note reads.[108]

This was not exciting stuff, perhaps; Soper complained that, to the RF, the romance now lay entirely in laboratory experimentation. But to him, the eradication concept was exciting and new; it implied a new goal, and a new public health morality. To accept eradication in public health implied a fundamental shift in psychology, or attitude, towards disease, especially low-incidence disease, when a disease has almost gone, and people tend to lose interest in continuing on to complete eradication. To Soper, though, mere reduction to *near* invisibility of a disease in a population would not do; it was only at this point that the serious work of eradication actually began. Eradication had to be absolute. Here was where the language of 'perfection' and absolutism, so evident in the eradication campaigns after the Second World War, entered into eradication discourse.

Soper took a lofty view of this absolute, believing it to be a morally superior form of public health compared to mere disease control; this was because whereas with mere control or reduction of disease, one could ignore or bypass the health of certain groups altogether, and settle for an overall low *per capita* incidence, without concern for equity, in eradication there could be no exceptions – by definition it included everyone. There could not be a 'partial eradication', or 'virtual eradication'. When Soper's predecessor in yellow fever work in Brazil, Michael E. Connor, in commenting on the failure of the yellow fever programme in Brazil in the late 1920s, had started speaking in terms of the 'irreducible minimum' of yellow fever, Soper would have none of it.[109]

One consequence of this view of eradication is that, for it to work, the eradicationist had to constantly expand eradication efforts from smaller to larger areas of the world. Soper referred to this as 'Soper's law', which he described as the general principle of the innate power of disease and vector eradication programmes to spread beyond their original starting point. As he saw it, once eradication of a mosquito species that transmits a human disease is achieved in one country, the right of that country not to be re-infected by its neighbouring country is recognized, with the effect that over time eradication has to expand from its point of origin until it becomes worldwide.[110] Of course this was not really a 'law' of public health, describing some inevitable development or outcome, but rather an expression of wishful thinking, or a logical deduction derived from the absolutist definition he had given to eradication.

If Soper's idea about eradication seemed 'democratic' in coverage (in that to work, eradication had to include everyone, whatever their social position or economic status), its mode of operations was not. 'Eradication is possible', he wrote, 'without universal public health services in underdeveloped countries', because that is what he had found working in Latin America.[111] He thought that eradication needed to be backed by special laws or decrees, imposing penalties such as fines on individuals who refused to obey the regulations of the eradication campaign. These ideas reflected Soper's experiences working in Latin America, in poor countries with undemocratic and often authoritarian governments.

By Soper's lights, democracy made eradication campaigns much more difficult – more, 'if you have democracy you cannot have eradication'.[112] Many years later, after the Second World War, when he took over the direction of the Pan American Health Organization, Soper took the view that the democratically-expressed opposition to DDT-spraying in the United States, which led to the US failing to fulfil its commitment to yellow fever mosquito eradication, was simply irresponsible, since it placed the wishes of one rich country above the needs of all the other, desperately poor ones. John Duffy comments that Soper had spent so long in Latin America working with relatively autocratic governments, that 'he had lost a measure of perspective' on the United States.[113]

Confirmation: The Anti-Malaria Campaign

Before Soper left Brazil in 1942 to join the US war effort, he ran one other major public health campaign that greatly reinforced his ideas about eradication. This was the campaign against a massive malaria epidemic that broke out in the northeastern part of Brazil in 1938–9.

Malaria was the third disease that the RF got involved in after hookworm and yellow fever. As Gorgas had discovered in Panama, it was not an easy disease to eradicate. There was certainly no obvious or quick technical fix that could be applied; debates among malaria specialists about which methods to use were often intense, even bad-tempered. The RF tended to follow Dr Ronald Ross in treating malaria as essentially a mosquito disease, investigating anopheline vectors and experimenting with methods of mosquito control in a number of countries in the 1920s and 1930s. Once the effectiveness of the insecticide Paris Green in killing anopheline larvae was discovered in the early 1920s, it became a signature tool of the IHD. Yet even in the late 1930s the 'American' method, as it was often called, focusing almost exclusively on larviciding (killing larvae) was disputed by many malaria specialists in Europe.[114]

It is in this context of the sometimes heated debates about malaria control that we can begin to appreciate the historic impact of Soper's eradication of an entire malaria mosquito species from Brazil – his first 'eradication as an absolute'.

When in 1938 it became obvious that an epidemic was unfolding in northeast Brazil, causing intense hardship among already extremely impoverished populations, and high mortality rates, President Vargas turned to Soper to take charge of anti-malaria operations. Soper had no previous experience with malaria. Yet confident as always, he was not deterred. Since according to his lights eradication was largely a matter of correct administrative techniques, to him the eradication of one vector was, with some adjustments, fundamentally the same as the eradication of another. Malaria had many different anopheline vectors, but in the case at hand Soper had been for some time convinced the epidemic was due to presence of the species known as *Anopheles gambiae*. This was an unusual species because it was a recent import from West Africa, its native habitat, arriving in the northeast of Brazil probably by aeroplane or boat; thus it seemed to bear out the nightmare scenario of the international spread of vectors and diseases in an increasingly globalized world. Identified in Brazil for the first time by the RF scientist Raymond Shannon in 1930, the *Anopheles gambiae* species was estimated to have spread over some 54,000 sq. km (20,849 sq. miles) by the late 1930s and early 1940s.

The explosion of malaria in Brazil in 1938 was especially worrying because *A. gambiae* is an 'efficient' transmitter of malaria, being anthropophilic (that is, preferring to feed on human blood) and highly susceptible to malaria parasites. Soper made much of the idea that, if not stopped in its tracks, the gambiae mosquito might spread across the entire American continent, with potentially devastating effects. Soper had failed to rouse the Brazilian authorities to take action before the late 1930s; and in fact, the *Anopheles gambiae* species did not reach or adapt to forested areas in Brazil, nor did it thrive in very arid conditions. Unknown to Soper, ecologically speaking the mosquito was quite hemmed in by the terrain into which it had first been introduced. This allowed Soper to combat the mosquito as a semi-domestic species, since it bred in fresh water at distances not too far from human habitations. Soper's task of getting rid of it was made in this regard easier, if still not easy; the gambiae breeding sites were in freshwater deposits that were often quite small and widely distributed in the terrain.

Pinning responsibility on the mosquito for an epidemic that had resulted in some 100,000 cases and at least 20,000 deaths in 1938 alone, and ignoring all the social, economic and political factors involved, Soper decided to concentrate all his efforts on wiping out every gambiae mosquito, down to the last one.

In this goal he once again found support from President Vargas. Faced with a very visible crisis, Vargas had acted promptly by setting up a North

East Malaria Service (NEMS) in 1938 as an autonomous agency. Somewhat reluctantly, the RF agreed to support the campaign financially (though Soper was instructed by headquarters *not* to commit the RF to an eradication campaign as such). Once again, Soper set to; and by dint of determined organization; by mapping the areas to be tackled and setting up a rigid system of inspections; by concentrating all his efforts on chemical attacks on the gambiae mosquitoes, using the chemical Paris Green on larvae breeding sites, and pyrethrum for spraying inside houses to get rid of adult insects; by hiring several thousand personnel, many of them from the Cooperative Yellow Fever Service; by fumigating all vehicles entering or leaving the area, and all aeroplanes, Soper succeeded in getting rid of the mosquito species, down to the very last example.

He had won, in a calculated gamble. The gamble was to concentrate entirely on the vector; to spend very large sums of money on killing it, even when he lacked critical information on the biology of the species, such as the duration of the viability of its ova, or the length of its hibernation; and to put aside any consideration of the failure of previous efforts to eradicate insects by deliberate means (the exception being the eradication of the Mediterranean fruit fly in the US in the early 1930s).[115] Before the entire project started, Soper had thought the eradication would take as much as ten years and cost $10 million. The actual cost and time were in fact far less, the Brazilian government spending just under $2 million over four years (1939–42). It was still an enormous sum for the time.

At first the results were discouraging; malaria in fact increased. But slowly the number of cases declined. In May 1939, 105,567 cases of malaria had been registered; in May 1940, only 7,876. On 31 August 1940 the last laboratory gambiae colony was deliberately destroyed, to prevent accidental release. The last gambiae in the wild were found just over a week later, and destroyed too. The mosquito had gone, and all control measures against it were suspended as a crucial test; further searches failed to find a single specimen. By January 1941, the anti-gambiae operation was ended; field distribution of anti-malaria drugs was terminated a few months later.[116]

Once again, an eradication service had been organized independently of all other public health services, with control over its own budget, personnel and rules; and once again, specific and coercive legislation was passed to enforce compliance from the local population with all the anti-malaria regulations. Once again, too, Soper avoided all involvement in clinical work or the care of the sick, which was left to the Brazilians. He agreed to negotiate the price for the purchase of drugs and to use his personnel as they travelled across the states carrying out inspections and anti-mosquito work to distribute quinine and atebrine (a German anti-malarial drug that had come into use in the 1930s), but only because Vargas insisted on it.

Otherwise, everything was focused on eliminating *A. gambiae* mosquitoes. The termination of the malaria epidemic itself was, naturally enough, attributed by Soper entirely to his successful elimination of the species.[117] All traditional methods of attacking malaria – ditching, oiling, screening, even the introduction of larvae-eating fish – were put aside in favour of 'Paris Greening' and pyrethrum spraying.[118] Hackett was surprised to find, when he visited the malaria service in January 1940, that Soper had not a single malariologist on the staff. Soper told Hackett he was not preventing malaria, but eradicating gambiae. This was vintage Soper – a robust defence of methods that were not those of a classically trained malariologist.[119]

Recent research by Randall Packard and Paul Gadelha has drawn attention to a number of other contingent social and political factors that, in addition to the presence of an imported and highly efficient insect vector, played their part in the malaria epidemic of 1938–9. The area had seen several previous malaria epidemics, transmitted by other anopheline vectors; the epidemic occurred in a time of intense immiseration of the population in the surrounding areas, caused by the return of the drought that regularly devastated the scrubby, parched hinterlands of the northeast of the country; many families faced starvation. The conditions led to a large migration of desperately poor people into the towns, where they hoped to find food and water; many of them were herded into camps, where disease spread easily.[120] Their point is that malaria epidemics are rarely the result of a single biological factor but have multiple, social, ecological and political causes. The 1938–9 epidemic was no exception; it had been preceded by numerous shifts in human populations, impoverishment, droughts and previous waves of malaria.

Soper did not entirely overlook these factors in his account of the epidemic; but he certainly drew an over-simplified conclusion from his experiences, namely that the vector itself was largely responsible for malaria. Even epidemiological studies were overlooked. Instead Soper attributed his success entirely to the systematic and ruthless eradication of the anopheles vector. And he did have a very dramatic result: a major epidemic had apparently been halted by means of eradication of a biological species. The campaign set a new standard for success: zero tolerance. There was no such thing in Soper's vocabulary as 'partial success'. Almost immediately, Soper began to speculate about similar anti-gambiae eradication efforts in Africa, the 'home' of the gambiae mosquito.[121]

At the time Soper's achievement was considered to be remarkable, and it greatly increased his international reputation, even though his approach to malaria was at the time, as he acknowledged, 'in disharmony with that of the modern malariologist', who 'believed in taking the long view of the malaria problem, aiming for steady progress, slow and imperfect though it may be'.[122]

A contributor to the book *African Highways* compiled by the British malaria expert Sir Malcolm Watson called Soper's work 'one of the outstanding achievements in tropical medicine'.[123] In his 1946 book, *A Malariologist in Many Lands,* Marshall A. Barber, who had worked as a volunteer consultant to Soper for two months in 1939 during the epidemic, was equally enthusiastic, calling the extirpation of the gambiae mosquito 'one of the greatest accomplishments in all malariology'.[124]

Species eradication, it appeared, would be an idea to be reckoned with in the future.

The Withdrawal of the Rockefeller Foundation from Eradication Campaigns

One of the drawbacks of relying on international public health agencies for national programmes is that the agencies may change their minds and withdraw their support. This is what happened with the RF.

The RF had reluctantly stayed on in the cooperative yellow fever programme until the mid-1930s, when it decided to withdraw from yellow fever work altogether, drawing a line under its commitment to practical public health. The discovery of an animal reservoir of the yellow fever virus had put an end to the dream of eradicating the disease. By 1937 the RF also had an effective vaccine. RF field trials of the 17D vaccine began in Brazil in February that year. By the end of 1938 over a million people in Brazil had been vaccinated, a massive programme in which Soper was closely involved. However, serious post-vaccination problems in late 1938 and 1939, including deaths from infectious jaundice (22 deaths in 1,000 cases in one area) seemed to put a large question mark over the safety of the laboratory procedures being used in Brazil; but investigations ordered by the RF soon established that it was the use of small amounts of human serum in the vaccine and not lax laboratory methods that was responsible for the contamination of the vaccine. Once the serum was eliminated, the problem was solved, and the large-scale vaccination of people exposed to jungle yellow fever was then resumed.[125]

The RF's withdrawal from Brazil, planned since the mid-1930s, was delayed until January, 1940 for a number of reasons, one of them being Soper's determination to stay on course with his yellow fever mosquito eradication programme (Soper himself did not leave Brazil until 1942).

Soper was angry at the RF's change of direction. Vaccination arrived as a technique several years after his mosquito eradication programme had been put in place. To Soper, the vaccine made little difference to vector eradication, even though the immunity from vaccination appeared to be long-lasting and gave protection to anyone travelling to areas where there was a risk of yellow fever, because he thought the vaccine was expensive, and that demand would soon out-run supply. More importantly, he thought that there was no way that all the people living in areas near the jungle and at risk of being infected with jungle yellow fever could be vaccinated in time to prevent the transmission of the disease to urban areas which, if still filled with *Aedes aegypti* mosquitoes, risked epidemic outbreaks (in fact it takes ten days after the vaccination for protection to take effect, time enough for people to travel from forested areas into towns where the urban vector could be infected). Better to stay his course and wipe out the *Aedes aegypti* species! In 1942, just before he left Brazil, Soper presented his 'Proposal for the Continent-Wide Eradication of *Aedes aegypti*' at the Pan American Sanitary Conference held in Rio de Janeiro.[126]

To the RF, though, it was Soper who had strayed from RF's goals. Species eradication was never a goal that the RF set for itself; and it never felt comfortable about it, which was one of the reasons that RF and Soper eventually parted ways.[127] Eradication, more generally, was by now a 'rash word in terms of prophecy', the RF said.[128] Dr Wilbur A. Sawyer, the new director of the IHD, writing to Soper as early as 24 September 1935, remarked: 'The yellow fever service has grown to such size that you have practically become a Government official in charge of a larger division of the Health Department . . . it is hardly consistent with our general policies.'[129]

By the late 1930s, then, Soper and the RF's views on disease control had diverged considerably. As I have said, Soper was not by temperament a researcher or a laboratory scientist, and he disdained the growing emphasis in the RF on scientific research instead of practical public health administration. He had, he said, been 'sold by Dr Rose in 1919 the idea of taking what is known to the people rather than spending my life trying to learn new things that might delay any further channels for application'.[130] He concluded that, as the RF turned more and more towards medical research, they had come to believe that public health administration was not glamorous enough for its scientists. The IHD, he thought, had become nothing but a 'gentleman's diplomatic club', where his '"capacity for fanaticism" did him in'.[131]

This divergence of goals perhaps explains the relatively small space given to Soper in the history of yellow fever put together by the RF in 1951, which emphasized the epidemiological and especially the laboratory discoveries the RF had made about yellow fever in the 1920s and 1930s, culminating in the production of the successful yellow fever vaccine in 1937. 'In the end' says Farley, 'officers of the Health Division regarded their work on yellow fever as their greatest triumph and no other disease had as much impact on the organization'.[132] But in reality, the emphasis on the results of scientific research served to downplay the failure of the foundation's original goal, yellow fever eradication.

Luckily for Soper, by the time the RF withdrew from public health work in Latin America (closing the IHD completely in 1951, to the shock of many of its employees), a steady process of 'Brazilianization' of Soper's programme had occurred, both financially and in terms of its stated goals. By 1942, when Soper left to join the US war effort, the Brazilian government had taken over the entire financial responsibility for its National Yellow Fever Service and responsibility as well for the task of getting rid completely of the *Aedes aegypti* mosquito in its territory (as well as aiding neighbouring Latin American countries to do the same). Between 1930 and 1949, in fact, Brazil spent altogether some $26 million on yellow fever work (compared to the $14 million spent on yellow fever eradication by the RF over 28 years). The result of this effort was an almost complete, *but never absolutely complete*, removal of the *Aedes aegypti* mosquito from the territory of Brazil for several decades. Urban yellow fever itself disappeared.

Yet we still have to ask, was this a wise investment of the limited public health resources available in a country like Brazil, given its many other pressing health problems? Soper had no doubt that it was; and he took his eradication ideas into his next job, and into the post-war world.

4 Post-war: A Capacity for Fanaticism

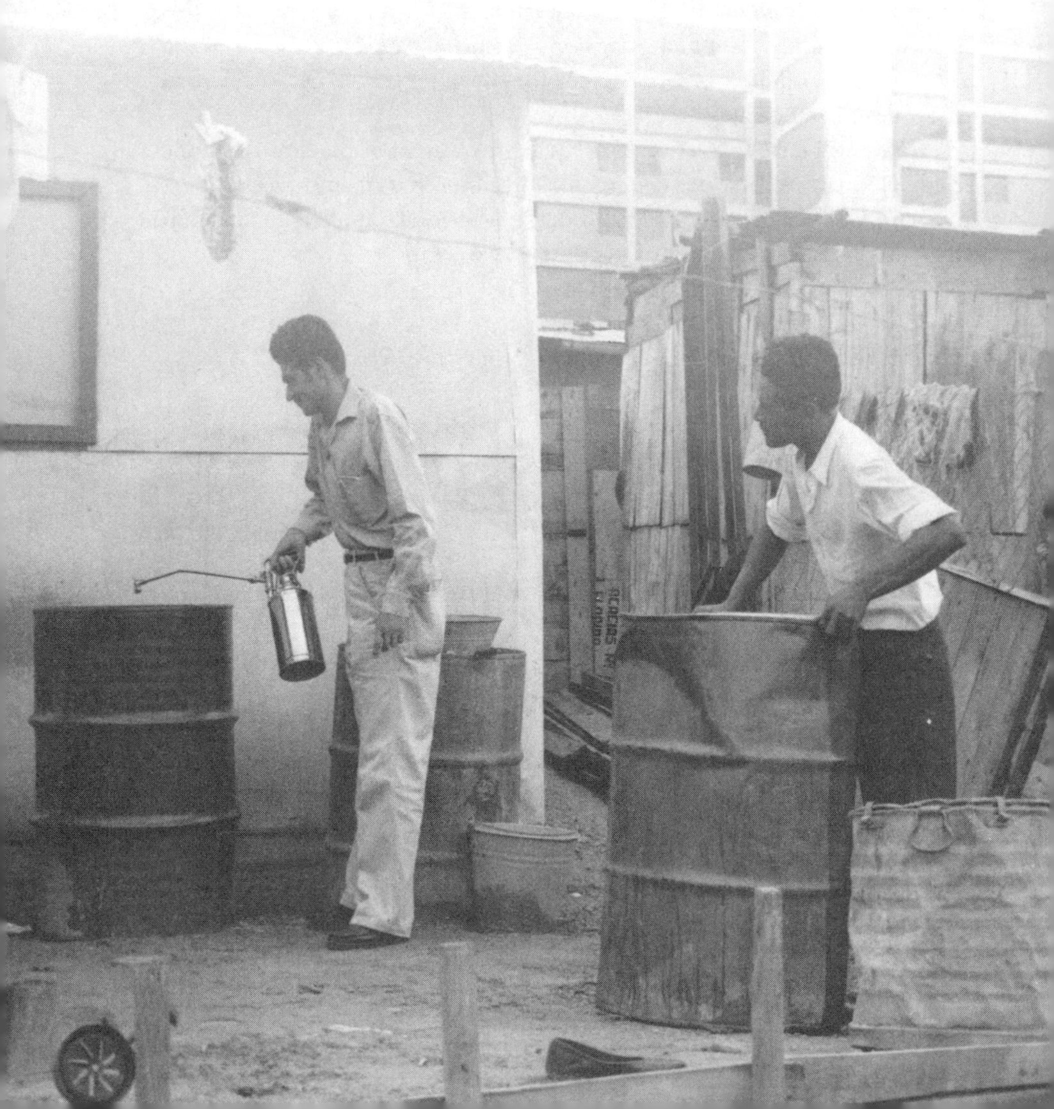

Soper's pre-Second World War enthusiasm for the concept of the complete eradication of disease was not shared by many public health officials. The Rockefeller Foundation told Soper not to use the term 'eradication' when discussing public health programmes; eradication had proven too difficult to achieve and the term only drew attention to its own failures in this regard.

Contrast this with the years immediately after the Second World War, when eradication became a key strategy in international health, pursued by the leading health agencies and supported financially by numerous organizations and national governments. Soper believed the revival of the fortunes of the concept had a great deal to do with him; he took pride, says Socrates Litsios, who worked for 30 years for the World Health Organization (WHO) in Geneva, and knew Soper personally, in 'almost single-handedly having resurrected the idea of eradication as a public health measure worthy of pursuit'. Litsios tends to agree with Soper's self-assessment, saying that Soper played 'a key, if not the leading, role in selling the idea that malaria could be eradicated worldwide'.[1] The malaria expert, Paul Russell, also became a strong proponent, calling Soper the prophet of disease eradication whose successes were due to an 'optimistic and fearless vision of the possible'.[2] Soper himself said that to be an eradicationist, one had to have 'the capacity for fanaticism'.[3] This he had.

Yet the change in attitude was obviously due to more than one man's passionate advocacy. What other factors brought about the shift in outlook?

To many people the Second World War itself was the key. As is well known, the war was associated with many technical and scientific innovations, from the atom bomb to wonder drugs such as penicillin and chloroquine (the latter until recently the drug of choice in treating malaria). Most notably, the war produced DDT, the long-lasting insecticide that had an extraordinary impact on the war effort, proving its worth in combating epidemics of typhus and malaria among the armed forces and civilians. Given the effectiveness of DDT in getting rid of the insect vectors of disease (as well as most other insects along the way), setting sights on the eradication of vector-borne diseases across the world once the war came to an end may have seemed to be simply a logical extension of new techno-scientific know-how.

Yet looked at more closely, the post-war adoption of the eradicationist strategy appears less straightforward. Why, for instance, was malaria selected by the WHO for its first global campaign of eradication? Malaria, after all, had long been understood by public health experts to be a very complicated disease whose control, let alone complete elimination, was likely also to be very complicated. The discovery that DDT was a cheap and effective insecticide of course made a difference to getting rid of mosquitoes, but we need to ask nevertheless why DDT over-rode the well-established view that malaria would not lend itself to the same technical solution everywhere – as the history of the effort to eradicate malaria by DDT eventually proved.

And why not try smallpox first? If the decision to eradicate was driven by the availability of technical solutions, smallpox was a logical choice. Not being a vector-borne disease it did not have to wait for DDT to make its eradication plausible. Unlike malaria, it had a vaccine, the oldest in existence, and by the middle of the twentieth century a safe and well-tried one. By 1950, the systematic use of vaccination had already led to the disappearance of smallpox from most countries in Europe, as well as from the Soviet Union, the Philippines, the United States and Canada.

Yet when Dr Brock Chisholm, the first director of WHO, selected smallpox as his first choice for a worldwide eradication effort, his suggestion was turned down. The delegates to the World Health Assembly in 1955 rejected the idea, on the grounds that smallpox eradication was 'too ambitious, too costly, and of uncertain feasibility'.[4]

A last example of the 'surplus' of factors influencing the post-war adoption of eradication strategies concerns yellow fever. Here Soper's role was all important; his idea about eradicating the urban vector occurred before the war, and though DDT and other new insecticides helped, they do not explain why Soper was able to convince *all* the American republics to sign up to the task of ridding the world of the urban mosquito vector of yellow fever, even though it could never be anything but a partial solution to the yellow fever problem. This was a Sisyphean task, given the number of countries that had to participate simultaneously for the campaign to work, and the sheer difficulty of deliberately exterminating an entire insect species – insects being among the most successful organisms in nature. Even the United States signed up, if reluctantly and belatedly. Was it DDT that made the difference? Soper's pre-war belief in the effectiveness of his methods? Or did post-war political factors play their part?

My point in raising these kinds of questions is to suggest that we should think of the triumph of the eradicationist philosophy in the post-war international health field not as an almost inevitable or pre-determined outcome of scientific innovation or new technologies (though these undoubtedly played their parts in the story), but rather as the result of many, often unanticipated, factors that were as much political as technical or scientific.

In this regard we have to take into account the Cold War and its rivalries, which made the international arena a political battlefield between the capitalist west and the communist east; the emergence of the United States as the hegemonic political power, and its ability to finance, and influence, new public health institutions; the growth of foreign aid, and its reliance on techno-scientific solutions to social problems; the emergence of development theory as the explanation of the problems of underdevelopment in Third World countries; and the influence of eradication advocates, as they acquired new positions of authority as the international public health field was institutionally re-configured in the aftermath of the war.

In this chapter, my focus is on what we might call the 'Soper era' of eradication, examining the impact of his wartime experiences in North Africa and Italy and then of his appointment after the war to the post of Director of the Pan American Health Organization (PAHO), which became part of the newly created World Health Organization. In this position, Soper championed his eradicationist views, capitalizing on Cold War rhetoric to get support, and leading eradication campaigns against many diseases. This chapter, then, is concerned with the continuities and the discontinuities in the eradicationist idea between the pre-war and post-war period. Special attention is given to the eradication of yaws, and to Soper's intense involvement in the continent-wide campaign to eradicate the urban vector of yellow fever in the Americas.

Soper's War

Soper had a 'good war', in that the Second World War led to further opportunities to test his eradicationist philosophy on new diseases and in new places.

When the US finally entered the war in 1942 Soper was in the process of closing down the anti-*gambiae* operation he had organized for the Rockefeller Foundation and the Brazilian government. He was 49 years old, and probably too old for regular army service (apparently he failed his army medical test).[5] It was at any rate generally realized that, as in every other war, disease would pose a serious challenge to the war effort and that medical expertise would be urgently needed in the armed forces.

After some uncertainty as to where or how Soper would contribute, he was seconded by the RF to the US Army's Typhus Commission, based in Egypt. Typhus was epidemic in North Africa as well as in Italy in 1942 and 1943; though the number of cases at the time was not great, the fatality rate was high and the military were concerned that wartime troop movements and civilian deprivation might lead to severe epidemics, as had occurred during and after the First World War. Typhus inoculations were available for the troops, but there was also the need to test new insecticides against the louse that transmitted the disease. Access to insecticides like pyrethrum, normally supplied by Japan, had by then been interrupted by the war in the Far East, and substitutes had to be found; the same was true of quinine, once the Japanese cut off Allied access to the Java plantations in Dutch East Asia.

Soper knew nothing about typhus, but was an expert on the use of insecticides in disease control, so his assignment made sense. He made a very difficult member of the Commission – he was opinionated and bloody-minded. He was after all, 'the commander', better suited to rule than obey.[6]

Typical of Soper's independence was his behaviour on arriving in North Africa in January 1943. Within one hour of getting to Cairo to meet up with the US Army's Typhus Commission, his attention was caught by the news that the *Anopheles gambiae* mosquito had apparently invaded Upper Egypt – the very mosquito he had just eliminated in Brazil. Immediately connecting the *gambiae* invasion to the devastating epidemic of malaria that he was told had occurred in a region close to Anglo-Egyptian Sudan the previous year, and appreciating the threat that the mosquito might travel down to the Nile Delta, which was the scene of British (and increasingly US) military activities, within a few days he arranged on his own to call on the Egyptian Under-Secretary of State for Health, Dr Aly Tewfik Shousha, and press upon him the urgency of carrying out an anti-*gambiae* eradication campaign before the species spread further into the country.[7]

Soper's brash assumption of superior knowledge thoroughly irritated the British military authorities who really ran the show in Egypt. The British medical doctors involved in malaria control also were very leery of the US butting in to a delicate political situation and complained of Soper's 'uncompromising personality'.[8] Soper later wrote, in part defence of the British attitude, that the devastating epidemics of malaria that the British were familiar with in the Punjab in India and Ceylon (now Sri Lanka) were not associated with the arrival of new anopheline vectors, but with a great increase in the density of the usual vectors; on the basis of their experiences, the British did not accept that the *gambiae* mosquito was a recent invader of Egypt nor that the mosquito could be eradicated. The British therefore rejected Soper's plan as impractical and unnecessary (though the reasons for their rejection were as much political as scientific).

Soper was able to convince the Egyptians, or so he says, that the *gambiae* species was indeed a newcomer to the Upper Nile area. 'Moreover', Soper said, 'I had made eradication appear so easy that there seemed to be no need of outside help'.[9] Permitted by the Egyptian authorities to visit the Upper Nile Valley, Soper saw for himself the appalling effects that the malaria epidemic had had on the local population. The return of epidemic malaria in 1943 was, as Soper had predicted, even more devastating, with serious economic losses and loss of food owing to the loss of harvesting; too many people were ill to attend to farming. According to one account, more than 180,000 Egyptians died in Upper Egypt in 1942 and 1943.[10] So certain was Soper that his plan for *gambiae* eradication would work that he arranged to have put in the

Egyptian officials' hands a manuscript copy in English of the *Manual of Administration* he had had drawn up for use during the *gambiae* campaign in Brazil, as well as a copy of the book he and his co-organizer, D. Bruce Wilson, had just written, giving a history of the detection of the gambiae, its spread, and the history of its extermination.[11]

This *Manual* proved invaluable when, in the spring of 1944, fearing another epidemic that might affect the thousands of allied troops based in North Africa, the British and the Egyptian authorities finally accepted Soper's suggestion that an eradication campaign against the *gambiae* species be launched with Rockefeller Foundation support and direction (the RF found the Egyptians had already translated parts of the *Manual* from Portuguese into Arabic). Soper, by then based in Italy and working with the Allied Control Mission on typhus control, went back to Cairo in May 1944 to survey the *gambiae* region and the effects of malaria once again. Malaria that year was already intense and criticism of the authorities for failing to contain it was mounting; though careful not to criticize the authorities publicly, Soper made evident his judgement that unless action was taken, a severe malaria epidemic would erupt in the autumn of 1944.

Once agreement between the Ministry of Health and the RF was worked out, with the Ministry paying for all costs except the salaries of the RF staff, several RF malaria experts were sent to Egypt to actually organize the programme. Among them were D. Bruce Wilson and J. Austin Kerr, with Kerr taking charge of the eradication service in Cairo and Wilson of field operations. They had both worked with Soper in Brazil, and throughout Soper served as 'advisor-in-chief' from Italy, where he was largely situated during the Egyptian campaign. The campaign was set up in classic Rockefeller or 'Soperian' fashion; it was placed within the Egyptian Ministry of Health, but as an autonomous *Gambiae Eradication Service* administratively independent even of the existing malaria service of the Ministry. The eradication service relied on the careful planning that Soper had worked out in his previous campaign in Brazil, such as detailed mapping of malarial areas and the location of houses; the systematic inspection of the work of the inspectors; and the large-scale application of the larvicidal chemical, Paris Green, supplies of which Soper had had the foresight to request be sent to Egypt.[12] The essence of the operation was 'a military discipline based on a system of punishments and rewards'.[13] Apart from the small RF staff the work was all carried out by Egyptian workers. As in Brazil, treatment of malaria victims was outside the remit of the eradication service (in the Egyptian case, it was left to the Ministry of Health).

By means of the application of many tons of Paris Green, supplemented by other insecticides and pyrethrum, by February 1945, the *gambiae* mosquito had apparently disappeared from Egypt and in November that year, the special Gambia Eradication Service was wound up. Since malaria in the Upper Nile Valley in 1944–5 was nothing like as bad in misery and mortality as it had been in 1942–3, Soper concluded that eradicating mosquitoes was indeed the way to get rid of malaria; to him, mosquitoes and malaria were one and the same. He thus overlooked, as he had in Brazil before, the many other sources of the epidemic, from the effects of the Aswan low dam in increasing irrigation and breeding places for mosquitoes, to the wartime disruption to the Egyptian population and economy, troop movements, the arrival of non-immunes in the region, crop failures and the consequent lack of food supplies and so on; and he overestimated the ease with which, in less urgent or non-wartime conditions, malaria could be dealt with.[14] But given wartime circumstances, and the devastation malaria had already brought to Egyptians, Soper perhaps understandably notched up the success of the mosquito eradication campaign in Upper Egypt as yet another mark of the correctness of his eradicationist philosophy (a view that the Rockefeller field officer who ran the programme did not share).[15]

The Beginning of the DDT Era

Note that the *gambiae* eradication campaign in Egypt did not depend on DDT; the chemical would not be introduced into the country for use in anti-mosquito work until 1946. But Soper got a chance to try out the DDT before this, when he became part of the wartime effort to test the chemical, first against typhus and then against malaria.

DDT (short for dichloro-diphenyl-trichloroethane) had been synthesized in 1874, but its exceptional insecticidal properties were not discovered until 1941 (by the chemist at the Geigy company in Switzerland, Paul Müller, who in 1948 was awarded the Nobel Prize for his work). The UK and the USA quickly conducted experiments in 1942–3 to test its potential.[16] DDT was found to work remarkably effectively on any number of insects; and insofar as it could be gauged in a short period of testing, it did not seem to be harmful to humans, at least in the doses required for public health work. Manufacturing of the chemical for distribution to the armed forces began in 1943, just as Soper arrived in Algeria from Egypt. Put to work on typhus, Soper became one of the first public health experts to appreciate the superiority of DDT over all other insecticides he knew. In using DDT to test its power in reducing lice in civilian populations (the French colonial authorities making available Algerian civilian prisoners for these tests), Soper found a method of modifying insecticide spray pumps in such a way that individuals could be de-loused without their clothes being removed (important in the case of Muslim women, and in emergency situations).[17]

This idea proved its worth when, as had been feared, in the winter of 1943–4, typhus became epidemic in Naples, where the Italian population was living in abominable conditions, demoralized and often starving after years of war. In December of 1943, Soper was sent from North Africa to Naples to re-join the US Army Typhus Commission just as supplies of DDT were about to be released for general military use. During the epidemic, some 83,915 kg (185,000 lb) of DDT were used to de-louse 3,266,000 people in the five-month period between mid-December 1943 and the end of May, 1944.[18] The chief virtue of DDT compared to other insecticides was that a little went a long way; it could be easily sprayed, and its killing power remained strong for weeks or even months (this is what is meant by its 'residual' effects). DDT was also found to work well against insect larvae, and could be sprayed in puddles or stagnant water. Soper recalled later that little thought was given at the time to the potential risks of DDT, and that those involved 'did not hesitate to pump it under the clothing of some 3,000,000 people and to assign workers to the pumps in rooms which were unavoidably foggy from the DDT dust in the air'.[19]

This wartime test of DDT was followed immediately by the first large-scale use of DDT against malaria, in a campaign in which Soper again participated, working under his Rockefeller colleague, Dr Paul F. Russell, a malaria expert serving in the US Army Medical Corps.[20]

The circumstance was an acute epidemic that occurred as the Germans in Italy retreated in the face of the northwards advance of the recently arrived Allied troops (Italy having switched sides and joined the Allies in the fight against Germany in September of 1943). As Frank Snowden has recounted in his superb history of malaria in Italy, when the Germans retreated north from Rome in the summer of 1944, they carried out acts of what he calls 'bio-terror', when they deliberately sabotaged the pumps that had been put in place by the Italian authorities in previous decades to drain the Pontine marshes and thereby control malaria. The main German aim was to slow up the advance of US and British troops by causing flooding, but it was also perhaps to cause a public health malaria crisis by creating the swampy conditions in which the local malaria mosquitoes would flourish. In any event, by 1944 a huge epidemic had engulfed the destitute and bombed-out civilian population – according to Snowden, a realistic estimate of the number of malaria cases was 100,000 in a population of 245,000 people.[21] This wartime upsurge in malaria in Italy undid decades of reductions.

Accepting the recommendation of Russell and Soper, the Allied Control Commission decided to spray DDT aerially over a large area to reduce malaria infection rates in the general population (household spraying was also used). The urgency of malaria in wartime conditions, and the potential of DDT to act swiftly to kill mosquitoes, once again overrode safety considerations (as Snowden says, the full effects of DDT were simply not known at the time). Mosquitoes began to disappear, and with them malaria transmission. The success of the DDT campaign in stopping the malaria epidemic had the immediate effect of converting the Italians to what was known as the 'American' method of dealing with malaria by exterminating mosquitoes; after the war, the Italians announced they would aim to eradicate malaria from Italy as a whole.[22]

A Post-War Re-Organization: Soper and the World Health Organization

These were the experiences that Soper brought back to the United States at the war's end, as he sought to re-position himself in public health. He returned to civilian life in May 1946 (though he in fact never joined the US Army, only wearing an army uniform without rank because it was convenient) after almost three and a half years of service. He was still on a Rockefeller Foundation salary (as he had been throughout the war), but the days of RF-sponsored, large-scale overseas public health campaigns, of the kind Soper had been associated with for decades, were almost over. The RF was moving away from practical programmes towards basic scientific research, in such fields as nutrition, agriculture and population studies. In 1951, the RF closed down its International Health Division; one of the RF field officers registered his shock, calling it 'one of the most shattering events in the story of American involvement in public health'.[23] Soper had to find a place for himself in one of the new institutions that were emerging in the aftermath of the war.

By far the most significant of these was the United Nations and its associated technical agencies. The defeat of the Axis powers in 1945 left the United States as the dominant, indeed hegemonic, power in the West, and the country put its political will and money behind the creation of the UN as an institution it believed was essential if world wars were to be prevented in the future. The UN was conceived as a revival of the League of Nations, but with the United States this time fully on board – in fact, as the major funder. It was seen as a means of ensuring collective security and a balance of power in a world that was already dividing into opposing political camps.

The idea that there should be established within the UN system a separate health organization, whose purpose would be to deal with the myriad problems of disease and ill-health facing the world, was put forward at the very first meeting of the UN, held by the victors in San Francisco in the summer of 1945.[24] At the suggestion of a Brazilian and a Chinese delegate, a resolution was passed to create a new international health institution that would be associated with, but organizationally independent of, the political structure of the UN. A technical preparatory committee made up of public health experts was given the task of drawing up a constitution. In 1948 the World Health Organization (WHO) was born.

The WHO represented a new outlook in international health. It reflected both the urgency of the health needs of huge numbers of displaced people in wrecked countries at the end of the war, but also an expanded sense of the possibilities opened up by the application of new techniques, medicines, insecticides – of science more generally – in improving the lot of mankind. WHO's charter defined health expansively, as a right for all, and as more than merely the absence of disease – as a state of 'complete physical, mental, and social well-being'.[25] The WHO in effect was a transmutation of the League of Nations Health Organization into a new, post-war setting; it retained its seat in Geneva, and League of Nations health staff were transferred to the WHO.[26]

The WHO's first director was perhaps a surprising choice – the Canadian Dr Brock Chisholm. Chisholm was a psychiatrist who had served as Deputy-Director of Health in Canada before the war. According to Farley's recent biography of Chisholm, the Canadian was selected over many others jostling for the post because he had the fewest opponents (Soper's name was one of several put forward briefly as a negotiating tactic, but with no real expectation that he would be appointed). Chisholm was committed to a social approach to medicine. He was somewhat of a visionary, and a man of controversial ideas, who wanted to associate the WHO with grand political movements, such as world peace and world government. In fact, given the WHO's limited budget and the huge demands made on it for help, it was infectious diseases, or their removal, that came to dominate the WHO's activities in its first two decades.[27] Outside the immediate post-war context, this focus on communicable rather than non-communicable diseases has come to seem a somewhat arbitrary preference; in the context, though, the emphasis was understandable.

The WHO was meant to be the single international organization responsible for dealing with international health; it was intended to replace or absorb previous international health organizations. This in fact occurred with two pre-war international health organizations, the Office International d'Hygiene Publique and the League of Nation's Health Office, both of which ceased to exist. But the one other organization that could claim an identity as a pre-war international health agency resisted such absorption. This was the Pan American Health Organization.[28] PAHO could rightly claim to be the oldest of them all, having been founded in 1902. Its founding had represented a recognition of new neo-colonial connections that were being developed between the United States and Latin America. PAHO's greatest concrete achievement before the Second World War was the passage of its 1924 Sanitary Code, the first such code to be ratified by all the members of the Pan American Union.[29]

Despite its neo-colonial character and the dominance of the US within it, PAHO had served over the decades to bring doctors, health officials and Ministers of Health from the Americas into regular contact with each other, creating among them a feeling of belonging to a distinctive community of public health experts which its members were unwilling to dissolve. Looking at the post-war situation, with a devastated Europe, mass displacements of people, and many countries demanding aid, the Latin Americans especially feared that the needs of their region would be subordinated to Europe if their agency disappeared. The wish to keep PAHO intact, as it reached out to WHO, was also felt keenly by the United States, whose influence (and money) was dominant within the organization; but pride in what the PAHO had accomplished was also felt by the Latin American members.[30]

Two other factors helped give a particular identity to PAHO and the idea of 'the Americas' in combating disease: first, the decades-long presence of the Rockefeller Foundation in public health in Latin America, and second, the more recent role of the US government's Institute of Inter-American Affairs (IIAA), which had been set up as an emergency war-time organization in 1942 within the State Department to promote health in Latin American countries in the period 1942–7, and to 'eliminate a fertile field for Nazi propaganda'.[31] The IIAA was involved in combating malaria (especially in countries where US troops were stationed, such as Brazil); aiding the organization of hospitals, health centres and nursing schools; and working on projects such as sewage disposal and water supplies. The charter of the IIAA was short-term, in keeping with its wartime focus, though it was extended at the end of the war for a further three years. In most countries, the IIAA worked through bilateral agreements, and executively through the setting up of cooperative health services. The work carried out by these services was quite extensive, the 'Servicios' surviving in many countries as health organizations long after the IIAA had been terminated, influencing the development of health planning and organization in a US direction. It was yet one more factor in the North Americanization of health in the Americas. The presence of the IIAA probably reinforced the idea of collaboration between Latin America and the United States, and strengthened the idea that the public health needs of the Americas formed some kind of unity.[32]

Soper learned about the plans for WHO and the discussions surrounding the terms on which PAHO might join when he made a tour of public health institutions in the US in the summer of 1946, as he returned to civilian life and sought a position for himself in the new post-war setting. In Washington he met the outgoing director of PAHO, Dr Hugh Cumming, who was due to retire in 1947, and the Surgeon-General of the US Army, Dr Thomas Parran. There the idea arose that Soper would put himself forward as a candidate for the directorship of PAHO (since by tradition, the director had always come from the dominant member, the USA). PAHO had a tiny budget, a very small permanent staff, and its continued existence in the future was still uncertain. Nonetheless, the position appealed to Soper. At the Fifteenth Pan American Sanitary Conference, held in Caracas, Venezuela in January of 1947, Soper was elected without opposition.

At the time Soper was perhaps the most Latin Americanized health expert from the US that PAHO could have chosen; he brought to the job not only years of working with Latin Americans, but his link to the Rockefeller Foundation and its resources (the Foundation agreeing to pay his salary for his first year at PAHO).[33] Soper had spent 22 years in Latin America, spoke Portuguese and Spanish well, and had many friends and colleagues in the region. His directorship of PAHO might be said to represent the transition of PAHO away from an organization completely dominated by the US, to one more responsive to and reflective of Latin American needs; the first Latin American to be elected as director of PAHO, the Chilean, Dr Abraham Horwitz, followed Soper into the office when Soper retired in 1959.[34]

As PAHO expanded steadily in size under Soper's direction he brought numerous Latin American public health experts into the organization. Among them was the Brazilian, Dr Marcolino Candau, who had worked under Soper in Brazil in the anti-malaria campaign of 1939–40, had joined Soper at PAHO for a brief period after the war before moving to the WHO in Geneva, only to be selected in 1953 as the second Director-General in WHO's history, a position he held for the next twenty years, thus giving Soper an important ally in Geneva.[35]

When Soper took over PAHO, he knew that many Latin Americans wanted it to stay intact as an organization; so did Soper, not because he feared WHO would put Europe's interests first, ahead of Latin America's, but because he worried that WHO would be heavy-handed and bureaucratic; that it would be stuffed with committees which 'handed down pontifical opinions', or spend its time 'sponsoring trips of hygienists from one part of the world to another', as he thought the League of Nations had been prone to do.[36] Soper's other concerns were to find some means of increasing PAHO's inadequate budget, to increase its executive capabilities and to launch new projects, among them eradicationist ones. In many ways, Soper saw PAHO as a new RF, but an RF completely dedicated to practical public health work.

As we know, Soper was a person of extraordinary energy and tenacity, who treated every problem at hand as the most significant in the world, and he quickly went to work to achieve his aims. Among the most delicate of his negotiations were those with the WHO. Although WHO's 1948 Constitution included the principle of regionalization, at the time no other regional organization like PAHO existed. Soper used the year-and-a-half interval of time between his election to PAHO, and the signing of a formal agreement with WHO, to solve PAHO's budget problems and expand its activities, thus presenting WHO with a *fait accompli* – an existing, regional organization that would be part of WHO and yet with considerable independence from Geneva.

WHO did not insist on PAHO's absorption because its own agenda, and above all its budget, was in fact very severely limited (at least before 1950, when the UN contributed additional funds).[37] Moreover, the US had a strong interest in PAHO keeping its inter-American and US-influenced character, especially as Cold War suspicion of the USSR intensified.[38] In fact, PAHO to this day has probably remained the most autonomous of the six Regional Offices eventually set up. Most of PAHO's activities were undertaken on its own initiative, and often prefigured actions WHO would take only later. In essence, PAHO ran its affairs with little reference to, or even support from, Geneva.[39] This suited Soper's ambitions very well, giving him the prestige and technical support of WHO but the autonomy to go his own way.

On 24 May 1948 Soper and the Director-General of WHO signed the formal agreement that made PAHO the regional, all-Americas office of WHO; this was ratified in Rome by the World Health Assembly (the annual meeting which brought together all the delegates to WHO) in 1949.

Soper's relations with Dr Brock Chisholm, the first Director-General of WHO, were generally polite but not, as noted already, ideologically close. The two men disagreed on a number of issues, not least political. Soper did not share Brock's interests in psychology and social medicine and was critical of Chisholm's lack of expertise in communicable disease. Chisholm agreed; he told Soper fairly early on in his tenure that he would not run for re-election, believing the post needed someone trained in public health, and he stepped down after only one term in office. One telling political disagreement with Chisholm of which Soper left a record in his unpublished papers, relates to the withdrawal of Hungary from WHO in 1950; this was part of the general withdrawal of the communist countries of Eastern Europe from WHO between 1949–56. Soper suggested to Chisholm, in part as a joke, that WHO might be renamed the 'Free WHO'. Chisholm objected, saying many countries remaining within WHO were in fact not free at all, but run by dictators. To which Soper rejoined that nonetheless he himself had 'lived and worked with the greatest freedom for 12 years under a dictator' (referring to President Vargas of Brazil); but Soper added that Chisholm got the last word, by saying 'there were always some people who had not done too badly under dictators'![40]

Once Soper was re-elected as director of PAHO for a second term in 1951, and his Brazilian colleague, Candau, succeeded Chisholm at WHO in 1953, the relations between PAHO and WHO became closer. Nevertheless, PAHO retained a great deal of freedom to pursue its own objectives in public health.

This independence depended on money, the next item on Soper's agenda at PAHO in 1947. The operating budget of PAHO was based on member countries' contributions, calculated in relation to their population size; in 1947, expenditures were 50 per cent higher than incoming resources.[41] By dint of increasing the *per capita* contributions of PAHO's member states, which immediately almost doubled the US's contribution, and by persuading Brazil and several other countries to make substantial additional voluntary contributions, PAHO's budget increased greatly, and as a result it became a more active and executive organization. By 1956, PAHO received $3 million from the US alone (according to Cueto, WHO's own overall budget in that year was only $13.4 million). PAHO's staff under Soper grew rapidly, from only 32 people in 1946, to 171 by 1950 and to 412 by 1954. By 1959, when Soper retired, the number had risen to 750.[42] Among the staff were doctors, scientists, veterinarians, nurses, sanitary engineers and administrative aides. Over half of the employees worked not in Washington, but in the field.

And there was a lot of work for them to do. Under Soper, an ambitious set of activities was announced. Farid, an Egyptian doctor who worked for WHO for many years, has referred to 'the missionary, crusading spirit still lurking in the psyche of most public health officials there [in the New World]. Being gifted with an adventurous and optimistic spirit, they attempt what seems to scientists of the Old World an impossible task.' This description seemed to fit Soper perfectly, and in fact Farid selected Soper as one of the brightest examples of such a missionary leader.[43]

Under Soper, PAHO launched activities in three main areas: 1) the development and improvement of basic and permanent health services; 2) the education and training of public health personnel; and 3) the fight against communicable diseases, 'particularly those for which adequate means for eradication are now available'.[44] The programmes included public health education; the improvement of nursing and the development of nursing schools; the establishment of a new institute of nutrition for central America and Panama, based in Guatemala, as well as a centre for the study of zoonosis (human diseases originating from animal diseases), based in Argentina; surveys of the health of populations, and the collection of statistics on morbidity and mortality; getting X-ray machines and the tuberculosis BCG vaccine distributed; and raising money for fellowships for doctors from Latin America to visit and study abroad (the majority for study in the United States, which contributed to the further Americanization of medicine and public health in Latin America and the further distancing from European, especially French, medical traditions). In addition, there were the endless meetings of the Executive Council, the Annual Reports to prepare; the organizing and running of PAHO's Sanitary Conferences, held every four years in a different American country, and involving hundreds of delegates; and the regular publication of PAHO's monthly news bulletin containing updates on epidemiological and other data and news of all the various health initiatives being undertaken.[45]

It was a busy life. Soper's diaries and notes from the period 1950 to 1959 give a picture of a peripatetic existence as he travelled endlessly throughout the Americas, to meetings to and from Geneva on WHO business, and on several extended visits to India, Pakistan, Ceylon and Africa, negotiating programmes, following with avidity all the developments in public health overseas and promoting his eradicationist philosophy.[46] A typical year sounds exhausting. In May of 1950, for instance, Soper visited Haiti, the Dominican Republic, Cuba, and then went back to Washington after a trip of several weeks; from Washington, he set off again for Geneva, where he met Chisholm, the Director-General of WHO, and among other things, told him it was wrong to try to force the Haitians, with whom Soper was planning an anti-yaws campaign, into a US mould. After his return to Washington, Soper departed once more in June to visit Haiti, Guatemala, San Salvador, Nicaragua and Mexico. He was back in Haiti in September, before attending the Pan American Sanitary Conference in Ciudad Trujillo, in the Dominican Republic, where DDT and how to use it was discussed; then in early January, 1951, he returned to Geneva yet again, returning via London to Washington, then from there yet again to Central America. On this trip, he went further south, on to Argentina, where he tried to persuade the government to set up a yellow fever campaign; from there he left for Rio de Janeiro, to discuss yellow fever vaccine production at the city's leading laboratory.

In 1955, Soper made a virtual world tour, lecturing on eradication in India, which was about to join the WHO effort and convert its malaria control programme into an eradication campaign, and meeting health experts from Pakistan, who were resisting such a move, arguing that complete eradication of malaria was not feasible, and was anyway simply not their country's highest priority.

To Soper, on the contrary, eradication of communicable diseases was the highest priority. Although PAHO had a broad agenda in health, it is also fair to say that, from the beginning of Soper's tenure in office, eradication campaigns gave a distinctive slant to PAHO's work. In short order, Soper persuaded PAHO to sponsor all-Americas eradication campaigns against the yellow fever mosquito (in 1947), yaws (in 1949), smallpox (in 1950) and malaria (in 1954). His ambitions in this regard were as absolute as the idea of eradication itself; at one time or another Soper wrote of ridding the globe of cholera, leprosy, influenza, rabies, polio, the plague and tuberculosis.[47] As far as he was concerned, all communicable diseases that could be eradicated should be eradicated. There was, in effect, a moral duty to aim for the ideal. The eradication campaigns stood out within the overall work of PAHO because they were the public health efforts Soper claimed most often as original; and because they pre-dated and influenced later decisions by WHO to endorse eradication of diseases on a worldwide scale.

Another reason for emphasizing the PAHO precedent in launching eradication campaigns concerns the Cold War and its impact on international public health. The post-1945 decades were deeply shaped by the rivalry between capitalist and communist countries that developed immediately after the Second World War. The UN and its technical agencies operated against a background of dramatic political events: the Berlin blockade in 1948 and the subsequent airlift by the west (and in 1961 the building of the Berlin wall by the USSR between the eastern and western parts of the city); the announcement in 1947 of the US Marshall Plan to rescue the battered economies of Europe (it soon became the centrepiece, says Gaddis in his recent history of the Cold War, of the western policy of containment and promotion of US objectives, the USSR rejecting participation for these reasons); the creation of NATO; the start of the Korean War in 1950; the first test of a nuclear device by the Soviet Union in 1949, and of the hydrogen bomb by the US in 1954; the Hungarian uprising and its defeat in 1956; the Cuban Revolution in 1959; the list goes on.[48] Throughout the period, a nuclear war was the ultimate nightmare; in the end, nuclear war was held off because the leadership in both the Soviet Union and the United States understood that, given the mutually destructive potential of their nuclear arsenals, after a nuclear Armageddon 'nothing would be left on the planet but the insects'.[49]

Instead, it was the insects (among other organisms) which the world aimed to eliminate, through disease eradication campaigns which several historians have come to view as essentially Cold War propaganda tools of the Western powers, especially the United States.

As noted already, the US became the single largest financial supporter of the UN and its specialized agencies, such as the WHO; unlike today, for several decades after the Second World War successive US Presidents looked to the UN as an agency capable of reducing international tensions, and more specifically as an organization through which to pursue the US's own interests and contain the spread of communism. After the immediate post-war years, during which war-battered Europe was the main focus of attention, the WHO shifted its main concern in international health to developing or 'third world' countries. PAHO was already focused on Latin America, which now got caught up in US perceptions of the region as one made up of poor, third world countries ripe for communist infiltration; in this context, the US directed its resources to health, in the conviction of the superiority of its science and technology (a conviction tested by the Soviet success with Sputnik in 1957).

WHO was directly swept up in these Cold War hostilities when, in 1949–50, just as WHO was getting started, the Soviet Union and the Socialist Republics of Eastern Europe began to pull out of WHO, accusing it of failing to respond to Eastern Europe's particular needs and of being a tool of western, capitalist and largely US foreign policy. The eastern bloc countries were not to return to the organization until 1957, following Stalin's death in 1953.

It was in this situation of Cold War conflict, and the absence of Soviet representation in WHO, that PAHO started its eradication campaigns, to be followed by the WHO, when it announced its first large-scale malaria eradication programme (MEP) in 1955. In addition to eradication campaigns identified as such, WHO and UNESCO organized and led some of the most massive health campaigns involving vaccines and drugs ever seen (for example, against yaws, using the new drug, penicillin, and against tuberculosis, using the BCG vaccine and new antibiotics, with the numbers of people being treated in countries like India reaching into the millions). It was a new era in global health.

Socrates Litsios draws attention to how the Cold War led western countries to abandon the pre-war idea that investment in agriculture and food production was a means to achieving malaria reduction, and to adopt instead the idea that malaria control, achieved via the application of DDT, would itself lead to social and economic prosperity. Litsios concludes that the Cold War 'kept the UN system on an emergency basis' throughout, leading it to focus on quick results, and avoid politically difficult issues such as social and health inequalities, or the relation of health improvement to land reform.[50] Along similar lines, Siddiqi, in a functionalist account of WHO, says the United States gave its support to malaria eradication in order to counter the influence of the Soviet Union.[51] Marcos Cueto, in his recent book, *Cold War, Deadly Fevers,* also frames his analysis of the post-war malaria eradication campaign in Mexico very much in these Cold War terms.[52]

Randall Packard, in several particularly trenchant articles, underlines the way in which the eradication of malaria was tied in particular to Cold War theories of 'development' and 'underdevelopment'. According to public health officials' understanding of development theory, disease eradication would lead to improved economies (rather than the other way around). Since public health experts believed they had the techno-scientific means to expunge disease, eradication campaigns could speed up the entire process, across the world, thereby unlocking the mental and physical potential of developing countries, and thereby too, forestalling political revolution.[53] This assumption – that removing malaria would unlock economic potential – was (and still is) deeply built-in to the 'disease and development' field, even though many malaria experts knew at the time that it was not so straightforward. Dr Wilbur Sawyer, who headed the IHD between 1935 and 1944, commented in 1951 that though it had long been 'surmised that improvement in health would be promptly followed by increased production, and a better economic position would result in fuller social development', in fact 'The problem is much broader than health, which cannot flourish in an adverse socio-economic environment.'[54]

The entanglement of eradication as a public health strategy with Cold War economic and political competition between west and east, and the early apparent success of malaria eradication, perhaps helps explains why, when the Soviet Union eventually returned to the WHO-fold, it came prepared with its own proposal for a worldwide eradication campaign, against small-pox; the Deputy Minister of Health, Dr Victor M. Zhdanov, presented this at the World Health Assembly in Minneapolis in 1958, along with an offer of 25 million doses of smallpox vaccine (a proposal that WHO accepted, though with reluctance, as we shall see later, having already judged the eradication of smallpox very difficult).[55]

Another Cold War effect of the absence of the Soviet Union from WHO debates over policy in the early 1950s may have been a weakening of support for broader, more social approaches to international health of the kind favoured, among others, by the WHO's Director-General, Dr Brock Chisholm. The US vehemently resisted any talk of socialized medicine and insisted on excluding such issues from WHO as a condition of its own membership; discussions on these and related topics delayed the US joining for two years, and even after it joined, the US insisted on reserving the right to pull out with a year's notice, WHO agreeing to these terms because it needed the US's technical and financial resources.

Instead the intellectual and policy space was cleared for more narrowly organized, technocratic, vertically structured eradication campaigns that did not require fundamental involvement in the political and economic life of the various nations involved. As I show later (in chapter Six), a 'social medicine' approach only emerged at WHO and its affiliated organizations in the late 1960s and early 1970s, partly as a result of the failure of the WHO-led global malaria eradication programme.

Without disputing the centrality of the Cold War context to the history of WHO and other UN agencies, I would argue that we cannot reduce the post-war attraction of disease eradication entirely to that context (which some people want to do). After all, both the Soviet Union and post-revolutionary China organized their own, vertical disease eradication campaigns outside of the WHO framework (for example, against smallpox and other diseases); such targeted projects produced rapid results and were highly suited to command economies and highly centralized governments, as Soper always said.

WHO, in contrast, lacked the centralized authority of the USSR; dependent as it was on its member states for funds and support, it was an organization with built-in limits to what it could achieve. Many imperial powers, Britain and France especially, resisted any 'meddling' (as they saw it) of the WHO in their colonial health affairs; advice was welcome, as long as it was technical and stayed away from more complicated matters such as the organization of health and social services.[56] In contrast, advising and providing support for campaigns against selected infectious diseases, based on new technologies, was something WHO could do. As Amrith says in his judicious account of international health after the war in newly independent India, WHO, 'born in the circumstances of post-war crisis, poorly funded and fragile, was hardly in a position to undertake interventions that depended on deep social and cultural knowledge, not to mention power'.[57]

As for Soper, his eradicationism does not seem to have been much motivated by the Cold War. As we have seen, his commitment to the absolutist idea that one could get rid completely of communicable diseases by deliberate public health interventions, without waiting for the social and political development of poor countries, pre-dated both the Second World War and the Cold War. He developed it in the 1930s, and based it on the idea of technical know-how, his pre-war successes as he saw them, and a Rockefeller-inspired belief that bridging the gap between existing knowledge and practical application was what public health was all about.

The Cold War figured in Soper's work, therefore, largely as an opportunity to draw new allies to his side. Commenting in his diary, for instance, on the Point Four programmne announced by President Truman in 1949, extending US technical and financial aid to developing nations, Soper wrote that 'although a great deal of money has been allotted to agriculture and other projects, it seems that everybody has come to recognize that the health field is the only one in which results can be gotten with sufficient rapidity and sufficient clarity to really serve as a holding operation against Communist penetration during the period when the general situation can be improved'.[58] In another unpublished document, called simply 'Eradication', Soper made a rare connection in his notes (perhaps in preparation for a lecture): 'Meaning of eradication – Revolutionary concept', and 'Rich and technically advanced countries have a stake in underdeveloped ones'.[59] The nearest Soper came to defining eradication in economic terms was to insist that achieving health was the first step towards economic well-being and a better way to achieve economic development than economic development programmes themselves.[60] He commented in his notes that 'The first measure of the economic burden of disease in the given country is the mean life expectancy of its population'.[61] There is no doubt, also, that he believed the virtue of eradication was that it *could* be achieved even in poor countries, *without* waiting for them to develop basic health services – a mantra of his.

In short, Soper's views resonated with post-war rhetoric, which provided him with a language for winning the wider support for eradication projects that he sought. His own commitment was, as always, not political, but technical. Eradication should be done because it could be done. Like a good RF man, he liked to think that public health worked well only when it was 'above politics'; he disliked the Institute of Inter-American Affairs, the US State Department's wartime agency involved in health projects in Latin America, simply because it was tied to US government directives and therefore not free of political pressures and US bureaucratic routines. Of course, Soper was very astute, in practice, about using political opportunities to pursue his own agendas. I suspect several of Soper's colleagues in public health were like Soper, not really Cold War hawks or warriors, but quite capable of using Cold War rhetoric to get support for projects they supported.

This does not mean that the Cold War did not have an important effect in stimulating successive US governments to provide lots of money to international health campaigns – it did.

As for Soper, as he saw it, what was good about the Cold War decades of the 1950s and '60s was that 'World eradication of such diseases as malaria and smallpox is no longer the dream of the idealist, but the most practical way to approach prevention'.[62]

He felt that, truly, a revolution was underway.

A Post-war Start: The Eradication of Yaws

Among the first health campaigns to be launched in the post-war era was one against yaws. Yaws and tuberculosis were chronic, widespread infections associated with poverty; both became targets of truly massive, post-war, campaigns involving UNICEF and the WHO, involving the treatment of millions of people over many years. Their outcomes were variable. Tuberculosis was dealt with by the BCG vaccine, whose efficacy in poor populations was uncertain or disputed; the mass campaign also involved case detection, drug treatment and, where necessary or possible, isolation of the sick.[63] Yaws was dealt with by the miracle drug, penicillin.

Yaws is a bacterial infection caused by a bacterial spirochete, *Treponema pertunue*, which is like, yet distinct from, the spirochetes involved in venereal and endemic syphilis. It is known by many names, such as *pian*, *buba* and *framboesia tropica*. Yaws is not sexually transmitted (so it is not a venereal infection); it is spread by skin contact among people living close to each other in over-crowded and unsanitary conditions. It is a particularly nasty infection of the tropics, whose development is favoured by heat and humidity. It produces disfiguring ulcers of the skin; if untreated, the infection can also lead to distorting lesions to the bones, and sometimes severe damage to the nose and palate. Painful ulcers on the soles of the feet can make walking difficult.

Soper got involved in yaws almost immediately on taking up the position as director of PAHO. His initial and most important initiative was in Haiti, the country in the American hemisphere most burdened by the infection; the rapid success against yaws in the country was so impressive that it led the Pan American Sanitary Conference (held every four years and where the members made broad policy decisions) to resolve in 1954 to eradicate yaws throughout the Americas.

The yaws campaign in Haiti was classic Soper in its single disease focus, its reliance on a specific technical intervention, the lack of engagement with the underlying socioeconomic determinants of the infection, the boldness with which he conceived the campaign and his insistence that the aim was eradication, and not just reduction.[64] In this latter regard, it differed from the ambitious anti-TB campaign, which was presented as a control campaign (though Soper, typically, held out hopes of eradicating TB as well).

The idea of eradicating yaws first presented itself to Soper two years into his new job, when in 1949 Haiti approached PAHO for help in planning an island-wide anti-yaws programme. Yaws was widely found in other countries in Latin America, but in Haiti it was considered among its most important health problems, with nearly a million cases in an estimated population of only about three and a half million people.

Yaws was not a disease with which Soper was at all familiar – indeed he confessed to complete ignorance of it; being Soper, this did not of course deter him, since to him all eradication campaigns were basically alike. 'The program developed for yaws eradication', he asserted, 'was essentially the same as that developed for eradication of Aa [*Aedes aegypti*] and later Agambiae [*Anopheles gambiae*] in Brazil and Egypt'.[65] This was so even though yaws is not an insect-transmitted infection, so the methods used to halt its transmission had to be quite different! But as we know, the issue for Soper was not the disease's social and biological ecology, but one of rigorous public health administration.

Soper learned over a dinner with a colleague in Washington that penicillin, which had been released for civilian use at the end of the war, was being shown to have positive effects on syphilis in its incubating stage, even at quite low dosages. Soper asked whether it would work on yaws. When told it might, Soper immediately set out a programme of intra-muscular injections, based on the complete coverage of an entire population, so there would be not only a cure of existing cases, but of potentially incubating cases, so that the disease would be eliminated entirely. He pressed forward, even as he admitted that the proper dosage of penicillin needed for treatment was simply not known.[66] With characteristic confidence, Soper 'dared to move rapidly, without waiting for years of detailed clinical studies'.[67] Since all previous efforts at yaws control in Haiti, including those using penicillin, had led only to a temporary reduction in incidence, followed by the disease's recrudescence, what was required, Soper thought, was an all-out, once-and-for-all effort.

To achieve this aim, Soper first had to wrest a pre-existing yaws project away from the Institute of Inter-American Affairs, which had been involved in anti-yaws work on the island since 1942. As mentioned already, the IIAA had been set up during the Second World War and had become an important agency of US policy in health in Latin America. Though the IIAA was destined to be wound up shortly, its officers were not at all ready to cede its anti-yaws work in Haiti to PAHO. Soper, on the other hand, was determined to establish a single chain of command under himself, which he eventually managed to do. He also insisted that the word 'eradication' be inserted into the agreement between PAHO and the Haitian government; in his unpublished papers he noted that the yaws service 'was sold to UNICEF and to WHO as an eradication programme and I am continuing to put this term in the agreement even though I know they are not as eradication-minded themselves'.[68]

UNICEF, the branch of the UN system dedicated to children's rights, was a crucial partner in the yaws campaign, as it would be in other eradication efforts. The agreement signed between PAHO, UNICEF and the Haitian government in 1950 was one of shared responsibilities – UNICEF would provide support in the form of supplies, such as penicillin, as well as laboratory equipment and the trucks needed to transport doctors and staff across the country; PAHO/WHO was to provide the technical advice and leadership of the campaign; and the Haitian government was to pay for all the local physicians and employees required to carry out the injections. Between 1950 and 1954, PAHO spent $200,055 on yaws eradication in Haiti, UNICEF approximately $580,000, and the Haitian government about $605,000.[69] These figures were typical of eradication campaigns, in that a large part of the costs, sometimes the bulk of them, were borne not by international organizations but by the national governments of the countries concerned. Sometimes, these costs represented a very large part of the countries' national health budgets.

On the principle of organization that Soper always insisted was essential to any eradication campaigns, the anti-yaws work was organized in Haiti in a special, independent service dedicated to yaws alone, with almost complete autonomy. This service at first set up a series of treatment centres or clinics to which patients were meant to come; but realizing that rural people were too poor to travel the distances necessary to get to them, resulting in the campaign reaching only 60 per cent of the Haitians affected with yaws, the service reversed direction in 1951, sending mobile teams out into the countryside to make house-to-house visits, where they aimed to treat not just those who were ill, but all those who had contact with the infected, thus achieving a saturation of the population.[70]

Another characteristic of the campaign derived from Soper was its administrative structure. The country was divided into zones, and the zones into further sub-zones, each of which was placed under the direction of an inspector who was responsible for epidemiology and for inspecting the work of inspectors below him, to ensure that the work of injecting the population was in fact carried out as specified and in the numbers claimed.

And in fact, the achievement of the campaign was remarkable. Between 1950 and 1952, almost 900,000 people were treated with penicillin (just under a third of the entire population). By the end of 1954, the programme had reached 97 per cent of the rural population, and by 1958–9 the overall incidence of yaws infection had been reduced to 0.32 per cent (compared to between 30 and 60 per cent when the campaign had started). Only about 40 infectious cases remained in the entire country.[71]

So impressive were the early results in Haiti that, when WHO and UNICEF held its first international symposium on yaws in Bangkok, Thailand, in 1952, the possibility of worldwide eradication was already being mentioned, and in that year WHO initiated a Global Yaws Control Programme (note that the term 'eradication' was not used).[72] Between 1952 and 1969 some 160 million people were examined for yaws, and some 50 million treated with penicillin in 46 different countries around the world.[73] These were massive efforts, in Indonesia, India and Africa, as well as Latin America. Globally, the results were extraordinary; yaws was reduced by 95 per cent.[74]

By the early 1970s yaws had declined so much, in fact, that it had become practically invisible as a public health burden. As a result, the urgency attached to getting rid of the last few cases began to diminish; the priority assigned it fell off, and with it the political will and the resources to continue. Countries turned their attention to new and more pressing problems, like malaria.

As a consequence, transmission was not interrupted, and yaws slowly came back, though not to the extraordinary levels it once had had. There were many reasons for this return beyond the familiar one signalled by Soper himself, namely that the last few cases are always the hardest to identify and deal with in an eradication campaign. But the combined effects of the factors impeding complete eradication demonstrated the danger of thinking of diseases in single factor terms, or in approaching eradication by a single technical intervention.

A first reason for the failure to eradicate concerned a lack of full appreciation of yaws epidemiology – incomplete knowledge once again. It turns out that, for every obvious or clinical case of yaws, there are many more latent cases of infection which if untreated can later become active; the wide prevalence of sub-clinical cases was revealed by later serological surveys of the population.[75] The strategy WHO had recommended to the anti-yaws campaigns was to treat the entire population with penicillin in highly endemic areas where prevalence was greater than 10 per cent. In areas where between 5–10 per cent of the population showed signs of active infections, all children were treated, but only those adults who showed signs of active infection, along with their contacts. Children and contacts were given half the dosage given to infected adults. When prevalence was less than 5 per cent only the active cases and contacts were treated. This strategy worked as a control strategy, but not as an eradication strategy. Many latent infections were missed, with the result that they remained foci of potential re-infection in the population, so that transmission continued.

A second reason for failure concerned the absence in most of the countries of adequate health services capable of taking over the anti-yaws task on a routine basis when the special service was disbanded. Eradication programmes by definition were vertically-organized, short-term and single-disease in their targets; routine health services, instead, had to address multiple health problems at the same time, and were meant to be continuous. In the 1960s, WHO began to emphasize the need to integrate the anti-yaws work into the fixed, everyday health services of the country. In this way, it was hoped, a mass health programme might act as a seedbed for improving health services and social development.

But in Haiti and many other very poor countries, everyday or basic health services were non-existent. As yaws disappeared, the mobile teams were disbanded, and nothing took their place. The routine surveillance systems needed to detect the few remaining foci and active cases were also missing.

In fact, the entire economic calculus of yaws eradication was just an assumption. Soper believed that yaws eradication, in itself, would have incalculable positive effects on economic productivity. But though the campaign brought huge benefits by ridding millions of people of an extremely nasty and debilitating infection, the actual economic impact of removing yaws from their lives was either negligible, or unknown. The idea that the virtual disappearance of yaws would translate into improved economic conditions for the rural poor, absent other changes in their fundamental economic and political circumstances, was naive, but was a basic assumption of nearly all eradication campaigns. Instead, the rural poverty, poor housing and poor sanitation that were the social and economic determinants of yaws went unaddressed; they had never been part of the eradication concept.[76]

By 1978 WHO had realized that control measures had lapsed in many places and yaws was returning. In some parts of Africa there were foci where the prevalence rates approached levels similar to those that had existed before the mass campaigns of the 1950s and '60s. The 31st World Health Assembly passed a new resolution on yaws in 1978, requesting member states to once more undertake programmes to interrupt yaws transmission.[77] In the workshops and conferences held in the 1980s, where public health experts began to discuss which other diseases to select for eradication following the success with smallpox, yaws was one of the first to be mentioned as the most amenable to extermination. The whole eradication cycle had to start again; in 2007, yet another consultation exercise was held by WHO to revive the effort to eliminate yaws by 2012.

So was the yaws eradication effort a great success, or a disappointing failure? It all depends, of course, on the goals being sought and the terms being used. Judged in terms of the reduction of a disease as a public health burden in some of the poorest and most neglected populations in the world, it had to be counted a great success. In the Caribbean and Latin America, yaws prevalence has remained very low, with cases confined to a few difficult geographical areas and vulnerable and marginalized populations. Worldwide, too, the prevalence is nothing like it once was – in 2007 the WHO estimated that there were 2.5 million cases of yaws (of which 460,000 were new cases), far less than the 50–100 million people estimated to have been infected with yaws in 1948.

But judged by the exacting terms of eradication that Soper had aimed for, the campaign had to count as a failure. Yaws is still here, and with it the burdens of poverty, social stigma and exclusion that yaws inflicts on those who are infected. In reviving a campaign against yaws today, WHO calls it a forgotten or neglected disease.[78]

Yellow Fever Again: The Continental Effort

The eradication campaign closest to Soper's heart, and one which we can only describe as quixotic, given what was known by then about yellow fever, and about the sheer difficulty of deliberately setting out to kill all and every example of an insect species, was the campaign to eradicate the *Aedes aegypti* from the entire American continent. This idea, which as we have seen in chapter Three, Soper developed in the 1930s, was in his mind his most original contribution to public health, and it remained the touchstone of eradication as he understood it all his life.

Before 1947 efforts to get all the countries in the Americas to pull together to get rid of the urban vector were sporadic and under-funded.[79] In Brazil, much of course had been done, and yellow fever incidence was low, but by the end of the war the government had stripped its National Yellow Fever Service down severely. In 1946 Brazil approached its previous benefactor, the Rockefeller Foundation, for help in the task of eradicating the *Aedes aegypti* mosquito, but the RF had already decided to get out of practical public health work, and refused. Soper's election to PAHO made the difference; within months, he had persuaded the organization to commit to a plan for a continent-wide vector eradication programme (voted on the basis of a Brazilian proposal in the autumn meeting of the Directing Council in 1947, suggesting Soper's direct hand in the project).[80] To accompany the declaration, Soper prepared an article, spelling out the implication that if eradicated across the entire Americas, the mosquito would not re-appear even when control measures were discontinued.[81]

Soper's argument about yellow fever vector eradication was that, if any one country managed to get rid of the *Aedes aegypti* in its territory, as some countries were already on their way to doing by the late 1940s, it remained at risk from re-infestation if any other country on its borders did not also get rid of the mosquito. Brazil, for instance, had frontiers with ten different countries and/or political units in South America; only if its neighbours also undertook to get rid of the mosquito species at the same time as Brazil would the country be spared the enormous cost of maintaining control services indefinitely – a financial rationale often given for aiming for eradication rather than mere control. Soper acknowledged the reluctance some people felt towards accepting eradication, owing to the 'traditional ingrained philosophy that a species eradication is impossible, that a species is something sacred and eternal in spite of the example of the dodo, the passenger pigeon and the dinosaur to the contrary, and that when species disappear they do so only in response to "cosmic" or "biological" rather than man-made factors'.[82] He had no such environmental or philosophical qualms.

The introduction of DDT did not alter the principles of the yellow fever eradication service as Soper understood it, only made it more efficacious, since DDT was superior to Paris Green as a larvicide, and to pyrethrum (used to kill adult mosquitoes in people's homes). The basic techniques of eradication were fundamentally administrative, and had already been spelt out in detail in the manual of operations he had published in 1943.[83] What was required was organization and political will.

Another argument Soper made in favour of eradication was moral. Soper maintained that once free of the *aegypti* mosquito, a country had the moral right to insist on protection from re-infestation, and its neighbours the moral duty to abide by it.[84] The supposedly inexorable widening of eradication efforts, from a single locale, to a region, to an entire country and then to an entire continent, was an exemplification of 'Soper's law' (as described in chapter Three). Of course, as he found out, there was nothing inexorable or law-like about it; instead, getting all the countries to rid themselves of the mosquito within their own national territories required almost superhuman exhortation on the part of Soper. It was not as if yellow fever was an active threat in the continental Americas at the time; in fact only one small outbreak of urban yellow fever had occurred in the previous decade and a half. Many countries had not seen a single case for decades. The decision to eradicate was not based, therefore, on an emergency or an overwhelming health problem, but was rather (in Soper's words) 'a deliberate effort to consolidate permanently the gains of previous decades and to guarantee future freedom from yellow fever to the cities and towns of the Americas'.[85]

Soper considered the decision a landmark in international health because it was 'the first official recognition by an international health organization of regional responsibility for the solution of a health problem involving an entire continent'.[86] But if previous control methods had done as well as they had, why aim instead for such a difficult goal as absolute eradication? Insect pests resist their elimination; reducing their numbers was much more practicable, and by keeping house infection rates under 5 per cent, yellow fever transmission ended. On the other hand, as Soper and other public health officials knew only too well, once a particular disease was reduced to almost invisibility, keeping control methods going year in and year out was also a challenge.

Having found what he thought was the secret to insect extermination, Soper set his sights on his lofty goal. A formidable opponent to those who questioned his logic, and a tireless worker, with an iron will and an ability to persuade, Soper worked on country after country, getting them to sign up to the campaign with PAHO, and then sending technical advisors on how to set up the services across the continent. Soper was dedicated, trustworthy and a man of conviction; presenting himself as above the political fray, the one political battle he cared about was to get the campaign on track.

As was the case with other eradication efforts, the anti-*Aedes aegypti* campaigns were conducted at the country level. In Paraguay the service was at first handled by the National Yellow Fever Service of Brazil; because the Brazilian yellow fever service was autonomous, said Soper, it could lend its technical staff to other countries and did so freely until PAHO became able financially to bear the costs itself.[87]

The work involved was tedious and meticulous, and Soper's diary recording his travels throughout the Americas for PAHO registers his tireless efforts to make the programme work, often against the odds. Soper pressed officials to attack the mosquito, even suggesting, against the advice of the US's own Food and Drug Administration, that DDT be put in water supplies, as a means to destroy mosquito larvae. 'We have let things stand before, now we have the money and the appropriation, let us do seriously what we are going to do', he commented in his diary.[88] Even when he recognized the growing problem of resistance of both *Aedes aegypti* and anopheline mosquitoes to DDT and other insecticides, he kept at it.[89] Resistance by people to having their houses sprayed was another difficulty that he acknowledged but did not let stop him; he noted in his diary that in Paraguay people refused a second spraying of DDT 'since they had not known how disagreeable it would be'. Combining paraffin with DDT, as he proposed, 'will to a certain extent be punitive', he added, but no matter, it had to be done.[90] In Argentina, where there had been no yellow fever for years, Soper persuaded the government to nonetheless mount a campaign against the *Aedes aegypti* mosquito.[91] He noted with satisfaction some years later that Argentina had indeed set up an *Aedes Aegypti Eradication Service,* where 'routine inspection by employees takes place in almost military style as it was the routine in north Brazil many years ago'.[92]

As an added incentive and regulation of the eradication effort, PAHO developed a procedure for issuing certificates to countries where the yellow fever urban mosquito had been eliminated; eventually this certification process required the absence of the mosquito from a region or a country for a year, as established by at least three surveys, the final survey being conducted in cooperation with PAHO technical staff. If certified free of the mosquito, the country was entered on a special registry established by PAHO. This method of international certification later became the basis for procedures set up by WHO to certify malaria and smallpox eradication.[93]

PAHO's journal, the *Boletin de la Oficína Sanitaria Panamericana* (*BOSP*) provided regular tallies of the sweeps against mosquitoes, and the organization investigated every case of yellow fever. Yellow fever had in fact nearly disappeared. In 1955, Soper presented to PAHO maps comparing all the areas in the Americas with yellow fever between 1900 and 1931, with those reporting yellow fever between 1932 and 1955. The maps showed that, whereas before the 1930s, most cases of yellow fever were coastal and of the urban-transmission kind, after 1931 and the introduction of systematic destruction of urban mosquito breeding, nearly all the cases were in interior areas of the countries, and were jungle yellow fever cases.[94]

'Nearly all' – this was the rub. In his 1955 report, Soper mentioned fatal cases of yellow fever in four American nations; a further five to eight countries had reported outbreaks each year during the previous decade.[95] The problem was that even a decade or more of negative observations (of recording no yellow fever cases in cities) was not sufficient to discount the possibility of the re-appearance of cases of yellow fever, especially since many countries simply did not have the resources to track down possible cases of deaths by fevers and do the necessary surveillance and epidemiological work to establish yellow fever's locations. Moreover, as urban yellow fever cases disappeared the only evidence of eradication was negative evidence – a difficult standard when many cases were silent or unrecorded.

Nevertheless, Soper remained optimistic. He admitted that progress was slower than he had anticipated, but found developments nevertheless gratifying. As he said in relation to his maps, now that everyone understood that jungle yellow fever was the source of urban epidemics, it was all the more important to get rid of the urban mosquito. To him, 'the eradication concept remained', even if yellow fever as an infection could not be eradicated. In twelve years (his years in office at PAHO, from 1947 to 1959) he claimed that eleven countries had been certified as completely free of the mosquito. By 1964, eradication of the vector had been achieved in most of South America and Central America.

But in 1967 Soper was shocked to learn that a large area in the North East Amazon region of Brazil was again completely infected by the insect.[96] In 1976, the PAHO countries were still at it, but with now only some ten countries in the Western hemisphere being certified by PAHO as apparently entirely free of the *Aedes aegypti* mosquito.[97] Brazil, the largest country in the South American continent, and the one with the largest endemic centres of yellow fever, was however no longer one of them; it had lost its certification, as had several other Latin American and Caribbean countries. In the Caribbean, DDT-resistant *Aedes aegypti* mosquitoes had appeared – a problem that haunted the malaria eradication campaigns also. In the 1970s, financial support began to wane, even as the first cost-benefit analyses of the effort concluded that eradication was worth it – that the benefits would exceed the costs 'at a discount rate . . . attractive even to the least developed countries', according to a report by economists.[98]

Aedes Aegypti Eradication and the United States

Responsibility for the waning support for *Aedes aegypti* eradication lay largely with the USA, or at least so Soper thought. Throughout the 1950s, the United States refused to do anything about getting rid of its yellow fever mosquitoes, despite having signed on to the project in 1947. This dereliction of duty, as Soper saw it, caused him intense irritation. The USA, he said, was a laggard, breaking its moral obligation to other countries, and acting selfishly, undoing the gains made in Latin America by risking the invasion of the countries by mosquitoes from the north. Where once the US had had its own medical inspectors based permanently in the ports of Cuba in order to report to the US all cases of yellow fever, now Soper imagined inspectors from Cuba patrolling the waters between itself and the US in order to prevent re-infestation of the island by US mosquitoes. 'I, as an American citizen . . . am repeatedly embarrassed when my Latin-American friends say to me . . . what is your country doing, and I have to say, well "just give them time, just give them time"', wrote Soper.[99]

The fact was that the US had decided Soper's goal of *Aedes aegypti* eradication was unnecessary and unachievable. The US had not had a single case of yellow fever for over 40 years; unlike South America, it also had no jungle reservoirs of yellow fever virus. To keep out yellow fever, it preferred to rely on the 17D yellow fever vaccine produced by Rockefeller researchers in 1937 (the 17D referred to the particular strain of the virus used in the vaccine). Its safety had been improved since its first tests, and by the 1940s it had been given to millions of people.[100] The US therefore relied for protection on vaccination certificates from travellers coming from yellow fever countries, and on keeping a stock of vaccine for emergency use at home in the event of a yellow fever outbreak.

Without denying its usefulness, Soper, however, continued to insist that vaccination was no substitute for mosquito eradication. The protection it offered only took effect a week or more after inoculation, in which interval of time a vaccinated individual could still transmit the virus to unprotected people if the *Aedes aegypti* mosquitoes were still present. Soper was convinced that the US would rue its decision – that one day yellow fever would return to the United States' shores and that, given the large presence of the *Aedes aegypti* , the country would have an epidemic on its hands before vaccination could arrest it. In addition, in Latin American countries with large rural populations and endemic pockets of the virus, everyone at risk in forested areas would have to be vaccinated, a task that Brazil, amongst other countries in the Americas, thought beyond its financial and administrative abilities.

The US did launch some pilot projects to test the feasibility of eradicating the mosquito and in 1962–3 began at least planning for a countrywide programme. By this time, re-infestation of Mexico along the border with the US was already occurring, putting the results of Mexico's painstaking controls in jeopardy. President Kennedy met with the Mexican President in June 1962, where the topic came up, but was taken aback when he learned the potential cost to the US was estimated at $125,000,000.

In 1963, the US did reluctantly, under pressure from PAHO and more as a 'good neighbour' gesture than because it believed in it (this was the period of the Alliance for Progress), take systematic action against the mosquito, in a programme barely lasting the five years promised. At the peak of the US effort, there were some 300 federal employees involved, working mainly at the Center for Disease Control in Atlanta, with thousands of other public health officials working under federal contract at the state level. But most of them did not think the programme worth it, nor did they think that mosquitoes being carried from the US into nearby countries were the main cause of infections of yellow fever in Latin America. Altogether, the US spent $53 million on mosquito eradication, 'only to decide that the insect was not that dangerous and probably could not be eradicated anyway'.[101]

The US programme also started at an awkward time; attitudes towards the large-scale use of pesticides were changing. In 1962 Rachel Ҫarson published what has come to be seen as a key manifesto of the environmentalist movement of the twentieth century, her book *Silent Spring*, and DDT came under attack as an environmental hazard. Carson's target was not the public health use of pesticides, but their large-scale agricultural use, which she argued left long-term, damaging chemical imprints on wild life and the balance of nature. Nevertheless, public health was caught up in the critique.[102]

Soper had left PAHO by this date, but he was still active in public health as a consultant.[103] He left an interesting account of a meeting he attended in Jacksonville, Florida, in August 1964 where the issue of insecticides and 'possible trouble with Rachel Carson' was brought up. The head of the local mosquito eradication effort, wrote Soper, 'is, I think, perturbed by the way in which the *Aedes aegypti* service is spreading insecticide in a high, wide, and handsome manner without limiting its application specifically to containers which may breed *Aedes aegypti*'. Soper's objection was not that DDT was itself bad, since his faith in DDT's usefulness in public health was almost unbounded, but that the US anti-*Aedes aegypti* programme was not being run in an effective and precise fashion, targeting the breeding sites of the mosquito: 'One gets the impression', he wrote, 'it [DDT] is being used in a shotgun campaign which will undoubtedly bring down the *Aedes aegypti* index but which will never bring eradication'.[104] In this Soper proved right. In 1968, David J. Sencer, the director of the Center for Disease Control which ran the US programme, called for a review of the entire eradication project, arguing that unless it was global, it was a waste of time. The next year, the appropriations by Congress were terminated by the new Republican administration, President Nixon having been reported as saying that the US could easily spend millions of dollars and yet be without a guarantee of success.

Soper very much hoped for an 'Answer to SILENT SPRING'; in his lifetime, however, the blanket, chemical, insecticide approach to vector-borne diseases became increasingly unfashionable and in 1972 DDT was banned for use in the United States.[105] Soper never forgave the US for failing to do its part in exterminating the *Aedes aegypti* from the continent when it could have, and as usual was not shy about making his opinion known. 'Failure of the United States to Eradicate *Aedes aegypti*' was the subject of the last chapter of his memoirs.[106]

'Eradication of *Aedes aegypti* is not easy', Soper had told the conferees at the Pan American Sanitary Conference in Puerto Rico in 1958 – his swan song as director of PAHO.[107] But he continued to resist any moves to dilute his absolutist ideal. 'Must force the issue of absolute definition of eradication', he wrote in his notes, adding cryptically and succinctly: 'Suggestion to redefine "eradication" is not acceptable. Must have courage of their convictions. *Capacity for fanaticism*.'[108]

At least the US's failure to follow through with *Aedes aegypti* eradication provided Soper with a convenient excuse for what was, in truth, a very difficult task, that of wiping out for ever from a continent an entire, well-established, biological species by chemical means.

An Impossible Project

The difficulty of sustaining Soper's mosquito eradication effort only began to be articulated more publicly and consistently at PAHO meetings once Soper had retired from the scene. The new director of PAHO, Dr Abraham Horwitz, who was elected in 1958 and took office early the following year, was initially determined to see the insect extermination project through to completion. But almost immediately after his election, for the first time, countries began to demand some end-point to their Herculean efforts. In 1961, for instance, at a meeting of the Directing Council of PAHO in Washington, the delegate from Mexico asked PAHO to pass a resolution setting a deadline for termination of the campaign – say within five years.[109] This suggestion was seconded by Brazil, which also was getting impatient waiting for other countries to complete the job.

The British delegate, representing the countries of the British Caribbean, demonstrated why the goal of vector eradication was so difficult to achieve. In the mid-1950s, he said, tests had already shown that the urban mosquito could breed in tree holes; this was a blow to the whole spraying regime, which was based on the idea that the *Aedes aegypti* mosquito bred close to houses and so larviciding was relatively easy. 'It became obvious at the start of the program that the method offered little or no hope of eradication, although it permitted reduction of the indices [of the mosquitoes].'[110] The British Caribbean was also one of the places where resistance in the mosquitoes to DDT was first observed. Shifting to another insecticide, dieldrin, at first seemed a solution; it was applied to the whole of North Trinidad between June and December of 1957, and then the entire island was sprayed in 1958,with a second spraying across the south of the island in 1959. By 1960, the mosquitoes had apparently disappeared again, but such profligate use of chemical insecticides could not go on forever, and anyway, resistance to dieldrin was not long in coming.

Horwitz was a director in a different mould from Soper. Once in office, he began to shift the focus of PAHO toward more social and economic approaches – to the delivery of clean water and better sewerage, and to overcoming the inequalities in wealth and health. Ecology also began to make an appearance in health discussions. 'The categorical nature of the target', Horwitz commented, referring to eradication and its setbacks, 'the dynamic and ecological processes involved, and nature's plan, which does not always coincide with what man can accomplish, explain the uneven course of the action taken – forwards or backwards'.[111] It was acknowledged in 1968 that 'the program for the eradication of Aa [mosquito] has remained stationary in the countries and territories where the mosquito was present and has regressed in others, which have become re-infested'.[112] The problem of getting to the end point in *Aa* eradication led to a convening of a conference in Washington in 1967 with representatives from twenty countries, who reiterated the need to complete the job of eradication as soon as possible.

In the circumstances, even when some countries objected to continuing spraying, Horwitz still thought there was no alternative to pressing forward to zero. He was also concerned that *not* completing the eradication effort would harm PAHO's reputation; he feared that giving up would infect people with what someone had called 'the disease of lack of confidence and discouragement'.[113] 'Over and above the dangers [of not pressing on]', Horwitz commented, 'there is a sense of defeat which is not in keeping with the outlook of the present generation in the Americas'. Some countries had put in so much effort that it was almost too much to contemplate what giving up on the eradicationist project would mean. Brazil, for example, had spent many millions of dollars on its *Aedes aegypti* eradication campaign alone; safeguarding such an enormous investment had to be brought into the picture. 'The thought of those who have not died . . . is what must be borne in mind by the reader when he reviews what has been achieved, though he does so in a highly critical spirit.'[114]

But as the French delegate to PAHO asked, was there really any chance that absolute eradication of a mosquito could ever be achieved? 'When could eradication be said to be complete and final', he asked, 'considering that a few mosquitoes were enough to cause reinfestation?'[115] This is what made the whole mosquito eradication programme so difficult to sustain; the disease had virtually disappeared; yet the goal of insect eradication had not been met. There was a growing sense that the cost-benefit ratio was questionable at this point; the costs on an annual basis were enormous, and the benefit was of eliminating a disease that 'had little importance as a cause of death'. Even the much-praised Pan American Sanitary Code had not been brought in to place sanctions against any country that created problems with the re-infestation of its neighbours.

By this time (1970) the US was unable to disguise its impatience. All pretence that the US would carry out its part of the bargain, for political or any other reasons, having been given up, the US delegate to the Regional Meeting of PAHO that year, Dr Ehrlich, suggested it was time for a complete re-assessment of the anti-yellow fever strategy. He pointed to the huge growth in the waste produced in increasingly urbanized countries, the vast residue of containers, cans and tires being produced, and the opportunities they provided for the endless proliferation of trapped water and therefore the creation of new breeding places for *Aedes aegypti* mosquitoes. He believed that satisfactory disposal of this waste to the point needed to achieve absolute mosquito eradication was beyond the resources of most nations, faced as they were with competition from other pressing health needs. He pointed to the improvements in the yellow fever vaccine and its delivery (such as the jet injector), which made mass immunization in early life feasible. Careful surveillance and monitoring was another method he thought needed emphasis. Speaking as a US government representative, he called on the member states of PAHO to participate in an appraisal of all the alternative approaches to the control and prevention of diseases transmitted by the *Aedes aegypti* mosquito.[116]

Many member countries in PAHO were ready to concede the point. The US delegate acknowledged that eradication efforts in his country had been discontinued, since *Aa* eradication 'did not have the same priority for the health of the American people as many other programs that were in the process of development'.[117]

And so, slowly, support for getting rid of the urban vector of yellow fever eroded away. At best about sixteen out of the 44 territories and countries of the originally infested areas had achieved complete eradication of the vector during the overall effort. Urban yellow fever, though, had practically disappeared.

Soper's Return?

Today we live in what Dr Wilbur Downs, who knew Soper well, called 'the unhappy present'.[118] With the abandonment of mosquito eradication in the 1970, the *Aedes aegypti* began to return and with them *Aedes aegypti*-transmitted viruses. Moreover, as the US delegate had predicted in 1970, the density of the *Aedes* mosquitoes is greater today than it was in past because of the greater density of urban populations and the opportunity city living provides for water-based breeding. In the vast urban slums that characterize twenty-first century cities in many developing countries, where piped water is scarce and rubbish collection often almost non-existent, abandoned containers of every description, from rubber car tires to plastic bottles, to water storage barrels, provide the perfect environment for the proliferation of *Aedes aegypti* mosquitoes.

Let us also not forget dengue fever. Dengue is in several respects the yellow fever of the twenty-first century. Like yellow fever, it is a viral disease of humans that can be fatal; like yellow fever in the 1930s, but unlike yellow fever today, dengue has no preventive vaccine. In the 1970s, when the anti-*Aedes aegypti* programmes were given up, no one was thinking much about dengue, which at the time only produced sporadic epidemics in Asia and the Americas. But in the early 1980s dengue began to appear more frequently, with several different variants of the virus circulating, including the deadly haemorrhagic variant. In 1981, a major epidemic, with an estimated 24,000 cases of severe haemorrhagic dengue, erupted in Cuba, requiring thousands of hospitalizations. Today, dengue is foremost in health officials' minds in many cities in Asia and Latin America. In 2002 and again in 2008, Rio de Janeiro had serious epidemics of dengue, and the whole process of careful mosquito control has had to be started all over again.

On the one hand, as we look back on the history of yellow fever and the attempts to control it, we have to ask whether, given the relatively low incidence of yellow fever when the continent-wide effort at eradication began, the pursuit of the extermination of a single species of mosquito was the best use of the resources, time, and energy of the often under-funded health systems of the poor countries involved.

On the other hand, it is hard not to feel a certain respect for the determination with which Soper led the PAHO countries in their more than 30-year quest to achieve urban yellow fever eradication, even if the campaign also reveals the utopian, even fanatical, aspects of Soper's agenda.

Nowadays, Soper's reputation among historians is generally low, owing to his intransigence over absolute eradication. His reputation among some public health practitioners, however, is on the rise; there are those who, like Downs, maintain that there is an argument to be made in favour of reviving the insecticidal and vigilant approach of Soper, in order to deal with potentially explosive epidemics of dengue fever and other infections.[119] Some even advocate his methods in relation to malaria as well. In the last chapter of this book (chapter Seven), following the chapters on malaria eradication and then smallpox eradication, I discuss several such 'Soperian' moments. The world today is very different from Soper's – indeed it has learned from Soper's mistakes. Outside of a few 'command' polities, the large, top-down and almost militant organizations in public health that Soper advocated are not possible. Goals short of eradication are preferred. But it is relevant to ask how far aspects of Soper's methods might be adapted to contemporary 'bottom up', community-based public health practices, in order to achieve sustainable control of infectious diseases in our current, globalized world.

5 The End of Malaria in the World?

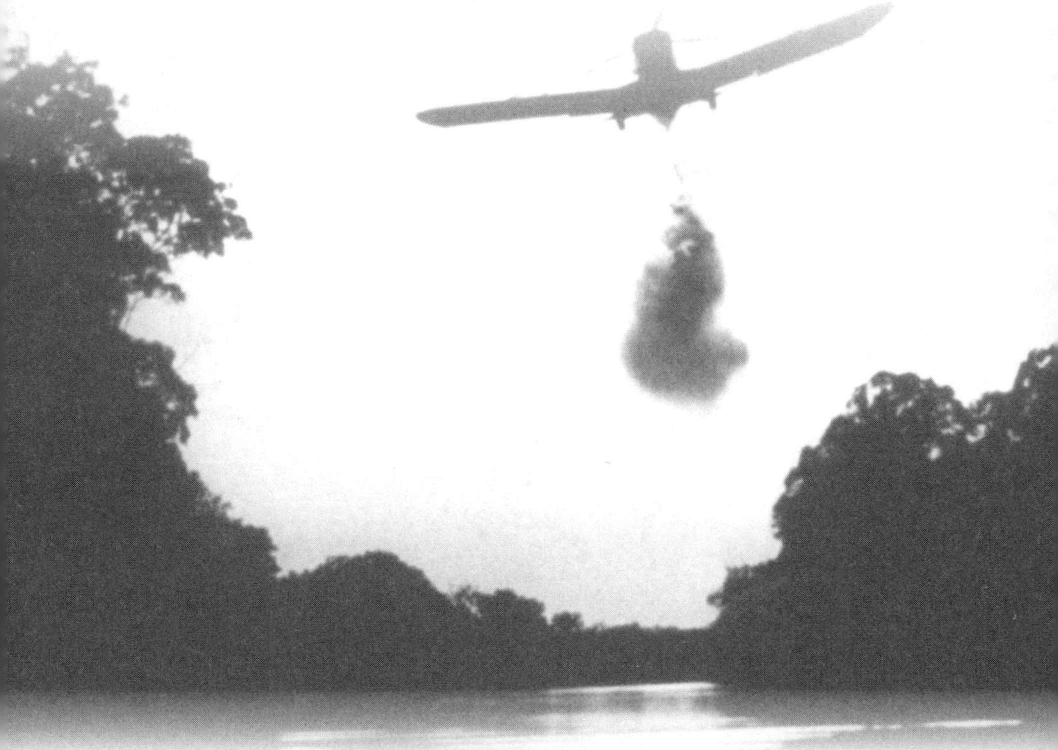

In 1947, Fred L. Soper travelled to Mexico City in his capacity as the just-elected director of the Pan American Health Organization. Speaking at a dinner attended by a large number of public health officials, he found himself, as he phrased it, 'forced into predicting the end of malaria in the world during the next 10 to 15 years'.[1] Rash words! But very characteristic of the man!

In promoting the idea of the worldwide eradication of malaria, Soper was taking up the disease which most pre-occupied international public health experts in the decades immediately after the Second World War. Malaria's disruptive impact on the war itself was of very recent memory, and the economic, social and physical burdens malaria placed on populations, especially poor populations, had long been recognized. In an era that would see an end to colonial rule in many places around the globe, would malaria remain a major barrier to development in newly independent nations? Could it really be banished forever?

Soper certainly thought so. Malaria had by this time almost disappeared from much of Western Europe and the United States. Why not use the new techniques born of the war effort to get rid of malaria in the rest of the world? True to his eradicationist convictions, Soper went to work to get PAHO involved; in 1954, at the Fourteenth Pan American Sanitary Conference held in Chile, the organization called for 'nothing less than the eradication of malaria from the Americas', and authorized $100,000 towards its costs.[2] The next year, malaria eradication became a worldwide campaign when the delegates attending the World Health Assembly (where WHO policies were decided) voted to endorse the eradicationist project.

Thus was launched the Malaria Eradication Programme (MEP), the most ambitious project ever undertaken up until that time by an international health organization. Born in a moment of post-war optimism and faith in science, the MEP was to be a demonstration of the power and promise of new technical solutions to disease. It was premised on the idea that systematic household spraying with DDT, the wonder chemical of the Second World War, would reduce the numbers of malaria insect vectors sufficiently so that the transmission of the parasites would be interrupted. Malaria itself would then disappear as a disease. The MEP was designed as a time-limited effort; five years, or perhaps ten, were what was predicted would be needed. The same methods were to be used across the spectrum of countries, rich or poor, wherever malaria was found. The MEP was specifically conceptualized as a universal, technical intervention that did not have to take on the almost impossible tasks of improving the social and economic conditions in which people in areas of endemic malaria lived. Instead, malaria eradication was to come first; socio-economic improvement was expected to follow.[3]

What happened to the MEP is by now well known in public health circles, if not more generally. After an initial period of immense enthusiasm and success, during which malaria rates plummeted even in some very poor countries with quite rudimentary public health services, the MEP began to run into difficulties that encompassed such a wide array of biological, social, political, economic and cultural factors as to make evident even to some of the most insistent eradicators that, though malaria could be dramatically reduced, complete eradication was not possible. Already by the mid-1960s WHO's confidence in malaria eradication was disappearing; money and resources started to run out. In 1969, WHO officially gave up the goal of eradication for most countries, recommending instead that they return to malaria control – a policy prescription that in many cases turned out to be a recipe for the collapse of anti-malaria efforts. Malaria returned, often in epidemic form.

The reason why this classic arc in disease eradication is so compelling is because so much was in fact achieved, and the falling off from the achievement was so dramatic. The MEP stands in many people's minds as the paradigmatic confrontation between Western biomedicine and disease, with the victory going to the disease. DDT and drugs proved to be no match for the wily mosquitoes and parasites of malaria, which were so much more able to adapt to new circumstances than the MEP itself.

And yet there are many people who would probably say that, if not measured in absolutist terms, but in terms of a massive commitment to malaria control, the MEP was a huge success – especially as we contemplate the current situation, with an estimated 350–500 million cases of malaria and two to three million deaths per year. Today, malaria is once again the object of a massive international effort at control. Even eradication is back on the international health agenda, promoted by the Gates Foundation, and supported, as well, by the current Director-General of the WHO. Will the techniques of contemporary medicine and public health, such as new drugs and insecticide-treated bed nets, this time around be enough to get it right? Is eradication a sensible goal to set?

The history of the MEP certainly offers some answers to these questions, but thus far it has been told largely from the perspective of the international organizations that led and supported it, like PAHO and WHO, and their Expert Committees and their prescriptive plans. These were certainly important in galvanizing political and technical will. But the de-politicized language employed in international public health – the language of parasites, vectors, drugs and DDT – did not include the political and social conditions in which people lived, the everyday difficulties their lives presented, their poverty, their other diseases, the variations in economic and technical resources in different countries, the degree of political commitment to the eradication agenda or even the differences in the scale of the operations required. These latter factors made up the true political geography of malaria; they were realities of underdevelopment. The MEP needs, then, to be examined not as a unitary whole, but as a mosaic of different national programmes – a shift in perspective we are now beginning to see in malaria studies which focus on how the MEP worked out in specific locations.[4]

In this chapter, I have selected one MEP, that of Venezuela, to serve as a case study of the interactions between the national and the international in malaria eradication. Venezuela merits attention because in so many respects its MEP represented the very best of what an MEP could do; it was run professionally, expertly and with great conviction. And yet it is also a cautionary tale about what an MEP could not, and perhaps cannot, achieve. Malariologists before the Second World War and DDT had come to think of malaria as essentially a local disease whose control would require local or place-specific solutions. There could not be a single plan for everywhere. This is also the lesson of Venezuela.

Malaria: A Very Different Disease

Fred L. Soper was not a malaria expert when he took up the cause of malaria eradication.[5] He was instead an expert, as we know, on insect vectors and how to get rid of them. Both yellow fever and malaria were insect-borne infections, and having discovered methods that would lead to the eradication of the insect vector of urban yellow fever, he found it easy to think of malaria in analogous terms.[6] Believing the essence of eradication was scrupulous adherence to public health administration, he thought that all that was required were disciplined teams of anti-mosquito workers and thorough supervision of the work done. There was, he said, 'an essential identity of the malaria program with that of yellow fever'.[7]

But analogies, as we know, are misleading as well as suggestive. And apart from being an insect-transmitted disease, malaria is not like yellow fever at all, and presents quite different challenges to its control.

To start with, malaria has many mosquito vectors, not just the three or four involved in yellow fever transmission; of the 400 or more species of *Anopheles* mosquitoes known to exist, at least 30 to 40 of them transmit malaria. This alone complicates the malaria picture. The infective agent of malaria is also unlike that of yellow fever, being a protozoan parasite rather than a virus.[8] There are four different kinds of malaria protozoa that infect humans – *Plasmodium vivax*, *falciparum*, *ovale* and *malariae* – each with its own complicated life cycle in the mosquito and the human host, and each producing a characteristic pattern of fevers and other symptoms in infected humans.[9] The *Anopheles gambiae*, widespread in Africa, is the most 'efficient' of the vectors, being anthropophilic (preferring to feed on humans rather than other animals); it is a 'species complex', meaning that it is made up of several races or variants with different transmission capabilities, which add to its differential impact. In addition, in Africa, the falciparum form of malaria protozoa, the most deadly to human health, is widely distributed. Put the efficient vector and the falciparum protozoon together, and you have very serious malaria indeed.

Clinically, though malaria is sometimes confused with yellow fever, since both diseases cause fevers, the symptoms are really very different. While yellow fever is an acute disease, malaria is largely a chronic illness, producing intermittent fevers, sudden chills, headaches, anaemia and general debilitation; once infected, people can harbour the parasite in their blood for months, or even years. Vivax malaria, once known as the benign variety of malaria, is benign only in relative terms; people with vivax infection feel exhausted and ill. Malignant (or pernicious) malaria, produced by infection with the falciparum type of parasite, is, as its old names indicate, a very dangerous form which, in the severest cases, can result in coma, brain damage and death.

Another difference between yellow fever and malaria concerns their distribution. By the mid-twentieth century, yellow fever was found only in the Americas and in parts of Africa; for reasons that are not clearly understood, yellow fever has never established itself in Asia, despite the presence there of the transmitting mosquitoes.

Malaria's distribution was far greater. In the nineteenth century, it was found in almost every part of the world, including most of Europe. In the course of the century, however, changes in the patterns of human settlement (for example, the movement of people away from malarial areas, such as the fens in East Anglia, England), together with increased urbanization and improved social conditions, led to the reduction of malaria in many temperate areas, largely in Europe and North America (without any deliberate efforts at malaria control). Meanwhile, malaria was simultaneously being 'tropicalized', that is, being spread into largely southern and tropical areas of the world. By the end of the nineteenth century, just at the time the role of anopheline mosquitoes was discovered in malaria transmission, malaria had become the paradigmatic disease of the new specialty of tropical medicine. Many factors were involved in the expansion and shift in the geography of malaria, the most important probably being the rapid development of export crop agriculture in Europe's overseas tropical colonies, which changed the environments of mosquitoes, parasites and human beings, increasing the breeding sites of insects and bringing them into close contact with large numbers of impoverished and non-immune labourers brought to work in the new agricultural zones. To understand malaria, then, we have to use what I have called a 'socio-ecological' approach, giving due weight to human actions, such as the development of new zones of economic activity and to the behaviour of mosquitoes in different ecologies.[10] The result of changes in land use, human migration and labour, and ecology is endemic and/or explosive epidemic malaria, depending on the circumstances. Randall Packard gives an extremely good account of this 'making' of a tropical disease (the title of his 2007 book).[11]

Emilio Pampana and Paul F. Russell, two malariologists who were involved in the post-war malaria eradication effort, judged that malaria reached its maximum world dissemination between about 1855 and the 1920s and '30s. As late as 1955, as WHO prepared to launch the MEP, it was estimated there were 250 million clinical attacks of malaria a year (in a total world population of approximately 2.5 billion people), with as many as 2.5 million deaths. Owing to the absence of malaria surveillance procedures in most countries, or indeed the most basic of health services, these figures almost certainly represented a huge under-count. They also did not include adequate information from the USSR or China.[12]

Malaria also differed from yellow fever in its social and economic consequences for communities. Though yellow fever could be fatal, people who survived an attack were left with a life-long immunity, with no impairment of functions. By 1937, in addition, a very good preventive vaccine was available. Malaria, on the other hand, though it did not kill most people directly (overall, about 1 per cent of those infected died, with a higher mortality rate among infants and children), was a chronic, repetitive disease that was associated with an increased number of deaths from other causes, a reduction in overall life expectancy, stunted physical and mental development, and high infant and child morbidity and mortality. Latent immunity to malaria was acquired through repeated bouts of infection, but was limited geographically, so when people moved their immunity was lost. Malaria's effects on the capacity to work, on economic development, and on demography were therefore very considerable. In epidemics, death rates soared way beyond the more usual one percent of those infected. In Ceylon (now Sri Lanka), the epidemic of 1934–5 killed 80,000 people in seven months; in Brazil, out of 100,000 cases in the epidemic of 1938, at least 14,000 people died. In India, before the Second World War malaria was considered the single most important health problem facing the country, affecting all aspects of life, threatening economic wellbeing, engendering poverty, reducing the birth rate and deeply harming pregnant women. 'The problem of existence in very many parts of India is the problem of malaria', wrote one malariologist:

'There no aspect of life in this country which is not affected, either directly or indirectly, by this disease.'[13]

Even in the United States, where malaria had begun a downward trend in the late nineteenth century, but persisted as a problem until the late 1930s in the southern, impoverished states, it continued to pose a serious economic burden; in 1909, its costs to the nation were estimated at $100 million a year, a figure that had risen to $500 million annually by 1938.[14]

Controlling Malaria Before the Second World War: Controversies

Malaria control before the Second World War tested doctors and public health officials. In fact, so complex is malaria that many experts had begun to think of it not as one disease, 'mal-aria', but as many different diseases, shaped in different ways in different spaces and populations, and posing different challenges to its control in different localities.

Efforts to control malaria were rarely systematic, and rarely tackled the rural areas where malaria was endemic. In most places, malaria was instead viewed as something people simply had to learn to live with – as an inevitable and chronic feature of everyday life. 'For the most part', said Pampana and Russell, 'malaria has quietly but consistently lowered the vitality of a community without causing sufficient alarm to stimulate effective control'.[15] Only in enclaves of economic or political importance, such as the Panama Canal Zone, mining and railway camps, or in colonial agricultural enterprises, were deliberate schemes put in place to control malaria.

The discovery in 1898 of the role that anopheline mosquitoes played in transmitting malaria, and the identification of the plasmodium as the pathogen, opened up the possibility of new methods of control, but also led to years of controversy. The control methods targeted either the mosquitoes, or the human host, or both. The first relied on a number of engineering, naturalistic or chemical methods to alter the environment in which mosquitoes live, so as to reduce their numbers; the second relied on drugs to suppress the worst symptoms of malarial infection in human beings.

Malaria had long been associated with swampy marshes (hence its name 'paludism', from the Latin for swamp, or 'mal-aria', Italian for the bad air given off by marshy and wet terrain), and this association led to environmental management. In ancient Rome, there were many efforts to drain the Pontine marshes in order to improve the area's healthiness and allow agricultural colonists to occupy otherwise disease-ridden territory; these efforts were largely unsuccessful until Mussolini made anti-malarial work a key feature of his fascist state in the 1920s and '30s.[16] In the twentieth century, environmental engineering was used to reduce malaria in the Panama Canal Zone, and also in mainland USA (for example, by the Tennessee Valley Authority).[17] But environmental engineering was expensive; the British colonies in Africa, for example, rarely found money to put to such work.

The British physician Sir Malcolm Watson, working in the Federated Malay States, developed a more ecologically precise method of manipulating environments in rubber and tea plantations in order to reduce the habitats in which specific mosquitoes thrived.[18] The malaria expert N. R. Swellengrebel introduced the method into the Dutch East Indies (today Indonesia) after learning about it from Watson, modifying it and naming it 'species sanitation'.[19] The method required a detailed knowledge of the ecology of the local mosquito vectors – one reason, probably, why the technique was not more widely taken up.

A more direct but environmentally brutal way to reduce mosquitoes or their larvae was to kill them chemically. The twentieth century was a century of chemicals, and petroleum, kerosene, and from the early 1920s on, the chemical Paris Green, were variously mixed and then dumped or sprayed on the breeding sites of mosquito larvae.

Chemicals could also be used to spray or douse adult mosquitoes in people's homes. Malaria had long been characterized as primarily a domiciliary disease, meaning that infection was the result of mosquito bites that occurred largely in people's houses, making the home an important site for control efforts.[20] After flying into a house to bite a human being for the blood meal the female mosquitoes require for reproduction, the mosquitoes usually rest on a wall or other surface for some time, and this provides the opportunity to kill them (and therefore the parasites they carry) with chemical insecticides of various kinds. In Brazil, the chemical fumigation used in houses during the 1903–6 campaign against yellow fever mosquitoes in the capital of Rio de Janeiro incidentally killed malaria mosquitoes at the same time, with the result that malaria incidence fell also.

House fumigation, though, was cumbersome and time-consuming, not very effective, and fell out of favour. Park Ross in South Africa introduced a more economic version of house spraying in the 1930s using pyrethrum, a powdered extract of the chrysanthemum flower that acted as an insecticide.[21] Soper happened to be attending a Pan African Health Conference in Johannesburg in 1935, where he heard Park Ross report on his success in spraying African huts against the deadly malaria vector, *Anopheles gambiae.* Soper was at first quite sceptical, since he remembered the failure of Gorgas to control yellow fever in Panama by house fumigation in 1904–5, as well as the failure of the Brazilians with pyrethrum sprays in Rio de Janeiro during the yellow fever epidemic of 1928–9. Park Ross therefore invited Soper to visit Zululand

and see the results for himself. The five-day, on-site visit led by Park Ross convinced Soper of its importance; in Zululand, the gambiae mosquitoes were highly domiciliary in habit, which made them susceptible to direct attack within the huts.[22] From the mid-1930s on, pyrethrum spraying in houses became an important addition to the anti-malarial chemical arsenal, at least until DDT entered the picture – the latter has a long-lasting effect that pyrethrum does not, so pyrethrum needs to be sprayed much more frequently.[23]

The other approach to malaria was to concentrate on the human host and treat the symptoms of the infection. Until the 1930s, the drug available was quinine.[24] The identification in 1817 of the alkaloid responsible for quinine's fever-quelling effects had made possible the production of quinine in commercial quantities; but variations in quinine's potency, its bitter taste and its strong side effects in the quantities sometimes required to treat malarial fevers, meant that it was not popular. In the early 1900s, when Italy instituted a progressive system of free quinine distribution, funding it through a tax levied on landowners, it was found that most of the quinine was simply not consumed.[25] Even in wartime conditions, officers and soldiers often avoided taking it. Because of such resistance, a quinine regime was sometimes imposed on populations forcibly, as when, for example, quinine ingestion was made a daily requirement in labour camps as one of the terms of employment.[26] But many malaria specialists had reservations about relying on quinine, since although the drug suppressed the disease's worst clinical symptoms, it did not destroy the parasites in the person's blood, and so did not interrupt malaria transmission.

A House Divided: Malaria and Complexity Before the Second World War

Somewhat paradoxically, as doctors gathered more and more knowledge about malaria in the 1920s and '30s, the issue of how to control it became more contentious, not less. In 1934, the Rockefeller malaria expert, Dr Lewis W. Hackett, described the world of malaria experts as a 'house divided'.[27] On one side were those who believed in the efficacy of mosquito reduction, even mosquito eradication, while on the other were those who thought of malaria in socio-economic terms, focusing on malaria as a human disease that occurred largely as a result of rural poverty, and aiming to control it by improving general standards of living, and by treating malaria cases by the regular use of quinine.[28] In rough terms, the Americans belonged to the first side, and the Italians to the second. As a Rockefeller expert, Hackett was firmly in the 'mosquito' camp; like Ronald Ross, he thought the role of the mosquito in transmission was a major discovery that was bound to affect how to control the disease. The Italians were less sure. They pointed to the lack of a clear relationship between the quantity of anopheline mosquitoes in any one place and the intensity of malaria, and to the failure to get rid of malaria by getting rid of mosquitoes.

In this latter regard, a major reference point was Mian Mir, a military cantonment near Lahore in India (now part of Pakistan), where between 1902 and 1909 the British authorities had conducted an experiment to test Ronald Ross's mosquito-reduction methods of malaria control. Obstacles had beset the effort from the start; drainage was more difficult to do than expected, and many irrigation canals were not touched because of the fear of causing any reduction in agricultural production; the mosquitoes also flew much further than expected, and so the irrigation canals provided a perfect breeding ground for further mosquito breeding; the operations against the mosquitoes were often interrupted, and not sufficiently systematic; and there was not enough money. Eventually, the project was abandoned.[29] Despite achieving considerable reduction in anopheles larvae, malaria incidence among the soldiers was hardly reduced at all. The results, in short, were simply not persuasive. Ross was furious, as usual, at what he saw as a deliberately half-hearted effort aimed at sabotaging his ideas. It was an important setback to anti-mosquito work; Sir Malcolm Watson, who was using mosquito control methods successfully at about the same time, said the lessons of Mian Mir 'had stopped practical anti-malaria work in many countries for a whole generation'.[30] Efforts at mosquito-reduction along the same lines in Puerto Rico and the Philippines were also less than satisfactory.

Even the introduction after 1921 of Paris Green as an effective anti-larval chemical did not allay the doubts many malaria specialists had about the connection between mosquitoes and malaria. The 'Italian school' of malaria experts continued to base their anti-malaria policies on draining swampy and unused lands, aiming to make them fit for settlement and agricultural development, rather than eliminating specific malaria-transmitting mosquitoes. The goal was to try to overcome the rural poverty, economic inequality, and lack of land and resources among agricultural labourers that they believed were the crux of malaria infection.

These differences of opinion about how to achieve malaria control were highlighted by the appearance in the 1920s of a series of reports produced by the Malaria Committee of the League of Nations. The majority of its members were generally sceptical that attacking mosquito larvae reduced malaria. Most controversially, in 1927 delegates from the Committee who were sent to look at the malaria situation in the United States took the 'Italian' view, reporting that malaria was slowly disappearing in the USA not because of deliberate public health policies or engineering works targeting the mosquito, but because of steady social and economic improvement: 'The history of special antimalaria campaigns', the report stated, 'is chiefly a record of exaggerated expectations followed sooner or later by disappointment and abandonment of the work'.[31] George K. Strode, head of the Regional Office of the IHD in Paris, writing to Frederick Russell, who directed the IHD, said he was very surprised to see the League of Nation's Health Committee say that anti-larval measures had a very secondary place in malaria work; in Brazil, where Strode had been posted previously, they had first place, and Strode maintained that the outstanding malaria experts of the day were not in accord with the League's ideas.[32]

Lewis Hackett, who had been sent to Rome by the RF in 1924 to study anopheline mosquitoes and devise methods which communities might use to control malaria, had also become thoroughly convinced that malaria mosquitoes and their larvae were very significant factors in the transmission and control of malaria. He challenged the conclusions of the Malaria Commission (of which he was a corresponding member), retorting that, on the contrary, 'only in a restricted sense . . . can malaria be considered a social disease'. Labelling it as such, Hackett said, 'has, it seems to me, been the refuge of those who have come to despair of direct action [meaning action on mosquitoes]'. He summed up: 'Malaria is an independent factor . . . the doctrine that social and economic uplift will ever obviate the necessity for laborious anti-larval campaigns and the meticulous mosquito-proofing of houses does not seem to us well-founded, either scientifically or in ordinary experience.'[33] The Dutch malaria expert, Swellengrebel, commenting on the socio-economic thesis of malaria, commented ironically: 'It is of little use to say to a country like Albania, for instance "Go and get rich".'[34]

These divisions between the schools of malaria control should not be over-stated. Several European experts gave due weight to the independent role of mosquito vectors, while members of the mosquito school also took into consideration the close inter-connections between climate, famine, general impoverishment and malaria. Though the RF experts did generally prefer anti-mosquito techniques, carrying out detailed entomological and epidemiological researches, and experimenting with new anti-larval chemicals, many of them were aware of the complexity of the factors involved in the secular decline in malaria that had occurred in many countries. They knew that in the United States, overall malaria, including the most severe falciparum malaria found in the southern states of the country, had begun to diminish by the late nineteenth century without coordinated anti-malaria policies, let alone anti-mosquito policies. This decline continued through the first half of the twentieth century, punctuated by rises, for example in the 1930s (the decade of the Great Depression); but between 1938 and 1942, malaria almost disappeared from the country.[35]

In reflecting immediately after the war on the causes of this decline in the US, Dr Marshall A. Barber concluded that most of the decline had occurred before anything was known about how malaria was transmitted. The use of screens in houses increased in the 1870s and '80s, but in Europe malaria also declined, and screens were not used, nor bed nets. Quinine was another significant factor, but Barber also mentioned increased prosperity, and perhaps increased drainage of malarial land, which reduced mosquito populations. He acknowledged that drainage improvements varied greatly from locality to locality, and that it was hard to assess their effects. In some places, agriculture reduced malaria, in others it increased anopheline breeding, depending on the species involved and their ecology; on the other hand, in some places where anophelines were abundant, the area was nonetheless not very malarious. On the whole, he concluded, social betterment or increased prosperity was itself anti-malarial. In the United States, 'an almost universal improvement in the way of life of the people brought with it more screens, more quinine, and more doctors prescribing quinine'. Better food and housing which followed the development of land helped people to resist all manner of disease.

In short, despite Barber's involvement with an anti-larval approach to malaria control (it was Barber who discovered that Paris Green was an effective mosquito larvicide in 1921, from which date it became the key chemical in RF anti-mosquito work), he tied malaria's virtual disappearance to numerous inter-acting social, economic, agricultural, technical and medical factors, in addition to anti-mosquito measures.[36] Writing in 1946, as the return of troops to the United States at the end of the war raised fears of the return of malaria, Barber saw no reason to 'de-anophelize' any country-wide area of the US (though the US pressed ahead, using DDT to eliminate mosquitoes).

In 1937, Lewis Hackett's book, *Malaria in Europe: An Ecological Study* appeared; this introduced an ecological perspective into the debate that Hackett hoped might bring a new consensus on malaria control. The new view was based on the fairly recent discovery that only certain variants, or races, within a particular species of malaria mosquitoes were actually successful vectors of the disease. This discovery, that some mosquitoes are in fact 'species complexes', solved the longstanding problem known as 'anophelism without malaria', that is, the problem of the prevalence in many areas of Italy of apparently malaria-transmitting mosquitoes, but no malaria. It was this problem that gave weight, Hackett thought, to the belief among many Italian malariologists that getting rid of mosquitoes was not the answer to malaria, whose origins, as we have seen, they attributed to poverty and socio-economic deprivation. But in the

1920s, malaria research showed that the main anopheline vector found in Italy, *Anopheles maculipennis,* was in fact divided into six different variants, not all of which transmitted malaria to humans (it was later discovered that *A. gambiae* is also a species complex). This explained why some regions of the country had lots of the vector but no malaria, while in others there was a connection, because of the prevalence of the transmitting strains.[37] To Hackett, knowing the malaria mosquitoes and their ecology was all-important to success in controlling malaria; the differences in vector species, their habits and their ecological niches meant that what might work in one area of the world would not necessarily work elsewhere. 'Everything about malaria is so moulded and altered by local conditions that it becomes a thousand different diseases and epidemiological puzzles', he commented.[38]

This growing appreciation of the ecology of disease also characterized the work of colonial scientists studying diseases other than malaria in the inter-war years, notably those involved with controlling epidemics of African trypanosomiasis (sleeping sickness).[39] Many of the researchers drew the conclusion that trypanosomiasis was too complex in its ecological determinants to be eradicated. Hackett was more eradication-minded, but his focus was on the insect vectors, not the disease.[40]

By the late 1930s, then, there was not yet a consensus about malaria control, only a consensus around malaria's complexity. It was both a socio-economic disease and a biological one, a widespread infection yet also local in its manifestation. The purely social approach of the Italians was beginning to lose its appeal, as it became part of Mussolini's fascist policies. Moreover, the Italian model could be misleading when followed in different geographical locations. In Argentina, for example, where strong ties to Italy existed because of the huge presence in the country of Italian immigrants, malaria control in the northwest of the country where malaria was a serious problem focused largely on drainage of wetlands, along the Italian lines; years passed before research showed that the main vector of malaria in the area was not a swamp breeder; malaria control was then re-directed to target the correct anopheline species, using an ecological model, separating the effort from the more ambitious and nationalistic agendas of social and economic uplift.[41]

Meanwhile, within Italy itself, several Italian malaria experts, such as Dr Alberto Missiroli, who had collaborated with Hackett on studies of mosquito control in the 1920s in Rome, and who after the war would lead the Italian malaria eradication campaign based on DDT, were also adopting the anti-mosquito approach. Mosquitoes, as Hackett had said, were important, as only some transmitted malaria, and only some strains in species, and understanding their habitats and habits was often crucial to successful control. But Hackett, always judicious in his views, realized that social and economic conditions also affected malaria. Human activities had to be recognized as factors, whether digging irrigation canals that increased mosquito breeding, clearing land, or introducing certain crops, all of which could alter a particular landscape, and with it the ecological niches affecting the breeding of mosquitoes, and thereby the incidence of malaria. The social and economic quality of life in populations also affected malaria, for instance in providing or not providing the conditions, and the means, for people to have adequate food, to live in houses that had windows and/or doors that could be screened, or to have access to quinine and other health services.

Snowden's compelling historical evaluation of the Italian approach to malaria likewise shows that the 'integral bonification' programme (meaning integrated agricultural improvement), which started in the first years of the twentieth century and became a centre-piece of Mussolini's fascist rule in the 1930s, was of fundamental importance to the decline of malaria between 1900 and the Second World War, and combined many approaches. Improvement involved land drainage, the settlement of reclaimed land by agricultural colonists, improved farming techniques and food production, the screening of houses, and the provision of rural health care services. The success of DDT in rapidly reducing malaria epidemics in Italy in the last years of the Second World War was significant, but Snowden argues that it needs to be put in the context of the relatively low overall levels of malaria already achieved in Italy by the war's outbreak. When DDT was first introduced in 1943, it was combined with other methods, such as the use of quinine, ditch clearing, the repair of drainage pumps and the pre-war infrastructure of health stations, as well as a massive distribution of food to the starving population. Snowden's history of malaria in Italy therefore indicates that a multi-factorial approach was responsible for the decline and in some places, disappearance, of malaria in Italy in the pre- and post-Second World War decades.

Probably this combined and nuanced view is close to how the majority of malariologists think today about malaria and its control. But before such a synthesis of ideas could be made, DDT was discovered, along with the anti-malarial drug, chloroquine. DDT shifted the argument decisively in favour of attacking mosquitoes, ignoring or bypassing the social context. A DDT-based programme would be a universal technique, to be applied everywhere, thus ignoring Hackett's idea of localism, and ignoring too the Italian school's idea of bonification and the need to improve social and economic conditions. The ecological knowledge was overlooked and the complexities forgotten in the rush to apply DDT. As Litsios remarks, this was 'a grave, but understandable mistake, in light of the circumstances that prevailed at the time'.[42]

What were those circumstances? One was the impact malaria had had on the war effort, on both the Allied and Axis side; in the Mediterranean, Pacific and Far Eastern theatres, at all times large numbers of soldiers were unfit to fight because of malaria. In this wartime context, the arrival of the super-insecticide DDT was seen as a godsend, and quickly put to use, without much respect, as we have seen, for worries about its potential dangers to human beings or to animals other than insects.

At the war's end, as the US troops returned home from overseas, and threatened to bring malaria back with them, the US Congress voted to fund an all-out malaria eradication campaign in the country based almost entirely on the application of DDT. The insecticide was represented to the public as the 'atom-bomb of the insect world' (the report published by the Malaria Control in War Areas agency, the forerunner of today's Center for Disease Control, even pictured the mushroom cloud on its cover).[43] The insecticide rapidly went into production. In 1944, the United States produced 4.2 million kg (9½ million lb); by 1947 the figure was more than 21 million kg (47 million lb) and by 1957, 71 million kg (157 million lb). The insecticide was cheap to make, long-lasting, and did not have to hit mosquitoes directly to kill them, owing to the residual properties of the chemical.[44] There was, says Humphries, a strong public demand for DDT, because it killed all sorts of bothersome insects; only 2 per cent of the households refused DDT spraying in the first year. By the late 1940s, more than a million houses were being sprayed annually. Even at the time, some malaria experts were uncertain about what DDT had really done; malaria was after all, already rare. The best that might be said of DDT was that, in the US at least, it 'kicked a dying dog'.[45] Most malariologists, nonetheless, remained very impressed by the potential of the new insecticide.

Another, very different, factor influencing the post-war malaria eradication debate centred on third world development, and especially food production. Malaria was a serious barrier to agricultural production in developing countries, where poverty was most severe and malaria incidence the highest. DDT recommended itself because it was apparently simple to apply, and DDT-spraying could be organized as a separate, expert service that did not have to depend on, or wait for, the setting up of basic rural health services (which in many countries barely existed). If anything, it was hoped that a malaria service would lay down the organizational seeds of such basic services. In addition, a simple equation was drawn between malaria reduction and economic growth; the expectation was that malaria could be eliminated without waiting for complicated reforms, such as land redistribution, which the WHO itself could not carry out, and which many countries, colonial and post-colonial, were unwilling or unable to carry out either.

Finally, framing the entire malaria eradication story was the Cold War. Of greatest importance here was the strong support the US gave to the UN system, politically and financially; its adoption of malaria eradication as a route to 'development'; and its use of public health to promote its 'way' over that of the USSR. The argument was that 'malaria blocks development'.[46] The malaria expert, Paul F. Russell, who in the 1930s had tested the effectiveness of various insecticides on malaria in Italy, reflected this outlook when he commented that the continued presence of malaria 'helps to predispose a community to infection with political germs that can delay and destroy freedom'.[47] Getting rid of malaria was, in this calculation, anti-communist. The departure of the communist countries of Eastern Europe from the WHO, starting with the Soviet Union in 1949, placed the United States in a dominant position to set the international health agenda for several years. The US had a historic bias in favour of technical fixes of social issues, the massive use of DDT being a perfect example.[48]

But though DDT changed a great deal in the malaria world, the actual decision to use the chemical as the key tool in a huge and expensive programme that was to include even the most malarious and poor regions of the world was not made overnight; in fact, ten years passed between the end of the war in 1945 and WHO's adoption of its hugely ambitious programme of malaria eradication.

To understand how the decision was actually made, we need first to look at the role of a core group of experts who formed what Haas has called an 'epistemic community', meaning by this a community of people who shared a cognitive framework and a determination to act on their beliefs. Members of the malaria epistemic community included: Fred L. Soper; Arnaldo Gabaldón, who headed the malaria eradication programme in Venezuela, the first to be organized on a national scale; Dr George Macdonald, a British malaria expert who developed a mathematical model of the spread of malaria infection that gave apparent precision and weight to the aims of eradication; Dr Emilio Pampana, an Italian malaria expert who became the first director of WHO's malaria unit; and Paul F. Russell, the well-known Rockefeller malariologist.[49] Several other prominent malariologists gave their support (for example, Sir Malcolm Watson and Leonard J. Bruce-Chwatt, both from Britain).

Soper was, of course, an arch-eradicationist when DDT came into the picture, and he found it easy to incorporate the new chemical into his outlook, considering it simply a very superior way to eliminate insect vectors. The point to him, initially, was the eradication of an entire insect species. This reflected his primary experience in public health, and to the end of his life he persisted in thinking that eradicating insects was a very useful thing, an original contribution.

When Soper attended the first international Congress of Malaria to be held since before the war, in 1948, he found himself being treated as something of a hero for his success in ridding Brazil and Egypt of the *gambiae* mosquito (though also gently teased for threatening to eradicate malariologists along with malaria).[50] What Soper did not acknowledge at the meeting, however, was that evidence was already accumulating in Sardinia that the complete elimination of an insect species was very costly, was very rarely feasible, and anyway simply not necessary in order to reach the public health goal desired. Instead, the mass application of DDT showed that by reducing the numbers of transmitting mosquitoes severely, the transmission of malaria would be so reduced that the parasites would disappear in human populations. The principle depended on the mosquito and parasite biology; after feeding by biting a human being, it takes ten to twelve days for the parasite ingested by the mosquito with human blood (which the female mosquito needs for reproduction) to develop inside the mosquito to the stage of infectivity to humans. Killing mosquitoes, which need to bite every two to three days, would therefore kill the possibility of the transmission of the parasite. Thus with eradication, transmission of malaria would be ended, but the presence of mosquitoes would not. The result would be 'anopheles without malaria' – the situation many places find themselves in today. It was a shift back to the old dream – eradicating a human disease.

An Experiment that Failed

But Soper's mind was fixed on eradicating insects, not parasites; at the war's end, while still stationed in Italy, he managed to persuade the Rockefeller Foundation, with the help of the United Nations Relief and Rehabilitation Administration (UNRRA) and the Italian government, to fund and carry out a very expensive test of his DDT-eradication theory on the island of Sardinia.[51] Sardinia was chosen because of the severity of its malaria situation, and because the main vector, *Anopheles lambranchiae*, was native to the island; one of the criticisms of Soper's previous work on mosquito eradication was that he had only succeeded in wiping out (and only in a region) a vector in Brazil and in Egypt that was an invader species and therefore un-adapted to the ecological landscapes of the countries concerned. Eradicating completely an indigenous mosquito species that was long-established in its native ecological landscape would, it was argued, be an important test of Soper's theory and of the efficacy of DDT.

Soper was confident, as always. Flying over the mountains and valleys of Sardinia, he saw no reason to change his mind about applying DDT in large quantities in houses and on the land, despite the geographical, epidemiological and other challenges the project faced, and the doubt expressed about the enterprise even by the very person Soper himself had selected to supervise the experiment, J. Austin Kerr. When asked why he had nevertheless recommended Kerr for the job in Sardinia, Soper replied he knew from working with him that Kerr had the administrative ability to do it, but that nevertheless he had warned George Strode, the director of the RF's International Health Division at the time, that Kerr 'was thinking of Sardinia as an opportunity to prove that eradication was unnecessary'.[52]

Kerr was right. It was unnecessary, as experience showed. Between 1946 and 1950, a truly massive assault using DDT was carried out on the vector.[53] The operation involved house-by-house spraying, as well as spraying from the air. Soper brushed aside suggestions for more ecological and epidemiological research to precede the assault; he thought it unnecessary.[54] Writing again to George Strode, in 1946, at the start of the Sardinia experiment, Soper said 'I do not believe the RF should undertake any long term detailed entomological or malaria studies there at this time', unless the DDT spraying failed to reduce the main malaria vector on the island (the *A. lambranciae*) densities, which, Soper added, with typical certainty, 'will be contrary to all previous experience'.[55]

But after five years of intense effort, involving the employment of thousands of workers and the application of thousands of tons of DDT, in a military-style operation, the *labranchiae* mosquito was still there, if in greatly reduced numbers. Malaria itself, however, had virtually disappeared *and did not reappear when DDT spraying was stopped.* This would seem to be a highly positive outcome; but given the experiment's original goals, it had to be counted a useful failure. Turning this around, the best that could be said was that it proved that eradicating a well-established mosquito species was impossible, at least via DDT, and was anyway simply not essential to malaria elimination.

From Soper's viewpoint, this was a hard lesson to learn – one reason no doubt why he barely acknowledged it as such.[56] In fact, he continued to refer to the eradication of the main vector in Sardinia as though it were a *fait accompli* – a rare lapse in a man otherwise given to accuracy.[57] Soper's work as director of PAHO kept him extremely involved in the malaria eradication effort, as his diary entries make clear (though it is interesting that he made no mention of the MEP in his published memoirs). He remained an enthusiastic eradicator, extending the idea to many non-vector diseases, and sticking with his absolutist notions. With malaria, he adapted his ideas to take on what would emerge as the new consensus, namely the need to use DDT not to eliminate mosquitoes altogether, but instead to diminish their presence sufficiently to interrupt the transmission of the disease and thus eliminate the parasite from the human blood stream.

As always in discussing eradication, Soper was blind to the many other factors, such as the improved nutrition and salaries that came, for example, with the Sardinia project and contributed their share to the dramatic reductions achieved in malaria on the island.[58] To him, DDT was everything, and allowed him to champion eradication's cause at PAHO and elsewhere, becoming indeed the most important spokesman for the eradication concept after the Second World War. 'Eradication of communicable diseases is a logical objective of modern public health practice . . . Once the eradication concept becomes firmly established, the public health attitude toward communicable diseases should become parallel to that of the fireman, who does not look at fire as something which must be reduced to a low level but kept burning just a little. Once the knowledge of how to prevent a given disease is available, the heath conscience of the world should no longer allow that disease to continue as a regrettable but inevitable affliction of mankind.'[59]

Soper would brook no doubt, no questions; DDT *would* work. 'How do these people manage to keep so backward in these modern times?', he wrote in his diary, after meeting some people who questioned the possibility of eliminating malaria.[60] His method was one of 'bulldog tenacity', says Wilbur G. Downs, a Rockefeller Foundation employee who describes how, in the 1950s, when Downs had already been working on malaria control in Mexico for several years, Soper came to the country to persuade the Mexican government to get on board with the idea of malaria eradication based on DDT. Soper summoned Downs to a meeting, where Downs had the temerity to speak up and tell Soper there were in fact many obstacles to eradication using DDT; one was the finding that DDT decomposed on the clay walls with which many Mexican houses were constructed, rendering DDT ineffective. On hearing this, Soper put his hands around Downs's neck, shook him vigorously and told him to shut up, since such talk impeded the commitment to malaria eradication.[61]

Other members of the malaria epistemic community also moved towards eradication.[62] By 1955, any hesitation had gone. In his new book, the malariologist Paul F. Russell proclaimed the new outlook in the title: *Man's Mastery of Malaria.* Declaring that 'this is the DDT era of malariology', Russell announced that 'For the first time it is economically feasible for nations, *however underdeveloped and whatever the climate*, to banish malaria completely from their borders'.[63]

This endorsement by expert opinion reflected experience with DDT already acquired in the field. DDT was made available for civilian use as early as 1944 in some places, and was rapidly taken up for anti-malaria work. By 1949, thirteen countries were involved in WHO-aided DDT pilot projects; by 1953 the number had grown to 29. In Italy, a five-year malaria eradication programme based on DDT was announced in 1946, and soon malaria appeared to be on its way out, presumably to disappear forever. In 1953, only twelve indigenous cases of malaria were registered in Italy, 'an amazing contrast to the 303,057 cases reported in 1919 and the 411,602 cases reported in 1947'.[64] Another test case was Venezuela, which initiated a nationwide effort in 1946. 'No other scheme up to that time had announced as its goal "total malaria elimination" by the new method', said Russell.[65] Venezuela was especially important because it was a tropical country – eradicating malaria in a tropical climate was believed to be a much greater challenge than in a temperate one. In this regard, Russell also mentioned Brazil's National Malaria Service, which was already engaged in 'one of the greatest DDT residual spraying project in the world', with some three million houses being sprayed annually.[66]

To take a last example of a country that helped move the debate from control to outright eradication, there was India. Within a year of independence in 1947, the Indian government had requested assistance from WHO and UNICEF in starting DDT malaria projects in four very endemic states, with very satisfactory results, some areas requiring only one spraying a year. In 1954, the Director-General of Health Services in India informed the World Health Assembly that the government had already started a national campaign aimed at protecting 125 million people by 1955–1956 (out of an estimated 200 million people living in malarial areas). Two-thirds of the $30,500,000 to be spent was to come from the Indian government, with bilateral aid from the US, and the rest from the various states in India's federal system. The Minister associated increased food production in certain states with the dramatic reductions in malaria infections.[67]

So impressive did these early campaigns seem that, by 1963, in the new edition of his book, *Practical Malariology*, Paul Russell was ready to declare that the goal of eradication was already on its way to being met. 'Man has at last mastered malaria', he said, so that it 'was well into its way to oblivion'. In the very first chapter he dismissed Soper's idea of species eradication, calling it 'rarely practicable or necessary'; the goal was not mosquito eradication, but disease eradication. Soper left his mark, however, in the language of absolutism and perfection that now characterized the entire malaria project. 'Malaria eradication is . . . an absolute, the total ending of transmission', Russell declared. 'It has perfection as the only acceptable standard of work.'

Eradication, he maintained, was altogether more exacting than control, 'exacting in clarity and honesty of thought, exacting in integrity of effort by all staff, and exacting in material demands, which means that so long as it continues it must be more expensive than a well-managed control scheme'. But in good Soper fashion, he also argued that the up-front high costs of eradication would be balanced out by the fact that eradication was to be a time-limited effort, a finite project, so that once done the public health staff could be 'liberated to make other contributions to public health and well-being'.[68]

In the space of ten years or less, then, Russell and other experts had moved to embrace malaria eradication by the new technique of DDT spraying in houses, and set themselves the most stringent goals. In the belief that there was now available a new method that would work in many different places, Russell felt confident in asserting that the strategy of eradication 'has remained unchallenged, and is likely to remain unchallenged, in so far as the great majority of eradication programmes are concerned'.[69]

Africa, Acquired Immunity and Eradication

The deliberations of WHO's Expert Committee on Malaria, which had been set up in 1946, followed the same path towards the adoption of absolute malaria eradication – not surprisingly, perhaps, since the key members of malaria's epistemic community served on it.[70] From its start, the committee saw the malaria problem in new terms, owing to the new techniques made available during the war. At its third meeting, held in Geneva in August 1949, the committee announced that 'the ultimate aim of WHO should be to eliminate malaria as a public health problem from the world'. DDT was discussed at some length, especially its potential hazards to human beings; but the experts concluded it was essentially harmless. This was certainly a global view of the problem, but it fell short of an outright endorsement of worldwide eradication as such. The committee noted that the malaria budget of WHO had actually been reduced since 1948, amounting to just under $375,000 for the coming year. Worldwide eradication was obviously not possible on these kinds of sums.[71]

A moment of clarification about malaria eradication occurred at the very next meeting of the Expert Committee in Africa immediately after WHO's *Malaria Conference in Equatorial Africa* in Kampala, Uganda, in late November 1950. This conference was significant to the story of malaria eradication because it raised the question of whether all the regions of the world would indeed be included, as eradication implied. Would the large malarial, poor and above all tropical countries, be suitable for eradication?

In the case of India, as we have seen, the answer already appeared to be 'yes'. Africa was another matter. The sheer scale and intensity of malaria in the sub-Saharan countries; the wide distribution of the *Anopheles gambiae* mosquito, the most efficient or deadly of the malaria transmitting mosquito species; the poverty of so many countries and the absence of even the most rudimentary health services; all presented a challenge to malaria control of a kind not felt anywhere else.

More than this, at Kampala there was a quite vehement argument over whether eradication should even be attempted in Africa at all. Present at the Kampala meeting were some experienced colonial Africa hands who worried that, in getting rid of malaria, Africans would lose the immunity they acquired through repeated malaria infections; this immunity did not protect individuals from malaria completely, but as adults many Africans were known to carry large burdens of malaria parasites without apparently suffering the clinical symptoms of malaria. The colonial doctors feared that if, for any reason, an eradication programme faltered before it was completed, malaria might return with a vengeance, to infect African populations who would then find themselves without any acquired immunity, and therefore be intensely vulnerable to endemic or epidemic malaria, with horrendous costs in terms of sickness and death.

This was the position taken by the British doctors, Bagster D. Wilson and P.C.C. Garnham, who opposed the idea of trying to start eradicating malaria; they wanted instead to start with some small-scale, pilot projects, to proceed cautiously. Their views were challenged by, among others, Dr Paul F. Russell, as well as their fellow Briton, Dr George MacDonald, who wanted to extend malaria control to all sub-Saharan Africa.[72]

This debate about African immunity to malaria was not new; it dated back to at least the early 1930s. But the caution about how to deal with malaria in Africa that had seemed appropriate before the war now seemed less so to many malaria experts in the era of DDT, when it was expected that following complete eradication, malaria would never come back to threaten African populations in the manner feared.

Which side of the debate the malaria experts lined up on depended largely on how they evaluated the costs, rather than the benefits, of acquired immunity itself. Yes, immunity was a form of protection, especially in areas of intense malaria endemicity; on the other side of the equation, though, it was acknowledged that the immunity acquired was only partial, was often highly local (being lost when people moved to other areas), and was achieved at a high cost in terms of mortality and morbidity from malaria infections. At the Fourth International Malaria Congress held in Washington two years earlier, where acquired immunity in Africans had also been discussed, a Dr

Alvarado, attending from Argentina, begged the audience to 'please try DDT; try, and try, and we shall see what happens'.[73]

The North Americans attending the meetings in Kampala agreed with this sentiment; they were taken aback by the idea of apparently leaving African populations mired in malaria. It went against the grain of their 'can do' political philosophy and their faith in the efficacy of DDT. Opposing the cautious views of the colonial British doctors, Russell took the line that Africans were not naturally immune to the most dangerous kinds of malaria, and that the costs to Africans, especially African children, in the sickness and death that came with the repeated malaria infections that were necessary to establish immunity, were simply too high; he argued forcefully that WHO should be in the business of saving lives.[74] At this point in what Garnham called the 'furious debate', Dr Leonard J. Bruce-Chwatt, interjected his own view.[75] Bruce-Chwatt had good credentials to do so, having worked since the end of the war on malaria in Africa as a member of the Royal African Medical Service in Nigeria. Bruce-Chwatt had 'entomological leanings', as Garnham put it, and took (perhaps to Garnham's surprise) the opposite position to the other Africa hands. According to Garnham's account, Bruce-Chwatt ended the debate by 'folding his hands and quietly saying "Let us *spray*"'.[76]

Thus, in principle, Africa was to be included in the MEP. Vector eradication schemes in Africa were recommended, without waiting for further experiments or trials to see what might happen. But in practice sub-Saharan Africa was virtually left out, except for a few pilot projects. The intensity of malaria transmission, the fears about loss of immunity and above all the lack of almost any health infrastructure in many of the newly independent African countries meant that the attack phase of the MEP, which was meant to interrupt transmission, might be endless and require an efficiency in spraying beyond what science and political will could achieve. Moreover, DDT was found to repel rather than kill the *Anopheles gambiae* vector and so was not effective. The sixth meeting of the Expert Committee on Malaria, which laid out the basic principles on which eradication was to be conducted, said it seemed 'premature' to undertake continent-wide eradication in tropical Africa.

Instead, various tests and pilot schemes were carried out from 1954–9, all of which showed that though malaria could be reduced very considerably by residual insecticide spraying, it could not be eradicated.[77] It seemed impossible, given the conditions, to interrupt transmission – the whole purpose of eradication. In 1964, recognizing the problems African and other developing countries were facing, the Expert Committee on Malaria proposed that countries with very poor basic health services begin with a 'pre-eradication' phase designed to improve the infrastructure before the 'preparatory' phase began.[78]

But in 1969 the global programme in effect came to an end. As Listios says, 'the 1950 Kampala conference placed Africa in a "no-win" position; neither was malaria eradicated, nor an independent control strategy developed in light of the "different" malaria that was and still is present in Africa'.[79]

The consequence of Africa's virtual absence from the MEP was that, from the very start, malaria eradication was not in fact going to be worldwide – and thus was not in fact capable of achieving the worldwide, absolute disappearance the programme promised.[80]

DDT: Safety and Insect Resistance

In all the discussions and sometimes-heated debates, the crux of the matter was always DDT and its effectiveness in anchoring a massive programme of complete eradication. Was DDT in fact safe? To humans, to the sprayers or the sprayed? To animals other than the targeted mosquitoes? To food?

That the answer was basically 'yes' was the consistent conclusion drawn by the other expert committee of WHO to play an important role in the malaria eradication effort, the Expert Committee on Insecticides. Meeting regularly from 1949 on, the main purpose of this committee was to keep track of any evidence of DDT's negative effects.[81] At various times, the committee reviewed DDT's potential toxicity in foods, the dangers of accidental poisoning to DDT-handlers, the safest ways of spraying or applying DDT, and the appropriate dilutions to use. It invariably concluded that the benefits of using DDT for public health purposes far out-weighed its risks.

The greatest worry the committee had was about the growing evidence of insect resistance to DDT. As early as 1942, two species of insects were reported to show resistance; by 1962 the number of species had reached 81, some of them the anopheles mosquitoes that DDT was supposed to eradicate.[82] The experts began to realize that there might be only a small window of opportunity for eradication to succeed – long enough for DDT spraying to interrupt malaria transmission, and yet not so long as to allow insects to acquire resistance. The recognition of the growing problem of insect resistance to DDT was an important factor in leading the Eighth World Assembly to decide on an all-out effort to get rid of malaria, before it was too late.[83]

It is striking that the potentially harmful effects of DDT on the overall environment were simply not high up on the Expert Committee on Insecticide's agenda. In 1961, for instance, just one year before Rachel Carson's book, *Silent Spring*, appeared and started the environmentalist debate about the long-term, residual effects of organic pesticides on wildlife, the committee instead stressed the *value* of insecticides to agriculture in getting rid of insect pests, citing the potential reduction in yields in citrus fruits and cotton if DDT use were to be curtailed.[84] In its 1967 report, it praised DDT's record in public health as outstanding.

The Problem of Incomplete Knowledge

It was against this backdrop of enthusiasm among the world's leading malaria experts that the worldwide malaria eradication campaign was launched in 1955. By 1961, some 66 countries were involved in malaria eradication programmes, involving more than 200,000 sprayers and targeting over 600 million homes. So dramatic were the early results that WHO estimated that, of 147 countries and territories that had initially been malarial, 45 had by this date completely or partially eradicated the disease. WHO was therefore confident that its goals would ultimately be met.[85]

But this confidence, as we know now, was misplaced. The reductions were not sustained; in some places where the decline in malaria incidence and mortality had been most dramatic, malaria began to return, sometimes in epidemic form. Why? What explains the failure of malaria eradication?

Though many reasons have been put forward, it is apparent in retrospect that a considerable part of the blame lies in that mixture of incomplete knowledge and absolutist ideals that had characterized all the previous eradication schemes. Put another way, we might say the failure lay in the gap between principle and practice – between the principle that the world could be thought of as a single geographic space, in which a single, universal method would work, and the practical reality of an untidy world, made up of many different spaces, with different political, economic and biological characteristics, and different requirements in public health strategies.

This gap is perhaps most evident when we compare the plan for malaria eradication drawn up by WHO's experts with the actual experiences in individual countries. Even in the most successful of national campaigns, the plan could not be made to map properly the circumstances in the field. On the one hand, we have a categorical, disarmingly simple, scientifically confident, scheme of action. On the other hand, we have tales of DDT supplies running out, trucks failing to be delivered, officials not showing up where they should, money not arriving, mosquitoes not behaving as expected, agricultural schemes altering the environment, people refusing to cooperate and politicians losing their will. Given the challenges, and the scale of the operations, it was remarkable that as much was achieved as it was.

The Expert Committee first drew up the plan in question on malaria at its sixth meeting in Geneva in 1956; the World Health Assembly having endorsed worldwide malaria eradication, a need was felt for overall guidance by the WHO.[86] The chief principles embodied in the plan were those of simultaneity, time-bounded-ness and urgency; simultaneity, because eradication had to be achieved everywhere at the same time, if the end result was to be absolute; time-boundedness, because after a few years of DDT spraying it was expected transmission would end, after which no further spraying would be needed; and urgency, because the growing threat of mosquito resistance to the residual insecticides meant there was only a small window of opportunity in which DDT could act. The plan defined malaria eradication as 'the ending of the transmission of malaria and the elimination of the reservoir of infective cases in a campaign limited in time and carried to such a degree of perfection that when it comes to an end, there is no resumption of transmission'.

These principles were laid out in a scheme of four distinct phases. First was to be a *preparatory* phase, involving an initial survey of malaria in the country, planning, recruitment and training of staff, a delimitation of the zones and districts, preparation of timetables and itineraries, and the operation of a pilot project. This phase was to last a few months, but not more than one year. Second would be the *attack* phase; this was the heart of the campaign and concerned the general insecticidal spraying of all houses in malarial areas until the discontinuation of transmission; generally speaking, this phase was to last three years, but it could well take longer, and involve a total of four or more years work. The third, *consolidation* phase, would mark the period from the discontinuation of all spraying to the declaration of eradication; in this phase, blood tests would be made to detect any remaining parasite infections, and steps would be taken to treat the last of the malaria cases with chloroquine or other drugs, in order to ensure that any remaining mosquitoes would not get re-infected with the malaria parasite. Finally, there would come the *maintenance* phase, in which a system of close surveillance of the population would be put in place, so as to make sure there was no re-introduction of malaria infections from outside the eradicated zone. The campaign would only end when malaria was 'substantially eradicated from the world'.[87] The WHO expected this to happen in five to ten years. Confidence in this scheme was boosted by the record of malaria spraying with DDT in Greece; launched in 1946, routine spraying was discontinued by 1953, without increases in the vector or malaria. The result seemed to indicate that the whole programme could work even faster than originally thought.

Many countries found reasons to embrace WHO's plan. The promise of financial and technical aid was one (in addition to US funds, from 1955 to 1958 UNICEF contributed many millions of dollars through a number of its technical agencies). Overall, an estimated $1.4 billion was spent on malaria eradication between 1957 and 1967, and a further $1–2 billion between 1968 and 1976. But as Amrith notes in his excellent study of malaria eradication in India, the resources that flowed to countries were not large enough, in themselves, to explain the rapid uptake of the eradicationist agenda. It is estimated, in fact, that in India external aid accounted for only 14 per cent of total expenditures on all health programmes between 1950 and 1959, when the malaria eradication effort took off.[88]

To fully understand the engagement of many countries in the international eradication campaign in this Cold War moment, then, we need to look at some of the broader political and ideological correspondences that existed between international agendas and country-specific ones – the shared belief in progress, in techno-science and in the economic returns that would result from the removal of malaria. In the case of post-1947 India, for example, Amrith shows how WHO's narrative of a malaria-free world was absorbed into the Indian narrative of independence and post-colonial national development, the adoption of the MEP in the circumstances representing a 'de-colonization of international health'. This is a rather different account of malaria eradication than the usual one, in which malaria eradication is presented as an imperial project imposed on unwilling subjects.

But if such correspondences helped make the international 'domestic' and persuaded many countries to sign up to the campaign, the path from principle to practice was not at all easy; as Amrith says, though 'On paper technical assistance was a finely honed machine', in practice 'everything was much more messy'.[89] And messy in each country in its own way.

This fact about the MEP was disguised by the universal scientific and programmatic language of parasites, vectors and insecticides employed, language which did not take into account the extraordinary variety of circumstances – economic, financial, technical and socio-ecological – that made up what I earlier called the 'political geography' of malaria. The Geneva view of eradication over-rode the politics of health, assuming that every participating country had the same stake in malaria and its eradication, and would make malaria one of its highest, if not the very highest, priority, regardless of the country's epidemiological and health situation. But the reality was that the MEP was not a unitary project, but a project made up of multiple MEPs that were organized at the national level. And even in the best of circumstances, the directors of national MEPs found at times that they had to deviate from the programmatic rules put out by Geneva and the Expert Committee on Malaria, to adapt to unanticipated problems of a biological or social nature, and in some key instances, simply go their own way in order to achieve their purposes.

Venezuela and the Malaria Eradication Programme

This was certainly the experience in Venezuela. I highlight Venezuela here because in many respects its malaria eradication campaign was indeed conducted under some of the best of circumstances. The country was not vast, like India. Economically and socially, it was 'developing', yet also, in comparative terms within the developing world, not desperately poor, being second in Latin America only to Argentina in terms of *per capita* income in the 1950s (though this comparative wealth concealed great social inequalities). Its tropical conditions made it of special interest. The anti-malaria campaign was led by one of the best-known Latin American malariologists, Dr Arnoldo Gabaldón; it was backed by the national governments of the period; and it was carried out to a level of perfection in technical terms that could hardly be faulted.[90]

If eradication could not work in tropical Venezuela, how could it work in other tropical areas of the world less favoured than Venezuela in organizational efficiency, epidemiological resources and financing? The answer seemed to be – it could not. Malaria could be made to virtually disappear; to disappear as a significant public health problem; to be greatly reduced; even to be eradicated over significant areas of a country. But absolute eradication across the whole territory? It was probably an impossible – and unnecessary – ideal.

By the early 1960s, Gabaldón was ready to admit this. Eradication as WHO had defined it was not possible in his country.

This admission was all the more significant because Gabaldón had been one of the architects of malaria eradication, being a key member of the epistemic community of malaria experts who helped steer WHO towards the plan.[91] The reasons for the failure were additionally significant because they were not, as was claimed in many other countries, the result of problems in administration, in personnel, in the supplies of materials or even in basic health services, fragile and fragmented though the latter were. They related, rather, to the nature of malaria itself in its geographical, ecological and social character. Gabaldón understood this. Yet rather than give up on eradication entirely, he redefined his goals and settled for 'partial eradication' – eradication of malaria (not mosquitoes) over a part of Venezuela's territory. For the rest, vigilant control of malaria was essential. Gabaldón kept the DDT spraying going even when WHO recommended it be terminated once three years had passed without an indigenous case of malaria. He kept his malaria service intact, ignoring WHO's change of direction when in the 1970s its experts recommended merging such a specialized service with the general public health services in the region.

His revised methods, Gabaldón said, preserved the dramatically low rates of malaria his campaign *had* succeeded in obtaining, while in the other tropical countries where WHO's revised methods were followed, malaria nearly always returned. Gabaldón thus carved out what Listios calls his 'independent path' in malaria.[92]

Two features stand out in the case of malaria eradication in Venezuela: oil and pre-DDT malaria control efforts. The first gave resources and priority to malaria, among the country's many public health problems. The second provided a basic organizational structure of services upon which the post-war eradication campaign could quickly be erected.[93]

Oil defined modern Venezuela as it did no other Latin American country. By 1928, the country was producing about 100 million barrels of oil a year, making it the leading producer in the world at the time. Though oil prices did not begin their spectacular rise until OPEC was founded in 1960, oil nevertheless enriched the country's political elite, especially from the 1930s on. The country's fitful development from the mid-1930s on was corrupt, and immensely uneven and unequal, the roughly three and a half million people making up Venezuela's population being sharply divided by class and ethnicity. In 1949, Gabaldón reported a population of just under four million, with 20 per cent being white, 8 per cent black, and 65 per cent mixed Indian-mestizo. Politically, the situation was highly unstable, with brief periods of semi-democratic government being constantly terminated by military-led conspiracies and strongman rule. Generally speaking, however, historians define the middle decades of the twentieth century as a period of at least some economic improvement and social modernization, financed by petroleum and agricultural exports.[94]

One outcome of an oil-and-export agriculture economy was an increased concern about the high incidence of malaria in the country. By the middle of the twentieth century, it was estimated the country had a million cases a year in a population of less than four million, with many thousands of deaths. In fact, malaria was considered the leading cause of Venezuela's high overall death rates (estimated at 21.1/1,000 in 1949); in the *llanos*, the vast, interior highland grasslands that made up one of the major geographical regions of the country, the mortality rate was greater than the birth rate, with the result that many of the towns were depopulated. The burden of malaria led the government in 1936 to pass a 'Law of Defence Against Malaria'. A special national Malaria Division (department) was created shortly thereafter. Malaria was seen as a threat to economic development, to agricultural exports, and to foreign investment. By 1949, government expenditure on malaria of $0.84 *per capita* was one of the highest in all of Latin America, consuming 25 per cent of the total health budget.[95]

By this date, Gabaldón had been running the malaria control programme in Venezuela for over a decade, and was the leading malariologist in the country, and perhaps even in Latin America as a whole. Qualifying in medicine in 1930, Gabaldón had entered the malaria field when the debates about how to control the disease were intense. As was, I think, more typical than not in this period, his approach combined features of both the 'Italian' and the 'American' schools. Gabaldón associated malaria with economic poverty, social misery and bad housing, as the Italians did; but he also absorbed the new entomological knowledge about malaria that was developing in the period. In 1931, Gabaldón spent some months in Hamburg, stopping off in Italy on his way home, where he visited the Rockefeller-funded experimental malaria station in Rome. There he was introduced to the anti-larval techniques of malaria control promoted by Hackett and other RF field officers. His orientation towards the mosquito side of malaria control was reinforced by two years of further study on a RF fellowship between 1933 and 1935 at the Johns Hopkins School of Public Hygiene, in Baltimore, from where he received a doctorate in hygiene.

In 1936, Gabaldón returned to Venezuela to take up the post of Director of the new Division of Malariology. There he began to undertake research into malaria epidemiology and malaria vectors. Eventually, the Division moved from Caracas to Maracay (a military town southwest of Caracas which was to acquire fame later, when in 1992 Hugo Chavez launched his unsuccessful coup against the government from the town's army base). Continued close contacts between Gabaldón and the RF, which had become active in the country in the 1930s and had sent a number of researchers there to investigate anopheles species, helped Venezuela become a training centre for young doctors in the region.[96] Such contacts accelerated the process of the North Americanization of public health. These ties were strengthened further in 1941–2 when Venezuela experienced a severe outbreak of malaria, just as the US entered the Second World War. The US's Institute of Inter-American Affairs (IIAA) gave $1 million to Venezuela to combat the malaria epidemic, with a special focus on controlling malaria in the Amazonian rubber fields.[97]

Gabaldón became well known as a meticulous researcher who published widely in his lifetime. But though Gabaldón focused on mosquitoes, he did not lose his interest in the social origins of malaria –in what he called 'integral sanitation'; he thought that the malaria stations he set up in the 1930s and '40s should in principle provide other services as well, such as vaccinations, building latrines and health education. Some of this agenda was put into practice later, when as Minister of Health from 1959–65 under President Betancourt, Gabaldón expanded the Malaria Division to embrace environmental health and committed the service to constructing model sanitary housing to replace the unsanitary (and difficult to spray) rural shacks that made up so much of Venezuelans' homes.[98]

Gabaldón had the virtue of being an excellent leader and public health administrator – one cast in the Soper mould, being energetic, determined, highly disciplined, and ready to impose his discipline on all who worked for him. As the chief malaria expert in the country, he was in charge of a wide range of malaria activities, from conducting surveys of malaria incidence, setting up experimental malaria stations, carrying out entomological and epidemiological investigations and putting in place practical anti-malaria measures. Before the Second World War, all the techniques then available to reduce mosquitoes were tried, such as engineering works to drain malarial land, the use of Paris Green and other anti-larval chemicals, and from 1943 on, pyrethrum spraying in houses.[99]

Slowly, Gabaldon divided the country up into manageable administrative zones, each with a doctor or an engineer as director; these in turn worked with the municipalities to set up anti-malaria brigades run by members of the local communities.[100] In 1937, a free quinine service was set up, using post and telegraph offices as distribution points; in one year alone 800,000 individual treatments were given.[101]

The actual impact of all these anti-malaria activities before 1945 is difficult to assess. Gabaldón himself acknowledged in a long paper he read before the Royal Society of Tropical Medicine and Hygiene in London after the war that the steady decline evident in malaria morbidity and mortality in Venezuela, from its peak incidence in the years 1916–20, was hard to explain purely in terms of public health efforts. Most of the measures, for instance, did not touch the rural areas, which received only 25 per cent of the total health budget, though they made up 50 per cent of the country's population. He speculated that part of the reason for the decline was the effect of slow improvements in economic conditions, which were reflected in improved standards of living. He also noted that in some Latin American countries where no nationwide campaigns against malaria existed, malaria death rates nonetheless showed a similar steady secular decline.[102] It is clear that the rapid success Gabaldón achieved with DDT once it was introduced in late 1945 owed a great deal to the fact that it was superimposed on this long-term decline in malaria (as was the case, already noted, in Italy, the US and elsewhere).

Gabaldón learned about the phenomenal properties of DDT in 1943 from a military officer when Gabaldón happened to be in Washington to lecture to US medical officers prior to their being sent to the Pacific Theatre on military duty. As soon as the war ended, Gabaldón arranged to have DDT supplied to Venezuela, making the country one of the first of six American Republics to start using DDT almost as soon as it became available in late 1945.

From the start in Venezuela, DDT was used on as large a scale as possible, ignoring initial tests as to its effectiveness, because Gabaldón was confident that full surveys of the distribution and epidemiology of malaria in the country had already been made, and provided an adequate background on which to judge the effects of treatment and DDT. The country's three main geographical-epidemiological zones were already understood, and their characteristic patterns of malaria endemicity had been established by prior research.[103] The habits of the main malaria vectors in the country were known; *Anopheles darlingi* was the most significant, because it was anthropophilic. A basic system of malaria organization was already in place, and could be adapted to the DDT era, and some rudimentary maps of human settlements had been made. Public health staff trained in malaria work were available. All of this led Gabaldón to skip WHO's recommended preparatory phase.

Despite this solid basis for the DDT campaign, Gabaldón emphasized the challenge eradication presented. House spraying would be no easy task, with the affected area of 600,000 sq. km (372,823 sq. miles) being about three times the size of Great Britain and involving thousands of homes scattered across a country that lacked good roads, communications and maps. The year-long pattern of malaria transmission in the country meant that spraying had to be year-round, a huge demand on resources and administrative efficiency; in addition, the chief form of malaria infection was falciparum malaria, the most deadly kind.

To launch the DDT campaign, the country was divided into zones, each of which was under the supervision of a zone engineer; DDT squads consisting of uniformed sprayers and their leader, and with auxiliary staff such as drivers, were organized; and an Operations Manual was prepared. By 1949, the number of staff involved had reached over 1,500 people. All the houses in malaria areas were targeted for spraying first; each area had its own plan of action based on the number of houses in the area and their distances from roads. The squad leader for the area would send a man a day ahead to prepare the population for spraying and advise them on how to protect things such as food from the DDT. Doctors sought and identified malaria cases using spleen examinations and sending weekly reports to the Division of Epidemiology at the Ministry of Health. Health visitors visited houses to take blood smears following the spraying, the slides being sent to field laboratories for examination and then shipped to a central laboratory for evaluation. The aim throughout was not mosquito reduction per se, but reduction in malaria prevalence. Gabaldón was very insistent that DDT was to be used as it was in *Aedes aegypti*, precisely and specifically, though its target was insects in the house rather than larvae breeding sites; he objected to the 'indiscriminate action' that untrained public health people sometimes went in for. Malaria needed specialized techniques – in this regard, Gabaldón was definitely on Soper's side.[104]

When DDT spraying in houses was started, targeting just under 500,000 houses, the spraying had to be repeated every three months; in 1947 and 1948, it was repeated every four months; and in 1949, every six months. By 1951, in about 70 per cent of the houses, spraying was being done only twice a year, the remaining 30 per cent being in houses in difficult-to-reach rural areas.[105] Quinine was used to treat malaria (mepaquine was substituted later) via 2,500 distribution posts.

Malaria death rates fell very rapidly, from 112.3/100,000 in 1941–5 to 14.8/100,000 in 1948.[106] By 1950, the figure had fallen to 8.5/100,000, and by 1955 to 0.33/100,000 (amounting to a total that year of 19 deaths and 1,209 cases).[107] The sharp decline in malaria had collateral health effects; there was a decline in death rates from other diseases, and an initial decline in infant mortality (but a rise in the rate in 1948 which Gabaldón attributed to the development of DDT-resistance in flies involved in the transmission of enteritis and diarrhoeas). As mentioned already, however, Gabaldón was honest in admitting that he also saw the effect on malaria of recent economic wellbeing in Venezuela, and that the respective part played by socio-economic factors and by DDT in malaria declines could not be disentangled from each other.

The quick results, however, led him to move from the language of control to the language of eradication.[108] By 1951 he was ready to argue that 'no goal short of malaria eradication should be aimed at'.[109] He predicted Venezuela would be the first tropical country to achieve this goal. In 1954, he claimed that malaria had in fact been eradicated in 20 per cent of the country, representing 49 per cent of the total population. Gabaldón believed this was the largest area of malaria eradication within the tropical zone following residual spraying, and he was the first to claim it as such. From this point on, the eradication programme in Venezuela began to turn its attention to searching out remaining cases of malaria, by collecting the results of blood tests to discover where infections still existed.[110]

These early results from Venezuela were so impressive that they were influential in persuading sceptics of the efficiency of DDT-spraying; Soper relied on them in getting a malaria eradication resolution passed by delegates at the Fourteenth Pan American Sanitary Conference in 1954.[111] When critics questioned the scientific credentials of complete eradication, Gabaldón was there to cite his own success, as well as the early results in Argentina and Ecuador, thus providing, says Litsios, 'concrete scientific facts' to back up the concept of absolute eradication of the disease.[112] At the meeting in Mexico in 1955 where WHO itself took up the matter, of the 28 countries submitting draft resolutions, thirteen were from Latin America; in this endorsement lay above all the example of Venezuela.

At Gabaldón's urging, WHO began to set up a system for certifying eradication, following the method already established by PAHO for certifying the eradication of the *Aedes aegypti* mosquito, eradication work which in many countries in Latin America was being carried out in parallel (though with different staff) to the malaria eradication effort. In 1959, Venezuela asked PAHO to begin the process of certifying just over 400,000 sq. km (248,548 sq. miles) of its territory for recording in WHO's Register of Areas of Malaria Eradication; the area was duly inscribed in 1961 and claimed by Gabaldón as the first such tropical area ever to be registered as completely free of malaria. By 1966, of the 26 countries or political units in Latin America, six had been granted such certificates, covering the whole or a large part of an area, and in three more countries the prospects for complete eradication looked good.[113]

Growing Problems

But despite the early successes with DDT like that in Venezuela, by the early 1960s malaria eradication programmes were beginning to run into difficulties. In the case of India, where the eradication programme dwarfed every other, employing some 150,000 people, the vast size of the country; the diversity of its regions; the complications caused by the federal structure of the government, which gave considerable independence to the individual states and sometimes caused state Ministers of Health to compete with the political centre; the problems of inspectors who were sloppy, or of DDT supplies running out; and above all, the absence of adequate basic health services, were among the many challenges the programme faced. So even though the malaria eradication campaign in India had had, by almost any measure, an amazing early success, with startling plunges in reported malaria cases, there was also growing recognition that malaria probably would not be, and perhaps *could not* be, completely eradicated. Vector resistance was a growing worry.[114]

In most of Latin America the story was the same. Dramatic early reductions threatened to be undone by difficulties that ran the gamut from inadequate financing, supply problems, administrative weaknesses, problems with mosquito resistance to insecticides and plasmodium resistance to drugs. Soper knew about these setbacks because he heard about them from the delegates that attended the various PAHO meetings that were held each year. Countries were critical of the absence of adequate funding from PAHO (though its budget of $2 million in 1954 did not allow huge sums for each of the eradication programmes). Many countries were spending large percentages of their total health budgets on malaria eradication, even as the goal of absolute eradication remained elusive. The US contributed an additional $1,500,000 to PAHO for malaria eradication in 1957 (and the US was already paying 66 per cent of PAHO's regular budget). Even so, the money was not enough. El Salvador, for instance, reported that 30 per cent of its entire National Health Department budget was being invested in the MEP, and one third of the personnel would be participating, even though malaria was not considered at this time to be its most serious public health problem (because of previous malaria control work). To defend eradication, the Minister of Health said he had to use of all the scientific arguments that PAHO and WHO had developed in promoting it, especially the argument that the cost of eradication would be smaller in the long run than maintaining control programmes indefinitely. 'The public health authorities had to promise that the eradication program would be rewarded with success in the following four or five years', he said. 'The Government, the public, and the medical profession are all waiting to see the results of a campaign in which so much of the nation's money is being invested.'[115]

Even countries with strong political motives for collaborating with international agencies and the US, such as Brazil, found it difficult to align their malaria work with the new eradicationist philosophy. Brazil had established its malaria control services and developed its own strategies after the war, combining DDT, which was introduced into the country in 1947, anti-malarial drugs, and in the Amazon, where the population was very dispersed and the vectors of malaria were not domiciliary, the innovative method of distributing chloroquinated salt – cooking salt impregnated with chloroquine (rather as iodine is added to salt to prevent endemic goitre). Between 1940 and 1958, the number of malaria cases per year in Brazil fell sharply, from an estimated eight million, to only 250,000 cases a year (in a by then much larger population). In these figures lay the evidence of a successful control programme. Only it was not an eradication programme, which is what the US, PAHO and WHO wanted. It was only in 1958 that the country finally launched its MEP, expecting the preparatory stage to last at least two years.[116] In 1964, Brazil was reporting that it expected to move on to the next, attack phase, in 1968; the number of cases declined rapidly as the MEP got organized, dropping to roughly 52,000 by 1970. But by the end of the decade, the numbers were on the rise again, reaching 170,000 by 1980; the rise was largely due to development projects in the Amazon, from highway building to mining, to agriculture, which opened up new areas for anopheline breeding while drawing thousands of vulnerable people, without immunity, into often chaotic new settlements lacking even the most basic of health services.[117]

In Mexico, the story was more or less the same; huge reductions in malaria were made, followed by stagnation in the programme and then the return of malaria.[118] A report from PAHO in the mid-1960s said it was impossible to tell *when* malaria would be eradicated in the Americas, because of unexpected biological problems that had not been foreseen when the venture had started.[119]

True to form, to the end Soper counted on malaria eradication being possible. In a 1965 lecture at the Johns Hopkins University School of Hygiene and Public Health, after his retirement, he declared: 'To the eradicationist, the demonstration of his ability to reduce the incidence of a disease constitutes proof of his culpability in not eradicating it.'[120]

In his book, control of malaria was morally not enough; whereas in many other people's book, eradication appeared to be impossible.

Then there was the matter of DDT. Soper was not unaware of the potential dangers of DDT. When the experiment with DDT in Sardinia began in 1946, Soper had written to the Rockefeller Foundation, which was funding a large part of the effort, to say there might be contra-indications to DDT's widespread use; he had heard reports that animals eating forage treated with DDT had high concentrations of the insecticide in their milk; he also relayed reports of animals dying from aerial spraying. According to Hall's recent account of the project, these worries were not conveyed to the public (and later tests on the population showed no damage to the human populations).[121] In Chile, in addition to households, all domestic animals were sprayed every three weeks as part of the malaria eradication effort. There were also many discussions about putting DDT routinely into drinking water to kill mosquito larvae.

The publication of Rachel Carson's *Silent Spring* in 1962 brought the question of the harm chemical insecticides were doing to the environment into the forefront of eradication debates, as we saw in chapter Four in relation to yellow fever. Carson was writing as a polemicist to draw attention to the silent, hidden, and long-term damage the massive use of insecticides did to plant and animal life, at a time when most experts maintained that they were harmless. 'It is not my contention that chemical insecticides must never be used', Carson wrote. 'I do contend that we have put poisonous and potentially potent chemicals indiscriminately into the hands of persons largely or wholly ignorant of their potentials for harm.'[122] At roughly the same time, new ecologically informed views about the balance between microorganisms and human beings in medicine were being put forward, and new, less military metaphors about health and disease were being used.

As the criticisms of DDT mounted in the United States, Soper remained largely, if more cautiously, positive about DDT, at least about its use for public health purposes (Carson's target, as we noted earlier, was primarily DDT's overuse in agriculture). His thoughts, however, he mainly kept to his private notebooks and diaries. In all his public comments, his main point, like that of the members of WHO's Expert Committee on Insecticides, was that the health benefits to humans from the use of long-lasting insecticides far outweighed the harm. He was also worried, *vis-à-vis* malaria, that if DDT-spraying were to be stopped prematurely, malaria would return, as happened in Sri Lanka in 1968, when following the cessation of spraying, the disease came back in a massive epidemic, with over 100,000 cases. The next year, Sri Lanka resumed DDT spraying.[123]

The topic of the safety of DDT would not, however, go away. Slowly, a scientific and citizens' consensus was building up that control, not eradication, was what had to be aimed for, at least in relation to agricultural pests, and that residual (long-lasting) insecticides had to be restricted except for the most necessary efforts to control disease vectors. This latter point provided an escape hatch for Soper and other disease eradicationists, but by the 1970s even this hatch was being closed, as a campaign was waged to ban DDT altogether. In December, 1970, Soper was contacted by a US doctor who was keen to get Soper involved in opposing what the writer described as the 'hysterical anti-DDT campaign' that was being waged. Soper, however, replied coolly; he was surprised, he wrote, by the 'unjustified attacks on the use of DDT', but added 'I may be even more surprised by the extent and serious nature of the findings on studies of the effect of DDT on many parts of the biological constitution of the world'. 'The toxicologists', he wrote, 'are coming up with data on the susceptibility of birds and marine forms which are very disconcerting. The present evidence is such that I believe the indiscriminate use of DDT should be abandoned. DDT should be used only when absolutely essential and preferably under conditions such that no heavy addition is made to the DDT burden of the earth.' He asked his correspondent not to quote from this letter, as he was still reading the literature on DDT; he ended by saying he was convinced that we had to continue with its use in malaria prevention, 'or suffer tremendous epidemics in areas now relatively free of malaria'.[124]

Finally, in 1972, responding to the growing pressure from environmentalists, the US government banned DDT altogether within the country (though dieldrin and other alternatives to DDT continued to be widely used, and of course, the US did not have any malaria). WHO's Expert Committee on Insecticides, however, continued to support the use of DDT as well as other insecticides in public health. It is a position that many public health officials defend to this day (indeed, DDT is currently used for malaria control in South Africa, among other places).

WHO Shifts its Strategy

By 1968, the situation had got to the point that the Director-General of WHO, Dr Marcelino Candau, who had been a staunch defender of the malaria eradication strategy, finally had to heed the growing criticisms from within WHO and undertake a re-evaluation of the entire project. The report WHO put out in 1969 in response acknowledged that in many places, eradication had not been achieved and probably could not be. It proposed that those countries where there was a good prospect of success should pursue the goal of eradication; but in countries where eradication did not seem feasible, or where eradication programmes had never started, they should instead return to malaria control operations.[125] The shift back to malaria control was, as Litsios says, an admission of failure that, in many instances, left many countries floundering. Not all eradication projects came to a halt, but many slowly deteriorated as funds began to disappear. The United States had at any rate already stopped the free shipment of DDT ten years earlier, long before it had halted DDT production. In India, for instance, free distribution of DDT from the US was replaced with a system of purchase via loans.

The rapidity with which malaria eradication and/or control programmes fell away in many places was a sign of the lack of real political support for them. Resurgence in malaria cases led to the imposition of controls again, and again, in a 'fire-fighting' approach to malaria, as Najera puts it. In reflecting on the question of the sustainability of malaria control and the record of the past 40 years (between the early 1950s and the early 1980s), Dr J. A. Najera, a malaria specialist with WHO, emphasized the importance of socio-economic factors in malaria control. He divided countries into three kinds; 1) countries that were fairly stable in terms of population and community organization, and had reached a required minimum level in health services and basic sanitation; in these countries, malaria was eradicated through the mixed effects of socio-economic development and the eradication campaign; 2) countries where malaria increased explosively, owing to socio-political instability and at times anarchic resource exploitation (for example, mining in forested areas); 3) countries intermediate between the two, where malaria transmission was greatly reduced by the MEP but not eradicated, and where the reductions were vulnerable owing to their dependence on external support which did not engage with the local communities or their health services. 'Seeing the global eradication campaigns of the 1950s and 1960s, with the advantage of historical perspective', wrote Najera, 'it appears as a reconfirmation of the judgement of the Malaria Commission of the League of Nations (1927)', quoting once again the sentence that had once so galled the mosquito experts: 'The history of special antimalarial campaigns is chiefly a record of exaggerated expectations, followed sooner or later by disappointment and abandonment of the work.'[126]

It was the abandonment of the work that Gabaldón in Venezuela was determined to avoid. In regard to the changes in strategy proposed by WHO, Gabaldón was in fact in a special situation. On the one hand, he believed the achievements in reduction in malaria reported by WHO in 1968 was 'an international achievement without parallel in the provision of public health service'. Of the 1,692 million people inhabiting originally malarious regions, 654 million now lived in areas where malaria had been eradicated. On the other hand, he conceded that his enthusiasm had been overdone: 'It is disheartening to have to reach the conclusion, contrary to my opinion of fifteen years ago, that malaria eradication worldwide has become at present an unattainable goal.' As a result, the eradication of malaria must be considered, he said, 'unstable, regional, and temporary'.[127]

Experience had shown him in fact that there were different kinds of malaria in his country, not all of which could be eradicated. They were the 'responsive', the 'refractory' and the 'inaccessible' malaria. Only responsive malaria was theoretically open to eradication because, as the term indicated, it referred to malaria where the vectors were responsive or susceptible to the effects of house spraying with DDT or other insecticides, because the habits of the mosquitoes led them habitually to feed and rest in people's homes. Systematic application of insecticide resulted in transmission being interrupted, as predicted by WHO's original eradication strategy. 'Refractory' malaria, however, referred to malaria vectors that were not responsive to DDT; they either learned to adapt to insecticides by avoidance behaviour (such as flying away from or off sprayed surfaces), or were simply out of reach of house spraying because they normally bred in inaccessible places, like the *Kertezia* anopheles vector that bred in bromeliad plants. 'Refractory malaria' also included malaria whose mosquito vectors became resistant over time to insecticides.

'Inaccessible' malaria referred to the all-important social determinants of malaria. In Venezuela, this meant malaria, which, owing to the behaviour or culture of different groups of people, such as their refusal to have their houses sprayed, or their migratory habits, could not be suppressed. Here Gabaldón had in mind especially the scattered Amerindian populations living in the Amazonian parts of Venezuela. Small pockets of populations carrying the malaria parasite in their blood meant there was a constant risk of re-introducing malaria transmission into eradicated areas; for this reason, he argued against WHO's recommendation that after the attack phase had stopped transmission, insecticide spraying be stopped. Instead he kept spraying continuously in highly endemic areas.

Gabaldón's 'independent path' to malaria control, in Litsios's terms, was thus three-fold. In the original WHO scheme, once eradication was achieved, DDT-spraying should stop. Gabaldón, as we have noted, disagreed, because he knew that as long as pockets of refractory or inaccessible malaria remained in his country, malaria could always be re-introduced and spraying would be needed on a continuous basis to stop its return to areas already cleared. He concluded that 'to insist upon eradication of refractory malaria from large areas without new and more efficient methods is a waste of energy, time and money'.[128] But he also argued that the term 'eradication' should still be used for those areas where malaria had been made to disappear. Why not make eradication a less absolute term? Why not settle for 'partial eradication'? His second divergence concerned WHO's emphasis on the need for active case detection work; Gabaldón thought blood testing except in certain zones where eradication was nearly achieved was expensive and laborious; concentrating on keeping up insecticide spraying seemed to him a better policy, and more cost-effective.[129]

Finally, Gabaldón parted company from the WHO when the organization began recommending in 1969 that countries begin to merge their malaria programmes with their general health services. Having built up a special malaria service over 30 years, with its cadre of specialist, technically trained epidemiologists and entomologists, Gabaldón did not intend to disband it. Better by far, in his view, was to expand the malaria service itself into a more generalized service with responsibilities for tackling other vector-borne diseases in the country.[130] Under Gabaldón's leadership as Minister of Health from 1959–65 this idea was partially put into practice when the Division of Malariology was enlarged, to become the Ministry of Malariology and Environmental Health. This took over responsibility for diseases like Chagas disease, in addition to malaria. The expanded Ministry also developed programmes, among other environmental sanitation projects, to construct model sanitary housing for the poor, to replace the shanty houses so many people lived in that were too rickety to be easily protected from insect vectors.[131]

It was a different model from that of WHO, but one that certainly had its own rationale.

To the end of his long professional career in public health, Gabaldón stuck to his guns, maintaining insecticide spraying and trying to make sure that areas where eradication had been achieved were kept free of infection. He took pride in Venezuela's accomplishment. Until the mid-1980s, malaria had in fact disappeared in Venezuela, except for a few marginal pockets. Gabaldón thought the premature withdrawal of spraying a mistake; that after the introduction of spraying in Venezuela, Mauritius and Guiana (all places where DDT had been systematically used), life expectancy had increased at a rate entirely unknown in public health until then; that the problem of insect resistance to DDT and other insecticides was due not to their overuse in public health but their over-use in agriculture; and that the recommendation by WHO that countries transfer their malaria control programmes to the general health services was another factor that had 'changed victories into defeats'. In 1983 he drew attention to the measures put in place in Venezuela; they were responsible, he wrote, 'for Venezuela today being the only continental tropical country which has not experienced severe recrudescences in its eradicated area'.[132]

Epitaph for Global Malaria Eradication?

Many others, like Gabaldón, regretted what they saw as the premature abandonment of malaria eradication. Dr Abraham Horwitz, who as Director of PAHO took a much broader, socio-economic view of the determinants of health than Soper, nevertheless criticized the 'overzealous champions of the environment' for threatening to halt production of DDT. Paul F. Russell agreed with Bruce-Chwatt's protest: 'We cannot lose all that has been gained over the past decade.'[133]

Soper, of course, was dismayed by WHO's abandonment of his ideal of eradication and its recommendation that countries begin merging their malaria services with their general health services. The latter, he said, did not exist in many countries, and where they did, they had no expertise with eradication techniques. In general, Soper published little on malaria (in his memoirs, only his Brazilian and Egyptian gambiae eradication campaigns are included, and the MEP is hardly mentioned).[134]

But he had, characteristically, his views on the matter. After retiring from PAHO in 1959, he spent the next two months on a tour of malaria eradication programmes in Taiwan, the Philippines, Sri Lanka and India, and was very disappointed with what he thought was a lack of commitment to eradication and deviations from the original methods. In the places he visited, he thought the problems were not due to growing mosquito resistance to insecticides, but to faults in administration. Like Gabaldón, Soper thought the most important thing was to *keep spraying* until every habitation had been covered; as usual, he thought identifying and treating everyone ill with malaria should not really be the main focus of the eradication campaign. Only too readily, he believed, people let interest and determination fade as malaria became less visible, and settled for 'partial eradication' – in his opinion, an oxymoron. He argued to the end that eradication of malaria was possible, even in Africa, but the effort could not be half-hearted.[135]

But by this date, the tide had turned. In tropical climates absolute eradication had been achieved only in a few island countries, or in partial areas of a country. Countries that had failed to initiate eradication measures posed a constant threat to contiguous areas where eradication had been carried out.

'Nature' itself presented an obstacle in the form of the development of insect resistance to DDT and its substitutes such as dieldrin. Seeking out and then testing the blood of people who were potentially carriers of the malaria parasite was another difficulty; this required a system of disease surveillance that was beyond the resources of many poor countries.

Paradoxically, adding to the sense of failure with the MEP was its very success. This was because, so great was the initial decline in malaria in some of the most malarial countries, notably India, that the huge increase in population resulting from falling mortality rates caused a growing concern among overseas donors, notably the US, about 'over-population' in the world's neediest places. Amrith describes the 'triumph of population control' that resulted; he notes the huge growth in US population studies in the 1950s, right when the malaria eradication programmes were launched.[136] Instead of disease reduction being tied to successful economic development, as the original "development" thesis predicted, now it was seen as being tied to over-population. The 1960s as a consequence saw the introduction of a new emphasis on contraception, which in India was introduced on a massive scale (and eventually, under Prime Minister Indira Gandhi, coercively).

But as population control became the new mantra in development circles, malaria control faltered in the face of the withdrawal of money and confidence at the heart of WHO itself. WHO's change of mind about the feasibility of eradication, and the new concern about environmental damage caused by the wholesale use of insecticides, sounded the death knell of the programme. In India, by 1964, malaria had been eradicated from 88 per cent of the area, but by that date was beginning to return.[137] In 1976 6.45 million cases were recorded, only to subside following the re-enforcement of controls for several years to about two million cases.

The experience of Sri Lanka (then Ceylon) was particularly important in the negative assessment of the MEP. The DDT eradication programme in Sri Lanka was built upon a good history of malaria control before the Second World War, and a systematic pyrethrum-based space-spraying effort during the war. A National Malaria Programme was organized in 1946, with spraying being extended to all areas where spleen rates were above 10 per cent (a rough measure of malaria incidence). Control became officially an eradication programme in 1958. Spraying was apparently so successful that already in the mid-1950s, it had been terminated, but then had to be resumed after a 1956 resurgence of malaria cases. Mortality and cases declined markedly, from over 275,000 cases a year in 1946, to just over 11,000 in 1955.

But as the effort met with difficulties, and enthusiasm declined along with spraying, malaria returned with a vengeance, leading to a huge epidemic in 1968–9 (with more than 500,000 malaria cases reported in 1969, compared to a low of only 17 cases in 1963). Gabaldón, sent to evaluate the situation in 1966, had the following advice for WHO: keep on spraying![138] The impact of the epidemic was especially severe because the earlier success in eliminating malaria had left the population without acquired immunity to the disease. The British colonial doctors' fears about what might happen if controls were not kept up were thus realized.[139]

How, then, shall we evaluate the malaria eradication effort? As Farley has said, public health opinion has tended to swing between two poles of a pendulum, between the belief that economic development is necessary to achieve a health transition, and the belief that a health transition is necessary to achieve economic development.[140] The truth probably lies in the middle, in the sense that what we see in the best cases is a virtuous cycle in which economic development brings improved incomes, better housing, schooling, and access to medicines, while public health interventions brings better health which in turn improves economic performance.

As I have said, the general consensus is that the MEP was a massive failure that, even though it resulted in many places in lowered rates of malaria cases and malaria deaths for many years, ultimately did not work because it did not take on board the complexities of the disease's determinants, and the dangers of relying on technical 'fixes' as an approach to health. On the plus side, by the end of 1974, of the estimated 1,945 million (nearly two billion) people living in originally malarious regions of the world, 73 per cent were free of the disease (leaving some 523 million people still exposed to infection in Central and South America, in Asia, in the South West Pacific and above all in Africa). By this date worldwide malaria morbidity accounted for about 100 million cases a year (today there are some 300–500 million cases a year), with mortality greatly reduced but still around one million a year.

On the minus side, there was a resurgence of malaria in several tropical countries where just a decade earlier eradication had seemed to be advancing – most notably in India, Sri Lanka, Thailand and Pakistan, the Philippines, Indonesia and the Indo-Chinese peninsula. Even in Venezuela, malaria would return.[141]

As the *Lancet* put it in its editorial, 'Epitaph for Malaria Eradication?' of 1975, the balance sheet was contentious.[142]

These mixed results, coming as they did in the midst of a re-assessment of WHO's primary mission and a re-dedication to basic health services in place of the one-disease campaigns represented by the malaria eradication programme, appeared to spell the end not just of malaria eradication, but of the eradication idea more generally.

Only the success, finally and belatedly, of yet another eradication campaign that had jogged along for years with little money and little attention from WHO until the last stages, rescued eradication as a public health philosophy, and gave it a new lease of life. This success was with smallpox. Wilbur Downs commented that: 'Smallpox certainly saved the day, and saved the skin, of the international agencies after the shambles of the malaria effort. Credibility was re-established.'[143]

6 The Last Inch: Smallpox Eradication

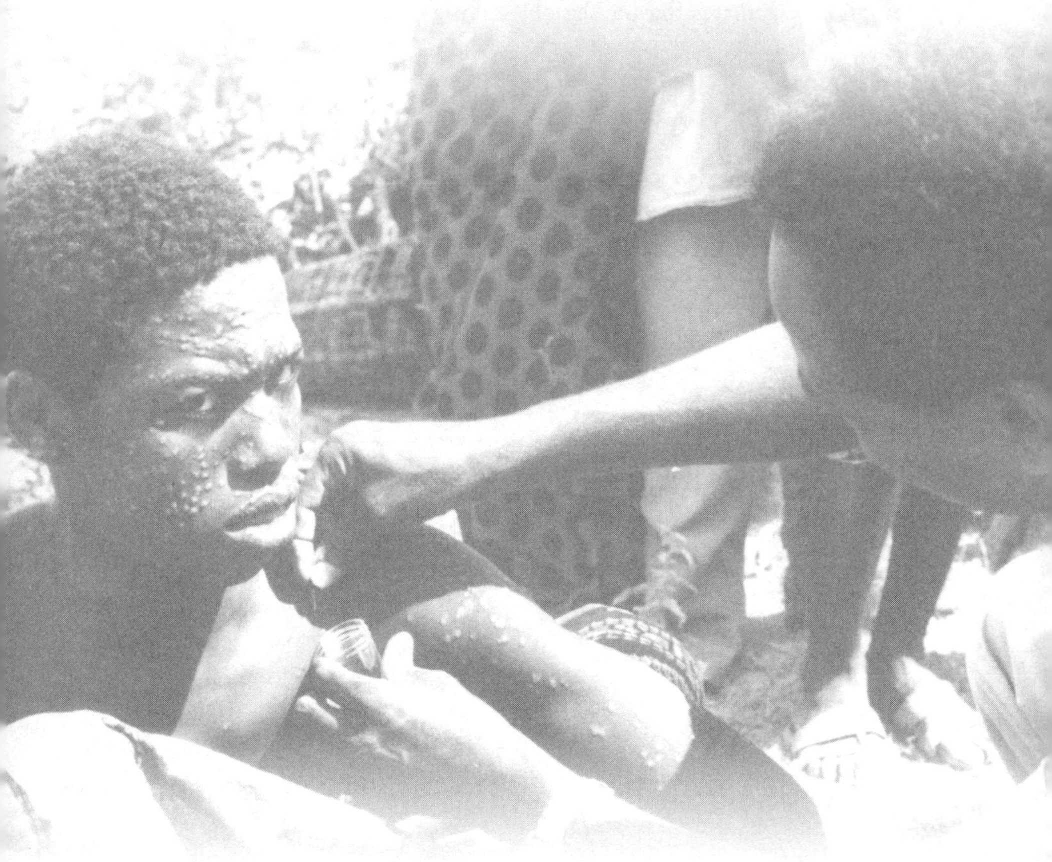

Smallpox eradication took a very long time – or a short time, depending on one's point of view. On the long side is the historian's view of the almost 200 years separating Jenner's discovery of the smallpox vaccine in 1796 and the elimination of smallpox as a human affliction. On the short side is the view of those who, in a final burst of intensified effort, took only ten years between 1967 and 1977 to finish the job.

The long history is a history of many efforts without success. Under Soper's watch, for instance, PAHO 'jumped the starting gun' on WHO and passed a resolution in 1950 calling on PAHO countries to eradicate smallpox in the Western Hemisphere. But the goal proved as elusive as Soper's other eradication efforts. After several years working to coordinate national mass smallpox vaccination campaigns throughout the Americas, Soper retired in 1959 with the job unfinished. Smallpox incidence was considerably reduced in the region, but it had not reached the magical number of zero. Only in 1966 did the World Health Assembly vote to bring to bear the technical and financial resources, and above all the political will, needed to complete the job. The last naturally occurring case of smallpox was found in 1977. In 1980, WHO certified formally that smallpox had indeed been vanquished – the first time a human disease had been extinguished by means of deliberate human intervention. It was a great achievement. Smallpox had been one of the most fatal and burdensome of afflictions for centuries, and now it was gone.

Given this unique outcome (thus far) in the eradication of diseases that infect human beings, public health experts have understandably scrutinized the smallpox story closely, in order to identify the elements that made for eventual success.[1] Some conclude the answer lies in large part in the biological and clinical characteristics of the disease itself. Though smallpox was a deadly and highly contagious viral infection, its transmission occurred only between humans, and it spread rapidly through susceptible populations, largely though the inhalation of the airborne virus. It involved no intermediate vector, such as an insect, and had no other animal reservoir. Clinically smallpox stood out because, after an incubation period of twelve to fourteen days, infection produced a dramatic and highly visible rash that eventually spread to nearly all parts of the body; this meant that smallpox was highly visible, and so easily detected and diagnosed. The lack of effective treatment for its victims, and smallpox's high mortality rate (20–30 per cent of those infected, but sometimes as many as 80 per cent in children, depending on the epidemiological and other circumstances), gave smallpox a high profile in public health, which in turn was an incentive to political action. Finally, and most importantly, smallpox had an effective vaccine that gave protection against smallpox 95 per cent of the time.

Yet when we put aside hindsight, and look at the history of smallpox prospectively, instead of retrospectively, these explanations of the success seem incomplete. For instance, the absence of an animal reservoir, essential for absolute eradication to work, was not established beyond doubt when WHO endorsed a worldwide smallpox eradication campaign in 1958, and as a consequence considerable effort and time were eventually put into proving a scientific negative.[2]

Epidemiologically, too, there were many things to be learned. Infected individuals were most infective to others between the onset of the rash, until the point at which the last scab fell off. It was widely believed that smallpox was one of the most contagious of all human infections. But in the 1960s, public health workers in Africa and India who were carrying out detailed studies of how outbreaks of smallpox passed from family to family, and from village to village, found that contagion from incidental contact between people was rare, and that it required very close contact over several days for infection to spread. This knowledge had implications for how vaccination should be employed, leading at the end-stage to a change in strategy.

Clinically, too, smallpox was not always obvious or easy to detect. The most dangerous form of smallpox, known as *Variola major*, was highly visible because it produced, after an incubation period of about ten days during which the person did not appear ill, a distinctive and terrible rash, first on the face, hands and feet, accompanied by high fever and severe pains; the rash then became pustules which covered the entire body and were extremely painful. Death when it occurred was from shock.

But there was another form of smallpox that was much less severe, known as *Variola minor* (sometimes called alastrim), whose rash was much less obvious and whose mortality rate much lower, killing about 1–2 per cent of those infected compared to the 30 per cent or more of those with the major kind. Appearing some time in the nineteenth century, the minor form of smallpox began to replace the major in much of the Americas and Europe by the 1930s.[3] This was obviously very good news for victims of smallpox, but it complicated the drive to eliminate the disease, because people learned to live with it, treating it as a minor affliction. Because cases were not necessarily identified, smallpox could spread before people could be isolated. The rash in the minor form was easier to confuse with other rash-like diseases, especially chickenpox. In general, it made the identification of smallpox cases difficult, unless you actively set out to look for them. It required a system of active surveillance that many countries simply did not have. It also meant that in countries where the minor form of smallpox dominated, the disease simply did not have the high priority that smallpox eradicators in Washington or Geneva assigned to it.

And the vaccine? Certainly, smallpox vaccine was fundamental to eradication. But throughout the eradication campaign the production of smallpox vaccine was very uneven; the techniques of application of the vaccine varied from country to country, and could cause considerable pain; and the potency of the vaccines used was unreliable and 'take' rates varied (and were often not evaluated or recorded). In Brazil, the vaccine used 'rarely met accepted standards of potency and stability', and was often contaminated with bacteria.[4]

There were, then, many barriers to success with smallpox eradication. Until the intensified stage, the campaign's financial resources were meagre and its conduct erratic. Many people, even those closely involved in the campaign, doubted the outcome until the very end. As Donald A. Henderson, who led the WHO's intensified eradication campaign from 1967–77, said, eradication was achieved by 'only the narrowest of margins'.[5] The retrospective sense of inevitability and triumph one sees in many accounts of smallpox eradication belie the reality of a much more uncertain and unsteady trajectory towards the final termination point.

My point, once again, is that retrospect is a powerful but often distorting lens on history; and history is what we have to deal with. The story of the world's greatest success in pursuing the holy grail of the absolute eradication of a disease – a real triumph of international cooperation at the height of the Cold War, and a result of the determination to finally bring a programme to its conclusion – serves at the same time as a cautionary tale in international public health policy. Eradication is a very hard goal to aim for. Setbacks are the norm; knowledge is always incomplete; the lessons of history get forgotten; and international coordination and cooperation are hard won. And yet, eventually, the job was done.

From Inoculation to Vaccination

Smallpox eradication differed from the other post-war eradication campaigns in that it was not the outcome of new, wartime technologies, like DDT and penicillin, but was based on one of the oldest technologies of disease prevention available, the first vaccine ever discovered. Today, when childhood vaccinations are routine and widely accepted, it is perhaps difficult to imagine how innovative a procedure smallpox vaccination was when it was first discovered in 1796 (the next vaccine against a human disease to be introduced, against rabies, was first used successfully by Louis Pasteur in 1885).

In the late eighteenth century smallpox had a worldwide distribution, and was a major killer. In Europe, in 1800, there were an estimated 400,000 cases a year; in the nineteenth century, perhaps 20 per cent of all deaths in urban areas each year were due to smallpox (and about one third of all children's deaths).[6] Smallpox left many people blind from the corneal ulcerations it caused (perhaps one third of all blindness was the result of smallpox infection); many of those who survived smallpox were left with deeply pock-marked faces.

Though there was no treatment for smallpox (and there still is not), smallpox could be prevented by variolation. This involved taking active matter from a smallpox pustule, and then scratching it into the hand or arm of an individual (or sometimes blowing it into the nostrils), in order to produce a mild case of the illness, with the expectation that the person would survive relatively unharmed, and with a lifelong immunity to any further smallpox attacks. Of ancient origin, by the eighteenth century the technique had been adopted in many parts of the world.[7] It was especially popular in the UK, having been introduced into Britain by Lady Mary Wortley Montagu in the 1720s, after she learned about it in Istanbul (and after she had lost her good looks to smallpox). Variolation had a much lower mortality rate than naturally occurring smallpox – about 0.5–2 per cent, compared to 30 per cent or more – and for this reason variolation was widely practiced, continuing to be used in parts of Europe until the end of nineteenth century, and in Africa into the twentieth century.

Variolation, though, had two serious drawbacks; it sometimes produced a serious case of smallpox instead of the mild case hoped for; and since it involved giving someone active smallpox virus, the procedure could inadvertently spread smallpox infection into the community and cause new cases of the disease.[8]

Jenner's vaccine was different in one crucial respect, and much safer than variolation. Jenner was a country surgeon practicing in Gloucestershire in the 1790s, when he decided to test an idea he had heard about locally, that milkmaids who had caught the cowpox were not susceptible to smallpox (hence their proverbially pretty, unscarred complexions). Cowpox was a somewhat uncommon animal disease that was known to farmers, especially those in the western counties of England. In 1796, Jenner decided to inoculate a boy of eight, called Jeremy Phipps, with matter from a cowpox pustule taken from the hand of an infected milkmaid; six weeks later, Jenner took the crucial second step, when he then inoculated the boy with matter from a smallpox vesicle, to see if he got ill. He did not. Further tests on other individuals confirmed his findings. Thus was discovered what Jenner called 'variola vaccinae' (from the Latin *vacca* for cow, and therefore meaning 'cow-related pox').[9] Giving people cowpox was the way to stop them getting smallpox.

Technically, Jenner's vaccination was a great improvement over variolation because it produced only a mild reaction in the healthy individual, and because the procedure did not risk spreading smallpox to others. For this reason, the medical innovation spread rapidly, eventually reaching every continent. Since cowpox was a relatively rare animal disease, its maintenance and transportation to new environments was a technical and social challenge.[10] In 1803, for example, the Balmis expedition organized by the Spanish Crown took a group of orphaned boys by ship to Spain's overseas colonies, using the boys to keep the cowpox vaccine alive through arm-to-arm transmission, passing it from one boy to another until the ship reached the New World. In this way, Jenner's vaccine was transported to Colombia, Ecuador, Peru, Mexico and, eventually, across the Pacific, to the Philippines and even China.[11] In the United States, vaccination so impressed President Jefferson that already in 1806 he was predicting that the universal application of the vaccine would one day eliminate smallpox from the world forever: 'Future nations', he wrote, 'will know by history only that the loathsome smallpox has existed'.[12]

But though overall smallpox incidence declined wherever vaccination was used systematically, its take-up rate was far from even, and many technical problems remained to be solved and misconceptions put right.[13] Jenner believed, wrongly as it turned out, that immunity to smallpox from a single vaccination would be life-long. It took a surprisingly long time before doctors recognized that re-vaccination was a necessary part of any smallpox vaccination regime (the British were especially slow in this regard; at the time of the 1867 Vaccination Act, most doctors still believed that re-vaccination was not necessary; even in 1898, re-vaccination was not made a requirement of Britain's new and comprehensive Vaccination Act, because of the fierceness of public opposition).

Problems with the quality of the vaccine were another matter. Over the course of the nineteenth century, Jenner's cowpox was somehow replaced by a different, but genetically related, virus now known as vaccinia; this virus forms the basis of our current smallpox vaccine. The replacement was not discovered until the twentieth century, and to this day the origins of vaccinia are unknown (and a certain mystery also surrounds the nature of Jenner's original variola vaccine as well).[14] The fact that the replacement occurred reminds us that vaccination was for a long time a very pragmatic affair, involving many different kinds of vaccinators, of varying degrees of knowledge and skill; that vaccine was being produced long before the bacteriological revolution provided the scientific and conceptual framework for an understanding of how vaccines worked; and that the vaccine was harvested and transported in a variety of ways (for example, on dried threads), which inevitably resulted in variations in potency and 'take' rates. The lancet method of application also carried with it the risk of contamination by other microorganisms that could spread disease to people through the vaccination procedure (for example, eczema and syphilis).

All of these issues qualified the enthusiasm for vaccination. Vaccination could be painful, since it usually required making a number of cuts in the arm with a lancet, after which cowpox matter was rubbed in, and a local inflammation resulted. The authorities often demanded the vaccination of very young children, sometimes as early as in the first three months of life (and sometimes regardless of the health of the infant at the time). Parents also resented the fact they were expected to bring back their child after eight days, so that the vaccinator could harvest cowpox matter from the vesicles to use in vaccinating others. These were serious drawbacks, and were good reasons for the refusal of people to subject themselves, but more especially their very young children, to the procedure. Smallpox vaccine production improved over the course of the nineteenth century. Jenner's original arm-to-arm method for maintaining the viability of cowpox was slowly replaced by a method of harvesting the vaccinia in the skin of living animals; calves were commonly used, but buffalo, sheep and other animals were tried in different parts of the world. This method allowed more commercial quantities of vaccine to be produced, but did not necessarily result in vaccine less contaminated by bacteria. The use of glycerine reduced bacterial contamination and prolonged the viability of the lymph (with refrigeration later helping to preserve its viability even further).[15] The main point is that there was no standard procedure for producing vaccine and vaccine quality varied greatly from place to place. Quality in tropical countries, where the hot climate caused glycinerated vaccine to deteriorate quickly, was a special problem. Even after a freeze-dried form of vaccine was introduced, the potency and quality of smallpox vaccine continued to be problematic right until the end of the final eradication campaign.

The Social History of Vaccination

To this day, vaccination defines, in a concentrated fashion, some of the fundamental challenges in public health, where the potential risks to an individual from a medical intervention have to be weighed against the potential benefits it brings to the larger community to which the individual belongs. Getting the balance right between these competing interests has been a major task of modern public health, and involves issues of competence, safety and trust.[16] For this reason, the two strands to the vaccination story, the technical and the social, cannot be separated.

Historically, the acceptance of smallpox vaccination has been a long, and sometimes contentious, process; there was no royal route to control via this particular technical means. Vaccination policies varied greatly from country to country, some countries introducing compulsory vaccination early, others very late (France had no compulsory vaccination until 1902).[17] Free smallpox vaccination was one of the first public health service offered by states (for example, the 1840 Vaccination Act in England, which offered free vaccination to the poor). However, when states passed compulsory vaccination laws (and enforced them), vaccination often met with resistance.[18] Many mechanisms short of outright compulsion also existed to ensure compliance. In this regard, Britain has been particularly closely studied because of its strong anti-vaccination movement. Compulsory legislation was passed in England in 1853, and tightened in 1867 and 1871, in response to outbreaks of smallpox, with penalties of fines and prison sentences to enforce compliance. Compulsion in turn prompted active resistance; by the 1880s some 200 anti-vaccination groups had formed. Eventually the state backed off from compulsion; the new Vaccination Act of 1898, though ostensibly making vaccination mandatory, in fact opened the route to conscientious objection, with the consequence that infant vaccination rates fell off rapidly. Whereas in the 1880s, about 50 per cent of infants were vaccinated against smallpox, by the end of the first decade of the twentieth century, only about 25 per cent of all children were.[19]

The impact of such low rates of vaccination might have been disastrous had smallpox epidemics been common, but by this time the era of major epidemics of smallpox was over. Past vaccination had given the population a degree of protection. But equally important was the contribution of various non-vaccination social interventions, such as improved overall sanitation, the use of the prompt notification of smallpox cases (legislated nationally in 1898), the tracing of all contacts and the placing of smallpox victims in isolation hospitals. In addition, there was disinfection of homes, clothes and bedding. The 'Leicester' method, as it has come to be called, after the town in England where it was first developed in direct response to the fierce anti-vaccination feeling in the area, was surprisingly effective in containing smallpox and was increasingly adopted by other municipalities in Britain, as a way to 'ring fence' outbreaks.[20] The replacement of *Variola major* by *Variola minor* as the dominant form of smallpox some time after 1920 was another factor in the continued fall in smallpox mortality in the UK. Hennock notes that the 'softer' English methods were never quite as effective in reducing smallpox as the more stringent, compulsory approach of a country like Germany – but both approaches worked. Thus though vaccination was important to the sharp reduction of smallpox, it was not the entire story, an insight that had to be re-discovered in the late twentieth century, when surveillance-containment methods were introduced during the intensified stage of the smallpox eradication campaign.[21]

The United States was if anything more resistant to compulsory smallpox vaccination than the UK, and as a consequence its vaccination rates, though varying from state to state, were generally low compared to most European countries, where compulsory legislation was the norm. In rural areas in the US, the vaccination rates were often less than 10 per cent. Smallpox incidence was as a consequence comparatively high in the United States until the 1930s. The fact that the minor form of smallpox had replaced the major form by the late 1920s only fuelled strong anti-vaccinationist feelings. Vaccination did not become routine in the United States until the 1980s, after smallpox had completely disappeared, and when a slew of new vaccines against polio, rubella, mumps, diphtheria and measles were introduced and became part of the normal 'package' of childhood immunizations.[22] The contrast between the *laissez-faire* approach to smallpox vaccination within the United States, and the mandatory policies the US imposed in their colonial possessions of Cuba and Puerto Rico after 1898, could not be more striking.[23]

Jenner knew that his vaccine meant smallpox could be eradicated. 'It now becomes too manifest to admit of controversy', he wrote in 1801, 'that the annihilation of the Small Pox, the most dreadful scourge of the human species, must be the final result of this practice'.[24] But, by the middle of the twentieth century, his dream of a world free of smallpox had still not been met. The technology was there; but if the social history of smallpox vaccination up to this point was any guide, achieving worldwide eradication would depend on a lot more than technology.

A Tipping Point?

By 1950, smallpox had declined in Europe and North America to such a point that many countries were engaged in essentially defensive policies – trying to stop smallpox from getting in from other places outside their borders. Vaccination rates had fallen off very significantly wherever smallpox had declined past a level of obvious visibility; this meant that populations in smallpox-free countries were increasingly vulnerable to infection from cases that somehow managed to slip past the system of border protections that were in place to keep the disease out, such as the requirement that visitors from overseas present international certificates as proofs of vaccination.

An incident of just this kind occurred in the United States in 1947, when a man travelling from Mexico to New York City became ill, and died in hospital; investigation showed he had died of smallpox. This one death caused a panic, and a rush by people in the New York area to get vaccinated. Within a month, several million had been vaccinated (the actual figures are hard to establish, though five to six million is usually cited). Altogether, this one imported case caused eleven further infections and two further deaths. It was later established that six people had also died from the vaccination itself.[25] This was not a sensible way to respond to a rare smallpox case, or conduct an exercise in public health.

The United States was in fact about to reach a tipping point, where the risks of sequelae (deaths and side effects) from vaccination would outweigh the risks from smallpox itself.[26] By the 1950s, the US was spending $15–20 million a year on defence against a disease the country had not seen for a decade and a half.[27] Thus though getting rid of smallpox worldwide was often presented as a generous, humanitarian act, a 'good' for the poor countries of the world, underlying the humanitarian rhetoric was an economic calculation that, if smallpox could be made to disappear from the entire world, the costs to the richer, smallpox-free countries of routine vaccination and its complications could be made to disappear as well. Eventually, the US spent a total of $32 million over a ten-year period on the global eradication of smallpox. This was actually a very small sum; if calculated in rational choice terms, the benefit-to-cost ratio was 400:1, making the smallpox eradication campaign, according to Barrett, 'the best collective investment the world has ever made'.[28]

Of course, people do not generally behave as rational choice theorists would have it, but rationally as historians would have it, that is, on the basis of all sorts of path-contingent considerations; as Henderson said, to the very end support for smallpox eradication was not generous, 'whatever the cost-benefit ratio may have been'.[29] When PAHO voted in 1950 to pursue smallpox eradication in the Americas, the decision reflected Soper's general enthusiasm for eradication, and the financial and administrative autonomy PAHO enjoyed within WHO. But WHO at large was not ready to follow Soper's lead. So reluctant were delegates to WHO to take on smallpox eradication, in fact, that when in 1953 the Director-General of WHO, Dr Brock Chisholm, proposed such a campaign, the delegates to the World Health Assembly (WHA) turned the project down, on the grounds it was 'too ambitious, too costly, and of uncertain feasibility'.[30] Instead, they voted in 1955 to launch what would seem, on the face of it, the much more difficult and even more ambitious task of eradicating malaria world-wide, with the results discussed in chapter Five of this book.

A few years later, the delegates to the WHA of WHO appeared to change their minds about smallpox when the organization was approached with a proposal for a worldwide eradication effort from an unexpected quarter – the Soviet Union. As we have seen, the USSR and the Eastern European communist countries had left WHO in a Cold War protest, almost immediately after it was founded; they only returned in 1957–8, following the death of Stalin. The next year, the Soviet delegate to the Eleventh WHA, Dr Viktor Zhdanov, then Deputy Minister of Health of the USSR, arrived at the meeting in Minneapolis, Minnesota, with a five-year plan for the worldwide eradication of smallpox. This plan was closely modelled on the 'command' model the USSR had used successfully to eliminate smallpox in the 1930s (through compulsory vaccination of the population). Eradication being the strategy of the day, the Soviet Union came armed with its own eradication project, to underline, perhaps, Soviet efficiency in public health. Zhdanov also offered to give WHO 25 million doses of vaccine to help launch the campaign.[31]

In an 'abrupt reversal of its views' the delegates to the WHA decided this time to endorse the proposal, which they did in 1959.[32] The delegates had not really changed their minds about the feasibility or desirability of a global smallpox eradication scheme; but they were persuaded to give at least the appearance of support – to give the go-ahead as a gesture of cooperation in the otherwise tense Cold War stand-off between the Western and the Eastern bloc countries. D. A. Henderson, who led the intensified smallpox eradication campaign between 1967 and 1977, later drew attention to this aspect of the campaign, calling smallpox eradication a 'Cold War Victory', which saw many smallpox and public health officials work together across the Cold War divide.[33]

Whatever the mix of political motives involved, the vote in 1959 did not translate into real support – to the irritation of the USSR. Smallpox at WHO 'had no dedicated budget, no deadline, organizational structure, or management structure'.[34] For many years, the entire staff in Geneva consisted of two people – a physician and a secretary. The first report by the Expert Committee on Smallpox, outlining the strategies to be followed to achieve smallpox eradication, did not appear until five years later, in 1964.[35] Even after 1966, when the WHO finally agreed to intensify the worldwide eradication effort against smallpox, and establish a separate budget for the purpose, the organization continued to rely on voluntary contributions, which meant that to the end, funding was never enough or to be relied upon.

As a backdrop to this apparent inertia, we have to remember that throughout the 1950s and '60s the worldwide malaria eradication programme was consuming by far the largest portion of WHO's financial and technical resources – one third of the total between 1955 and 1970.[36] The rise, and eventual fall, of the malaria eradication programme must be kept in mind when considering the history of smallpox eradication; not until WHO began to scale back malaria work from eradication to malaria control in the late 1960s did the organization turn its attention to other programmes and strategies, launching the intensified smallpox programme.

Until then, PAHO was on its own when it came to smallpox, at least for the duration of Soper's three terms of office between 1947 and 1958. From

1948–64 PAHO itself spent $600,000 on smallpox eradication in the Americas, a modest sum but a sizeable outlay from its overall budget.[37] Sanjoy Battacharya, who has written an excellent and detailed history of the long haul to achieve complete smallpox eradication in India, from the colonial period until the last case in the most smallpox-infected country in the world, is right when he says that for most of its history, the international eradication programme was not a well-coordinated campaign, and certainly not well-coordinated by WHO.[38] As with malaria eradication, we need to start telling the story from the bottom, or national level, up, rather from the international level down.

This is an important point to make in light of the sharp criticisms some of the PAHO countries later came in for from WHO experts – criticism of the slow pace of PAHO efforts to coordinate smallpox eradication campaigns across the South American continent where smallpox was still endemic; of the methods the countries had used, or failed to use; of the reluctance of many working on smallpox to accept new strategies when they appeared; of the unreliable quality of vaccine produced in the region's laboratories – in short, of PAHO's overall failure to eradicate smallpox in the Americas on its own. The most insistent critique came after 1967 and was directed largely against Brazil, by this time by far the largest source of smallpox cases in the Western Hemisphere, for being slow to shift away from the established method of mass vaccination campaigns recommended by WHO experts for years, and embrace the new 'surveillance-containment' approach that had emerged during the intensified period.[39]

As usual, hindsight makes judgement easy, and the criticisms are a bit unfair. Even Dr William Foege, who first discovered the method of 'surveillance-containment' in late 1967 while working for WHO in Nigeria, did not at first think it would be *the* crucial method which would put the final end to smallpox; like others, he saw it as a method that would work in conjunction with, not a substitute for, mass vaccination. It took some time before people realized that 'putting out a fire' by jumping on each smallpox outbreak, isolating victims in their homes, tracing all their contacts and concentrating on vaccinating them, rather than the entire population, might be the most efficient way to get rid of smallpox. It was, in effect, a re-discovery, or better, a modification of the Leicester method, as many people have subsequently recognized.[40] In Leicester, identification and notification, followed by isolation of smallpox patients, was devised as a method to contain smallpox without forcing people to be vaccinated, and it worked pretty well. Vaccination was used in the intensified phase of eradication after 1967, but the 80, 90 or even 100 per cent coverage originally recommended was found not to be necessary to stamp out the transmission of smallpox virus.

But as the authors of WHO's semi-official account, *Smallpox and its Eradication* acknowledged, if systematically carried out, 'it would appear that mass vaccination alone resulted, or probably would probably have resulted, in the elimination of smallpox in South America and most African countries' even without the new surveillance-containment methods, if not in the very high incidence countries like India, Bangladesh, Indonesia and Pakistan.[41]

PAHO on its Own: Soper's Smallpox Years

When Soper took charge of trying to implement PAHO's resolution to eradicate smallpox in the Americas, he was of course fully primed on the cost-benefit arguments in favour of eradication over mere control, having in effect defined the terms himself. He had not shown any particular interest in smallpox as a candidate for eradication before, but his election to head up PAHO in 1947 happened to have occurred just before the 'ill-advised, chaotic' mass vaccination campaign in New York City erupted in response to a single imported smallpox case.[42] These events drew his attention because they made evident to him the complete failure of the Pan American Sanitary Code, under which PAHO operated, to prevent the spread of smallpox from country to country in the western hemisphere.

Soper's first thought was to do something about the glycerinated liquid smallpox vaccine generally used at the time; it was known to deteriorate rapidly in the tropical or neo-tropical environments that existed in many areas in Latin America. Learning about a freeze-dried vaccine that had been used extensively by the French and Dutch authorities in their overseas colonies in the 1920s and 1940s, but which had never been taken up in the Americas, Soper turned to the National Institutes of Health in Washington, to see if they could find a way to produce such a vaccine for use in the Americas. They in turn farmed out the problem to the Michigan State Laboratory, which by the end of 1949 had 50,000 doses of freeze-dried vaccine ready for field tests. The tests were carried out in Peru, where it was found that the freeze-dried kind was indeed superior to the liquid glycinerated vaccine.[43] The availability of this new tool was a significant factor in the decision by the Pan American Sanitary Conference in 1950 to announce a hemisphere-wide campaign to eradicate smallpox. The main work of PAHO was to set up freeze-dried equipment and technical training.[44]

In terms of the numbers of cases involved, smallpox eradication in the Americas seemed a feasible proposition. The long history of smallpox vaccination in Latin America, from its introduction early in the nineteenth century, to the middle of the twentieth century, was a history of sporadic and usually unsystematic implementation. Over the decades, a mix of rapid vaccination when smallpox threatened to be epidemic, with some routine vaccination and/or nation-wide occasional mass vaccination campaigns, had resulted in a steady secular decline in the number of smallpox cases in the region. While tens of thousands of cases had occurred annually up through the 1930s, vaccination services, erratic and varied though they were, had by 1950 eliminated smallpox from Central America, the Caribbean islands, the Guianas, Panama and Chile, while Mexico had managed to reduce the number of cases drastically (and got rid of the disease by 1951). In Venezuela, a national vaccination campaign in 1946–7 had ended smallpox transmission there.

At the same time, smallpox was still endemic in several countries – for instance, in Peru, Colombia, Argentina, Paraguay and, above all, in Brazil. These countries presented a constant source of imported cases into the other countries in the region. Sudden epidemics could break out in countries that had not had cases of smallpox for decades. Cuba, for instance, had been free of smallpox since 1904, but over the decades the island's vaccination rates had fallen steadily, and vulnerability to imported cases of smallpox went up. In 1949, the almost inevitable happened – there was an outbreak of three cases, all imported; in a reprise of what had happened in New York City two years earlier, these few cases led to the rapid vaccination of 1,500,000 people. Then, once more, complacency returned, such that by 1959 only 10 per cent of Cubans were vaccinated out of a population of seven million.[45]

Thus getting rid of smallpox in the few remaining endemic countries seemed a sensible thing to do. The standard and recommended method for eradicating smallpox completely in the space of a short period of, say, a few years, was mass vaccination, backed by some form of compulsory legislation. The target figure was usually set at coverage of at least 80 per cent of the population within three to five years. In 1964, the first report by WHO's Expert Committee on Smallpox Eradication set the figure even higher, indicating a coverage rate of 100 per cent of the population.[46] The recommendation was based on experience with smallpox in India, where, in situations of extremely dense populations and very high incidence of smallpox, vaccination rates even above 80 per cent were deemed simply not high enough to halt smallpox's spread. But it was realized later that even the 80 per cent coverage rates asked for were not backed up by sound epidemiological evidence; India's vaccination coverage rate was actually much lower than 80 per cent. The figure of 80 per cent was 'an arbitrary one, intended to indicate what could be reasonably expected in a well-conducted campaign'.[47] Many countries in fact managed to interrupt smallpox transmission with coverage levels far lower than this. The rationale for the high coverage was that the vaccination rates in populations in countries where smallpox was still endemic were either low or unknown; in the circumstances, aiming to vaccinate absolutely everyone was the safest and easiest way to achieve the ends desired.

Soper was not a man given to research; as we know, to him public health was all about bridging the gap between existing knowledge, and its application. Approached this way, the problem at hand no doubt seemed fairly straightforward: a vaccine that worked in tropical conditions was available, whose application was a matter of planning and rigorous supervision of the work being done. Carrying out further epidemiological or other research into smallpox did not seem necessary. Soper had some experience managing large-scale vaccination efforts, having supervised the testing and then the widespread introduction of the yellow fever vaccine in Brazil in the late 1930s and early 1940s. He was also a superb administrator, demanding discipline, accuracy in reporting, and constant inspection of the inspectors.

But at PAHO the circumstances were very different from those that had existed when he was running yellow fever eradication in Brazil before the war. Apart from the fact that the executive budget was small, and PAHO was engaged in promoting many other health programmes in the region, Soper had to coordinate smallpox eradication at second-hand – with results that were not always what he wanted, as we have seen with yellow fever. He had to accept that PAHO itself did not have the funds or the appetite to join directly in intensive, mass vaccination campaigns. His role as Director had to be to persuade national governments to sign up to the task of undertaking mass vaccination campaigns, to urge cooperation between them, and advise where possible on technical matters.

His greatest challenge was to try to coordinate the roughly simultaneous conduct of numerous national mass vaccination efforts. The difficulty was that these national efforts did not and could not amount to a unitary campaign. Even more, perhaps, than in malaria eradication, they were instead separate endeavours, each shaped by local contingencies, each of them taking place within a country's distinctive political and economic circumstances, and reflecting its particular political struggles with inadequate technical resources and financing, lack of continuity in public health administration and inadequate vaccine supplies.

Several other problems challenged smallpox eradication on Soper's watch. One was getting an accurate picture of the actual scope of the smallpox problem. The small numbers of smallpox cases registered in the Americas gave confidence that complete eradication might be feasible. The WHO, for instance, received official notification of only 88,618 cases from fifteen countries and territories in Latin America for the entire period between 1949 and 1959.[48] The trouble was, the figures were wrong; they represented a serious under-count, because of failures in systems of reporting or checking, or the failure of many rural areas to report at all, owing to the complete absence of rural health facilities. The problem was not unique to Latin America; in India it was estimated that probably less than 2 per cent of all smallpox cases ever made their way into the official statistics, even though in India, most cases were of *Variola major*.[49] The problem was compounded in Latin America by the fact that the less severe variant of smallpox, *Variola minor*, had by the late 1930s replaced the severe form almost everywhere in the continent. This lowered the risk of deaths from smallpox, but also lowered the disease's visibility, both as a public health priority, and practically, in that it made cases harder to track down. Because the symptoms were usually mild, the infection had a low death rate, and in many cases people simply lived through their infections, without coming to the attention of public health authorities. Eradication required systems of surveillance and detection, something missing in most countries until the very end stage of the eradication effort. Usually, in the rush to meet their quotas, vaccinators had no time to spend on searching out every last case in an area. Not until well after 1967, when the intensified phase of the smallpox eradication effort began, did rigorous systems of surveillance and reporting begin to get put in place to ensure that all smallpox cases were indeed discovered and ring-fenced with vaccination.

Given the character of smallpox in Latin America, governments were in effect being asked to devote resources and personnel in a massive way to eradicate a disease that was simply not their greatest disease burden or highest priority. Many of these governments were also simultaneously involved in running other eradication campaigns, such as the campaign against the *Aedes aegypti* mosquito of yellow fever, and after 1954, the campaign to interrupt malaria transmission. We have to remember that the bulk of the costs of all these eradication campaigns was being borne by often impoverished national budgets, siphoning resources and personnel from what the governments thought were more urgent health needs. Cooperation between national governments and the Regional Office at PAHO was not always easy.

Three other issues plagued the smallpox eradication campaigns in Latin America (and elsewhere): vaccine production, vaccine quality and vaccine delivery. Vaccine was eventually put into production in several national laboratories in Latin America, but for a long time supplies remained inadequate, as did quality. Some countries continued to use liquid vaccine despite its problems, because they could not get hold of the freeze-dried form; the freeze-dried vaccine, in turn, was frequently contaminated with bacteria.[50] Later, many laboratories failed to send their vaccines for testing at the reference laboratories that were designated by WHO in 1966 (in Canada and the Netherlands) to ensure basic standards of potency and purity; when they did send them, they were often shown not to meet international standards. The Oswaldo Cruz Institute in Brazil, the leading biomedical institution in the country and one of the main producers of smallpox vaccine for the entire region, 'never did succeed in producing a consistently satisfactory product', according to the official WHO history of smallpox eradication.[51] The facilities were often lacking in equipment, supplies, and adequate staffing.

The method of applying the vaccine was also not satisfactory. Initially, the old-fashioned rotating lance was used, which could be painful. In the 1960s, an electric jet injector that allowed far more vaccinations to be made per day was tested and then employed in Latin America, but the device proved at times too elaborate for use in the field (even after a mechanical model was adopted to overcome problems with electricity supply in rural areas). Much more effective was the simple, bifurcated needle which was introduced in 1965, several years after Soper had left PAHO; this was designed so as to place exactly the right dosage of vaccine between its two prongs, thus allowing much more efficient use of the available vaccine, and much less loss. Yet even to the end, there was considerable variation in how vaccine was delivered, and much of the vaccine was wasted.

Year after year, Soper reported to the PAHO Directing Council on the status of smallpox eradication in the Americas; he tried to put a good face on PAHO's efforts, but increasingly had to acknowledge the lack of overall progress towards the desired goal of elimination. In 1957, in a quadrennial review of the work of PAHO presented to the member governments, Soper cited the Colombian case to epitomize the problems national campaigns faced. Colombia was ranked one of the most smallpox-burdened of the Latin American countries in the 1950s; since 1948 vaccination programmes, as well as other public health services, had been interrupted repeatedly owing to the quasi-civil war that wracked the country. It was not until 1955 that Colombia was able to launch a mass vaccination campaign, basing it on compulsory vaccination for every person in the population over three months of age. At the time it was estimated that ten million people were without vaccination and susceptible to smallpox (luckily the form was 'alastrim', the name given in the region to the mild kind). But in a country of great rural poverty, poor transport and poor communications, the barriers to rapid success were considerable. Starting in October of 1955, by the end of 1957 only 2.5 million vaccinations of the 10 million needed had been carried out (compare this with the several million people vaccinated in New York in a few weeks in 1947).[52] During the campaign, no effort was made to ascertain the 'take rates' of vaccination or to register which people were receiving their first, or primary vaccination, and which their secondary or re-vaccination. The goal was to simply vaccinate everyone who showed up, regardless of their vaccination status.

To achieve maximum coverage, a system of assembly points was used rather than the more painstaking and costly house-to-house methods adopted later in India. Via radio, posters and newspapers, people were informed about when to get themselves to an assembly point, established as a distance of not more than a few miles by foot from where they lived, on a designated day, in order to present themselves and their children to visiting teams of vaccinators. These vaccinators were sometimes the only health visitors the local population met. Where possible, re-vaccination of everyone was supposed to be conducted three or four years later.

Vaccination was not then the routine part of basic health services that it is now – indeed, there were no basic health services as such in many impoverished and rural areas; so smallpox eradication was an exceptional measure, done by special teams of vaccinators organized for the job. Everything depended on their thoroughness and reliability. Unfortunately, vaccination was often a hit and miss affair, with little record keeping, or follow up. Given the history of resistance to smallpox vaccination in Europe, and worries about its side-effects and risks, it is interesting how silent the official PAHO accounts are on these aspects of the mass vaccination efforts. There appears to have been little coercion, unlike in India in the final phases of the smallpox eradication campaign, perhaps because there was also little urgency in the approach to smallpox in Latin America.[53] No mention appears either about fatalities from vaccination itself. In a rare reference to this in the massive 'official' account of worldwide eradication, it was stated that in smallpox endemic countries where eradication was being carried out, the risk of smallpox usually outweighed the risk of post-vaccination encephalitis; moreover, though cases of post-vaccinial encephalitis 'undoubtedly occurred', there were anyway so many other prevalent illnesses that could produce cerebral symptoms, such as malaria, that it was difficult to attribute such sequelae to smallpox vaccination itself, or other causes – a rather casual approach to the issue, it would seem, given the seriousness with which such post-vaccination sequelae were taken in Western countries.[54]

As Soper attended his final Pan American Sanitary Conference as Director of PAHO in 1958, he reiterated his confidence in the possibility of smallpox eradication – but had to admit that thus far smallpox was still only very partially achieved. He could report sharp reductions in incidence in Mexico, Peru and Venezuela – but in other places mass vaccination was far from over, and in Brazil, the place with by far the highest incidence, a smallpox eradication campaign had not even started (and would not start until the 1960s).

If only smallpox had involved insects in its transmission! One feels this would have given greater zest to his endeavours. On leaving PAHO for good at the end of 1958, Soper nonetheless tried to put a good face on the matter, emphasizing that the financial expenditure required for the completion of the eradication of smallpox in the Americas 'was relatively modest when compared to the enormous cost of eradicating other diseases'.[55] In this, at least, he would be proved right.

New Outlooks in International Public Health

The Chilean physician Abraham Barak Horwitz (1910–2000) was elected in 1958 to succeed Soper as director of PAHO – the first Latin American to hold the position in PAHO's more than half a century of existence. Horwitz went on to serve four consecutive terms in office, more than any other person before or after him.

Horwitz was a very different man from Soper, with a different orientation in public health. With him, in fact, came a new tone and new ideas in international public health work. As the 1950s gave way to the 1960s, new narratives of 'health and development' emerged, replacing eradication in popularity. Horwitz was very much in tune with this new trend; his background was in both clinical medicine and public health, and this gave him a concern for the routine problems of people's general ill-health, the clinical effects of malnutrition, and the socio-economic sources of sickness that Soper lacked. His main interests lay in epidemiology, nutrition and basic sanitation. Like many other Latin American doctors of the period, he had trained in public health at Johns Hopkins University in 1944 on a Rockefeller fellowship, returning from there to head Chile's School of Public Health. He also worked as assistant director of standards for Chile's national health service, as well as on the smallpox eradication effort in Chile.

Horwitz brought a different emphasis to PAHO, stressing in his reports and speeches the importance of developing systems of basic health care, of improving nutrition and children's health and of taking a broader, more social and economic view of the causes of ill-health than the purely biological or medical. Tying these together was the concept of 'development' and how it could be made to meet Latin America's basic needs. Development had of course, many meanings; in the United States, as noted already, the concept was closely tied to the Cold War and to policies aimed at countering communist influence in the US's 'backyard'. Without shedding these Cold War links, the new emphasis on social and economic development in PAHO discourse represented a concern within a more Latin-America-inflected organization to move beyond the post-war emphasis on the control and/or eradication of communicable diseases, and towards a greater effort to grapple with the problems of basic, routine health services.

One reason for the shift was the rapid growth in WHO's membership, which nearly doubled between 1948 and the late 1960s. Given the voting structure of the organization, this meant that the voices of post-colonial and developing countries began to be heard more often in WHO's deliberations. As Godlee points out, the change probably inevitably meant a more political and/or politically contentious WHO.[56] Eradication campaigns could be presented by the Western funders as a-political technical initiatives that would somehow float above or outside the political fray (though of course they never did). But trying to devise fundamental health services in poor countries was another matter and was bound to be very controversial, given the divisions of the Cold War. The United States, for instance, was vociferously opposed to anything it viewed as socialized medicine. But recommending, devising or planning basic health services from Geneva meant making political choices, however one looked at them. There was a growing consensus within WHO that this was the direction WHO had to move in – that something more fundamental had to be done to meet the health needs of poor nations than supporting a series of eradication campaigns.

Horwitz was attuned to this shift in emphasis. In 1961, for example, he singled out for praise the Charter of Punta del Este, an agreement signed by representatives from around Latin America at the resort town in Uruguay in August that year. The Charter was part of President Kennedy's *Alliance for Progress* (announced in March 1961) and was therefore very much a product of the Cold War and America's determination to keep Latin America in its sphere of influence. The aims were large – to increase the economic growth of Latin America, to reduce inequality, to transform agriculture and to improve health. Needless to say, most of these vaunted goals remained unmet. Nevertheless, to Horwitz and many Latin Americans, the Charter did at least seem to signal new attitudes and new initiatives in public health policy, laying out specific targets of a broadly social nature, such as providing potable water and sewage disposal to not less than 70 per cent of the urban and 50 per cent of the rural populations; to Horwitz, this represented what he called an historic effort to accelerate social and economic growth in Latin America.[57] In the 1970s, a more radical notion of 'social medicine' emerged, signalling a more profound change in outlook within WHO that culminated in the well-known *Declaration of Alma-Ata* of 1978, which placed Primary Health Care squarely at the centre of WHO's philosophy. These later changes in international public health are taken up more fully in chapter Seven.

The Charter of Punta del Este included the eradication of disease among its various goals. But how was eradication to be achieved – through separate and autonomous campaigns, as Soper had always insisted, or as an integral part of the basic health services of a country? Horowitz thought the latter.

Many people at WHO had hoped that the malaria eradication campaign would leave a legacy in the form of a core organization with technical expertise that could provide the framework for building more general health services; but experience was already showing that, on the contrary, it was the pre-existence of such basic health care services that allowed eradication campaigns to succeed.[58] This was particularly true of malaria, a chronic, rural disease closely connected to poverty and local environmental factors.

Soper, of course, objected to any such talk of merging eradication campaigns with what he said were often non-existent basic health services, calling the idea a 'definite attack on the special mass campaign dedicated to the eradication of a given disease'. He thought that waiting while such services were built up, and postponing tackling communicable but preventable diseases, was unacceptable. He acknowledged there was a fundamental conflict between the two philosophies, but saw only the advantages of the mass campaign, with its single disease focus, its clearly defined objective, and its national coverage. He referred in disparaging terms to the 'smug satisfaction' rich countries took in their superior health services and low incidence of communicable diseases, and the block he believed this put on their awareness of the needs of poor countries, which had no basic services and a high incidence of communicable but preventable diseases.[59]

In the unpublished document from which I have drawn these remarks, Soper made a rare reference to René Dubos, signalling his awareness of another current of thought that was leading many people to reject his eradicationist philosophy – the ecological.[60]

Dubos was a French-born bacteriologist working at the Rockefeller Institute for Medical Research (his isolation of anti-bacterial substances from microorganisms in the soil led to the discovery of antibiotics), who over time had become increasingly interested in the more general problems of human health in relation to ecology and the environment. His popular books, such as *Mirage of Health: Utopias, Progress and Biological Change* (1959) and *Mankind Adapting* (1965), coincided roughly with the publication of Rachel's Carson's *Silent Spring* (1962) but had a different focus. They were widely influential in the biological community for introducing a dynamic view of disease in human populations that linked the social and the biological within an ecological and evolutionary framework. Over time, Dubos became a visionary public figure, and a radical critic not only of public health as it was practiced at the time, but of urban life and of capitalism more generally. The hallmark of Dubos' ecological viewpoint was complexity: there were, he argued, multiple points of inter-connection and influence between all living things, their natural environments, and also their social environments (human beings and their activities). From his ecological point of view, it was impossible to extract one element – a vector, say, or a pathogen – and try to deal with it in isolation from all the other organisms in its ecological niche to which it is connected.

To Dubos, this ecological outlook necessarily undermined projects such as disease eradication or vector eradication, since they failed to take into account the dynamic and continuous processes by which pathogens (and therefore diseases) interacted and adapted through genetic and behavioural modifications. Dubos was critical of eradicationism precisely because it overlooked the biological and social dynamics of diseases in human society: 'Eradication of microbial disease is a will-o'-the-wisp', he wrote, and 'pursuing it leads to a morass of hazy biological concepts and half-truths'.[61]

This was not just a matter of saying 'diseases are always with us', or that pathogens and vectors are hard to eliminate. It was suggesting that a method of public health that did not engage with the ecological aspects of disease was inadequate and misguided. Control or reduction of disease, in this regard, was far preferable to eradication. Detailed knowledge of ecology allowed subtle manipulations of the environment (such as planting shady trees to stop sun-loving anopheles mosquitoes from breeding) that would help control disease, without the brutal sledgehammer of chemicals. To Dubos and others like him, Soper's style of eradication was a blunt instrument that paid no attention to ecology at all. In Dubos's view, eradication was doomed to fail.

In this he was shown to be wrong – the eradication of at least one disease, smallpox, was in fact achieved. Other ecologists, some of them the founders of the discipline, were also more open to disease eradication than Dubos – the idea that there was a hard and fast opposition between the two outlooks is historically incorrect.[62] Nevertheless, the ecological approach tended to stress the complexity of diseases and their control, and helps explain why so many eradication campaigns failed; they overlooked the changing, dynamic character of local environments and the need for constant adjustment of policies to altered circumstances. A generation of physicians and biologists were alerted to the limitations of the eradicationist approach by Dubos's writings; they 'held the opinion that it was impossible to separate a wild microbe from the ecological web it lived in'.[63]

Soper, as we know, had little patience for such views. One young RF scientist, David E. Davis, describes how, on arriving in Rio de Janeiro in 1942 to explore whether birds might be involved in the long-distance spread of jungle yellow fever, Soper requested from him a plan of action. Presented with one for the study of ecology, Soper asked, 'What's ecology?' He then proceeded to demolish Davis's ideas 'unmercifully', but in response to Davis's stout defence of his plan, Soper, with typical generosity, proposed first a game of ping-pong, and then invited him home to dinner.[64] This catches the assertive nature of Soper, but also his good humour. A few years later, in

1946, Soper wrote to John Logan, who was then in charge of the Sardinia eradication experiment, that he regretted that the very word 'ecology' had ever been invented. Logan countered (in a letter to the Director of the IHD), 'We would have been better off if we had not heard of Egypt and Brazil' – referring to Soper's early successes in vector eradication which set so much of the stage for his wholesale adoption of absolute eradication in the post-war years.[65]

Horwitz, as we have seen in chapter Four, was much more receptive to the ecological outlook, but nevertheless, as Director of PAHO, and having inherited several eradication campaigns, he thought there was no other course but to press forward, rather than give up, in the face of delays and setbacks.[66]

The question remained: how was the smallpox eradication effort to be made to work? Here Horwitz took a more critical stance towards the ongoing smallpox eradication efforts in Latin America than Soper had done, anticipating in fact some of the criticisms that others at WHO involved with the intensified phase would make later. Horwitz, for instance, recognized that the official figures from Latin American countries on smallpox cases were inaccurate. Reporting on the status of smallpox eradication in the Americas at a Havana meeting of PAHO in the summer of 1960, less than two years into his job as director, Horwitz informed the delegates that it was widely known that the official figures on cases in the Americas were lower than the true figures, and that smallpox in the region was 'inexcusably high'.[67] He realized there had to be systems of detection and retrospective reporting; unlike Soper, Horwitz was a trained epidemiologist, who in 1964 was already calling for epidemiological surveillance services in places where smallpox eradication had been completed or was still in progress.[68] He also continued to urge governments to integrate their smallpox vaccination services with their basic health services wherever it was possible.

Horwitz was also concerned about the lack of adequate smallpox vaccine to run the eradication campaigns. He estimated Latin America needed a total of 45 million doses a year – whereas in the year of greatest production thus far, only 23 million doses had been produced. Since few countries had donated smallpox vaccine to the WHO apart from the USSR (whose vaccines went mainly to India), the laboratories in the PAHO countries had to step up production if they were to meet their targets. Horwitz pointed out that there was also little reporting on 'take' rates, that is, the efficiency of the vaccines being used; compounding the vaccine problem was vaccine wastage because of a lack of technical skill. In the circumstances, no one should be surprised, he said, if the region of the Americas saw continued outbreaks of smallpox.

From Mexico, however, Horwitz had better news to report, as well as an interesting shift in strategy. The country was still performing general smallpox vaccinations, but it had begun to concentrate its efforts in places where smallpox cases actually occurred, rather than aiming for blanket coverage even in areas where there was no evidence of smallpox. Many places did not meet the 90 per cent immunity indices deemed necessary, yet they had no smallpox – suggesting that perhaps mass vaccination was not the answer to smallpox eradication. 'If the countries that still have foci concentrate their attention on them, surely they will soon be free of the virus. Then they can put vaccination on a regular basis in all those other places where smallpox virus no longer exists.' Here, in germ, were some of the elements of what later became the 'surveillance-containment' strategy, namely concentrating vaccination around the hotspots first, in order to interrupt transmission.[69]

But things continued to move forward only slowly. Like Soper and other Regional directors of WHO, Horwitz found getting cooperation between PAHO and the various Ministers of Health was not always easy; 'mutual collaboration', he reported, 'had not yet been attained'.[70] Reasons of priority, and political, financial and administrative factors, singly or in combination, he judged responsible for the failure to move faster. Brazil at this point had only *proposed* to vaccinate 46 million people in six years; but in the first nine months of 1964 it had managed to vaccinate just over five million – not a lot. Moreover, the figure of only 300 cases of smallpox Brazil reported for the previous year had to be later corrected to over 6,000 cases, that is, twenty times more cases than had been originally stated. By this point, in 1965, sufficient vaccine was apparently being produced to undertake or complete systematic programmes of immunization of 210 million people in the region – but only about 21 million were actually vaccinated that year, that is, only 10 per cent.[71] Given the small total number of smallpox cases and the vast size of the population, we can see in retrospect that targeted vaccination, ring-fencing just those areas where smallpox was most likely to be transmitted to others, would have been much better than vaccinating millions, but mass vaccination was the sanctioned method at the time.

Horwitz, one feels, was growing weary with the persistently unresolved character of the smallpox problem. By 1969, thirteen different smallpox eradication resolutions had followed PAHO's original resolution in 1950 – with yet no end in sight.[72] A Dr Watts, attending a meeting of the PAHO in 1967 as a US delegate, agreed; he was discouraged, he said by the numerous resolutions that were 'essentially repetitive in nature and promising little progress'.[73] Dr Marcolino Candau, the Director-General of WHO, seconded the general complaint; they could not go on like this, he said, 'each year producing beautiful resolutions which offered goodwill but gave little promise of solving the basic problem'. The time had come, he said, 'for countries to decide what they were willing to do to eradicate smallpox, a disease which is, along with other quarantinable diseases, the chief reason for the existence of the international health organization'.[74]

But this was a bit disingenuous; Candau had never been enthusiastic about a global smallpox eradication campaign.[75] Though many national governments since 1958 had committed a considerable proportion of their scarce resources to their national smallpox vaccination programmes despite having other health priorities, WHO itself had not been able to find the money or the political will to fulfill its pledge; between 1960 and 1966 it put only 0.2 per cent of the organization's regular budget, and 0.6 per cent of its disposable budget, into smallpox eradication.[76] Something more than this had to be done if smallpox was going to be made to disappear.

The Intensified Eradication Campaign, 1967–79

Something was. In 1967, WHO finally launched what came to be known as the Intensified Smallpox Eradication Programme, with the result that smallpox disappeared completely throughout the world in what seems in retrospect a remarkably short time. The last naturally occurring case was identified in 1977. Two further years of careful surveillance were needed before all the different WHO regions were formally certified as being free of the disease, with a worldwide announcement being made to that effect in 1980.

Yet even with the intensification of effort, the money was often inadequate, and the eradication campaign was buffeted by political events, conflicts, and poor vaccine. Success depended on many factors, some serendipitous; as Henderson, who led the intensified campaign said, the outcome was in doubt until the very last case.

The turn in events started in 1966, when for the first time delegates to the Nineteenth World Health Assembly voted narrowly to set up a dedicated budget for smallpox eradication. This was followed in 1967 by a vote in favour of launching a real global eradication programme, with an expected duration of ten years. At this point, there were still 44 countries reporting the presence of smallpox, and 21 in which smallpox was endemic. The worldwide total number of smallpox cases reported officially each year was small (131,000 in 1967), but the number was known to be a tremendous under-count; the actual annual incidence was estimated at being somewhere between ten to twenty million cases.[77]

The suspected incidence of smallpox was so high in places like India, in fact, that many experts still believed smallpox would never be eradicated – that the vote for the programme was just another rhetorical exercise. No epidemiologist opposed smallpox eradication in principle, one scientist commented, but it had to be recognized for what it was, 'a hope, a laudable ambition, a goal to which to aspire but which, for even the first infection in man, is a long way ahead'.[78]

Meanwhile the actual money set aside for smallpox eradication remained small, far too small to do the job. The bulk of the money (estimated at a cost of $180 million to eradicate smallpox worldwide in the next decade, starting in 1967) was expected to come not from WHO's regular budget, but from the outside. This meant voluntary donations, with the bulk of the costs being borne by national governments – 30 per cent from donations, and 70 per cent from the countries carrying out the campaigns. For the first several years of the intensified campaign, the voluntary donations were tiny – Barrett gives a grand total of $79,500 donated in cash between 1967 and 1973. After 1974, voluntary donations increased, eventually just under $1 million dollars being donated from international sources.[79] In the end smallpox eradication was achieved at a cost of $300 million.

One outcome of World Health Assembly's vote was to bring in a talented director and an increase in technical staff. According to Tucker, Candau, the Director-General of WHO, was quite annoyed with the decision by the delegates to go forward with smallpox eradication, as he remained convinced it would fail and further discredit the WHO's reputation. At Candau's insistence, Dr Donald A. Henderson was seconded from the US's Center for Disease Control (CDC) in Atlanta to lead the intensified programme from WHO's headquarters in Geneva. Henderson had been working at the CDC as the head of surveillance in the Epidemic Intelligence Service, and had already been involved in smallpox issues. Acting swiftly, Henderson arrived in Geneva in late 1966, and by November of 1967 already had the programme up and running.

Henderson's appointment to lead the intensified campaign from Geneva indicates the special role the CDC was to play in the final smallpox eradication effort. The CDC, which had been established by the US government during the Second World War as a branch of the United Public Health Service in charge of malaria control, had become the leading domestic agency responsible for epidemiological intelligence and disease investigation within the US after the war. Its work also led it to various short-term projects overseas (for example, in testing the jet injector in Jamaica and Brazil), but its role in smallpox was on a different scale and was the result of an unexpected development.

In May 1965, President Johnson's White House announced that the US would support the effort to eradicate smallpox worldwide, aiming to achieve it within a decade. This announcement provided an opening to transform an existing USAID-funded programme of measles vaccination in Western and

North Africa into a measles and smallpox vaccination project; Henderson, for one, had not thought measles was an eradicable disease, whereas smallpox, in principle, was. Ogden, in his history of the CDC's smallpox 'crusade', notes that President Johnson's endorsement of US involvement in worldwide smallpox eradication was the result of 'patient persuasion' by the US Public Health Service, led by Henderson.[80] Once a financial commitment by the US government was forthcoming for a five-year project, with a launch date of 1967, smallpox eradication picked up steam. Soper, busy as a consultant, was thrilled. Writing to thank President Johnson for his support, he made the point that smallpox eradication was already so far advanced that smallpox-free countries could not fail 'in their own interest, to see the job through to the finish'.[81] Here was an implicit reference to a cost-benefit calculation.

And in fact the US at this point had more than enough reason to put real money into smallpox eradication, since the burdens, financial and medical, of maintaining routine smallpox vaccination were already clearly outweighing the benefits. This point was brought home to the CDC by a clinical pediatrician, Dr C. Henry Kempe, who ran a pediatric department in Denver, Colorado, which served as a national referral centre in the US for all cases of side-effects from smallpox vaccination. Kempe had been corresponding with the CDC on this subject for some time. He had already advocated terminating routine smallpox vaccination of the civilian population in the United States because, according to his calculations, between 1948 and 1965 there had been some 200–300 deaths in children as a result of complications, such as encephalitis, following vaccinia vaccination, but only a single death from smallpox itself in the same period. The CDC, after thinking Dr Kempe a bit of a fanatic on the subject, concluded, after their own studies, that he was, in fact, right.[82]

But to give up routine vaccination in smallpox-free countries, when smallpox was still endemic in many places overseas, carried risks; hence the need to complete the job of global eradication. In his letter to President Johnson, Soper added a further Cold War argument; the USSR, he told the President, 'has registered disappointment with the limited support given to smallpox eradication in the last seven years' – all the more reason, he seemed to be implying, for the US to step up its contributions and get the job done, presumably winning allies in the third world in doing so.[83]

With the US decision made, Henderson quickly assembled a number of short-term consultants to work in the field, giving technical advice. Many of them had acquired operational experience in West Africa, which gave them a good introduction to the challenges of running mass vaccination efforts in countries where there were poor communications and transport systems, and difficult geographical terrain. Like Soper and Horwitz before him, Henderson learned that coordinating eradication efforts across such a wide spectrum of countries was not an easy job; each country had its own way of organizing mass vaccination campaigns, and faced its own problems, which ran the gamut from disputes over turf, to technical difficulties, to floods and famines and to outright war (for example, the Biafran War in Nigeria that lasted from July 1967 to January 1970, and the war between March and December 1971 between East and West Pakistan that resulted in the creation of Bangladesh as an independent state). Getting the cooperation of the Regional Directors of WHO was another task, and not always an easy one, as they were semi-autonomous and not used to simply accepting instructions from Geneva.

At this point, no new strategies to achieve eradication were put forward, mass vaccination of populations in the endemic countries being the accepted method. It was felt there was a need for better reporting and surveillance (along the lines developed by the CDC's Epidemiological Intelligence Unit), but otherwise the goal was to reduce smallpox to zero incidence through vaccinating 80 per cent or more of the population. Using the assembly point-method, it was hoped that a programme of many national campaigns, conducted in all the remaining endemic countries, could result in the vaccination of some 220 million people in 1967 alone.[84] Henderson wanted to act quickly, and as a result says Ogden, the Intensified Smallpox Eradication Programme was based 'not on time-tested certainties but on best available assumptions', some of which proved to be wrong (as they so often did in eradication campaigns).[85]

Henderson understood the need for operational flexibility, and proved to be a resourceful coordinator who introduced several important changes to the procedures over time. He rejected the charge made by some critics later that WHO's smallpox eradication programme was run in a military, or authoritarian fashion, from the centre out, and insisted that, on the contrary, everything depended on cooperation and the adaptation of procedures to new circumstances. In his account, he emphasized especially the importance of research, something hitherto almost entirely absent in the standardized mass vaccination campaigns. Actually, little money was set aside initially by WHO itself for basic or laboratory investigations – only $20,000 in the 1967 budget.[86] Again, the SEP depended on the nationally funded work in several different laboratories situated in the US, the UK, India and the USSR, among other places. A main concern was to find out whether there were any natural animal reservoirs of variola virus (which of course would have made eradication virtually impossible). The answer was 'no', but only a tentative 'no'.[87]

Epidemiological studies were more significant for the actual work of vaccination. Smallpox had always been considered one of the most contagious diseases in existence, spreading rapidly through populations; but field studies in Africa and in Asia, tracing how smallpox actually passed from person to person, or from village to village, showed to people's surprise that smallpox actually spread rather slowly (it was less contagious, for instance, than measles). It required repeated close contact with a smallpox victim for infection to be transmitted, not just casual contact. Another surprise finding was that in many countries, vaccination rates were much higher, and protection from vaccination longer-lasting than had been thought. Past vaccination efforts, though not eradicating smallpox in many places, had given some community protection against the infection. At this point nearly all the cases of smallpox in an outbreak were in people who had never been vaccinated; young children were especially vulnerable, and eventually they were given priority in vaccination campaigns.[88] Finally, it was discovered that when smallpox epidemics erupted, cases tended to cluster in certain villages, rather than spread out everywhere. This meant that the outbreaks could be terminated by rapid vaccination of all the contacts in the clusters, rather than by saturating a huge population with vaccination. Epidemiological investigations, in short, were going to change how smallpox eradication was actually brought about.

When the intensified programme was launched in 1967 attention was focused especially on what were considered the remaining 'key sites' of smallpox. In Latin America this meant Brazil; if this country got rid of smallpox, the entire Americas would be smallpox-free. In Southeast Asia, Pakistan (and Bangladesh, after its independence in 1973), India and Indonesia were the critical places. In Africa, the key sites were many, including several countries with very high incidences indeed of smallpox.

Yet once the campaigns were launched, progress to the zero point was remarkably rapid. By January, 1969, the number of countries with endemic smallpox had already been reduced to five; the huge country of Nigeria, which was being torn apart by the Biafran War, somehow managed to keep its smallpox eradication campaign going, the country registering its last indigenous case in May 1970. By the end of 1972 a population of 153.5 million people had been vaccinated in the African continent (many more than the estimated total population at that time, indicating that many people had been re-vaccinated). Others countries had similar success; Brazil, for instance, started a federally organized, special service vaccination service in August of 1966, and registered its last case in the country, in the state of Rio de Janeiro, on 19 April 1971. Certification was achieved in Brazil in 1978.

By the autumn of 1973, only four endemic smallpox countries remained in the world – India, Bangladesh, Pakistan and Ethiopia. At various points, each of the four appeared to reach the zero point – only to see smallpox return.

Bangladesh was a particularly difficult case – a major endemic centre. After a tremendous effort, vaccinators thought they had eliminated the disease in 1971 – only to have it explode in epidemic form later that year, during the country's war of secession from Pakistan. The war caused thousands of people to flee Bangladesh for safety in the adjacent Indian state of Bengal to the south; the end of the war then led to their chaotic return to Bangladesh at the end of year, under terrible social and economic conditions, including flooding and famine. The result was a serious epidemic of smallpox, which spread through refugee camps crammed with poor and vulnerable people. It took a year of intense work before smallpox was, once again, eliminated in the country – this time for good. Compulsory vaccination was used at the end-stage, for instance, as a requirement for entry into refugee camps, where food and other goods were distributed to returning refugees. The very last case of smallpox in Asia actually occurred in Bangladesh, in October 1975.

The same pattern of 'almost eradication', followed by unexpected outbreaks, also occurred in India, historically and to the end the country with the highest overall incidence of smallpox. It was, in effect, the world's critical endemic centre of smallpox.[89] Luckily we have several accounts of how the smallpox programme was conducted in India, including an excellent, very detailed, and revisionist one by Sanjoy Battacharya.[90] My purpose here is not to go over this story in any detail, but to comment on a few of the salient features of what was, after all, the single largest smallpox programme in the entire WHO-sponsored eradication effort.

India was a very large and diverse country, ethnically, religiously and linguistically; in the 1960s its huge population was still overwhelmingly rural, very poor and scattered across its various states in thousands of small villages and towns. Politically, the country was organized federally, with the major responsibility for public health lying with the individual states, each with its own public health and medical bureaucracy, and each operating semi-autonomously, sometimes in ways that were at odds with the federal centre. Approaching smallpox as a single 'eradication campaign' was, in the circumstances, impossible. Furthermore, at the federal level, the successive Ministers of Health were not all convinced that smallpox was their most important public health problem (compared to tuberculosis, malaria, respiratory infections and diarrhoeas), even though by 1973 the country had 57.7 per cent of the world's smallpox cases.[91]

Battacharya's book describes numerous points of conflict that existed between the Indian authorities and WHO in Geneva, as well as between Indian officials at the state level and the Indian Ministry of Health in Delhi. For instance, Henderson's call to centralize the Indian operations under the federal government was opposed by WHO's Regional Director of WHO for South East Asia (SEARO). WHO consultants sent by Geneva to work on the Indian programme often felt frustrated by events, sending Henderson scathing internal letters and memos, complaining about everything from poor vaccination coverage, the poor conditions of vaccine storage, unreliable reporting and even forged records.[92]

But there was cause for complaint on the Indian side too. As Battacharya says, official accounts by WHO officials tend to give the impression that their administrative apparatus was sufficiently powerful to result in well-executed programs; this 'seriously undermines the huge number of indigenous officials and agencies involved in the day-to-day running of the different elements of the eradication programme'.[93] His point is that the work was done, and the policies were largely set, by local Indian officials, and involved continual adaptation to local conditions, such as the available supply of people to carry out vaccinations. Identifying cases of smallpox was not as straightforward as was often said after the fact; even though the majority of infections were of the severe or major form, there were many kinds of smallpox infections, with different kinds of rashes that were not always easy to distinguish from other diseases (eventually photographic and diagrammatic cards were used to help vaccinators identify the smallpox cases).

In the period 1973–4, the Smallpox Eradication Programme in India was employing about 135,000 workers of all kinds, ranging from public health officials, to private physicians, officials seconded from the anti-malaria programme, and even people involved in family planning, all of them aiming to vaccinate 90 per cent of 129 million households in over 600,000 villages. Setbacks almost inevitably interrupted progress. In 1974, for instance, there was a bad outbreak of smallpox in the extremely poor northern state of Bihar, which was only contained with difficulty. Battacharya refers in fact to the 'faltering approach to "Smallpox zero" status', rejecting any idea of inevitability towards an end-point.[94] The final years of the campaign coincided with the political 'State of Emergency' declared by the then Prime Minister, Indira Gandhi, in 1975, a political intervention by the centre that led to the cancellation of national elections, the imprisonment of many opposition figures, press censorship and authoritarian rule. Henderson seized the opportunity of the emergency and the centralized authority of Indira Gandhi to try to keep up the pressure on eradication and surveillance, so that the job of smallpox eradication could finally be completed. The emergency also allowed compulsion to be used under certain circumstances.[95] By 1975, India still had some 115,000 health workers involved in house-to-house searches for cases of smallpox in each of the country's towns and villages. The last known indigenous case in the country was detected on 17 May 1975.

The very last case of naturally occurring smallpox anywhere in the world was found in Somalia, just over two years later, on 26 October 1977.

'The Realm of the Final Inch'

The phrase, 'the realm of the final inch' was appropriated (and modified) by Henderson from the Russian Alexandr Solzhenitzyn's novel, *First Circle* (1968); Henderson used it to indicate the critical moment that Soper had always singled out in his discussions, when a disease or a vector targeted for eradication has almost disappeared; at this point, the costs per case detected and eliminated go up, just as the visibility of the disease practically disappears.[96] Almost invariably, the urgency of the pursuit vanishes too, vigilance diminishes, controls peter out, and the disease on which so much time and effort had been expended eventually returns.

But absolute eradication was defined by absolute absence. And as Soper knew to his cost, this was very hard to achieve. So what had it taken to push the smallpox campaign on to the magical number of zero? Was it political persistence, better financial and technical resources, better coordination between the different levels of organization, better understanding of smallpox, or new eradication techniques? Were there any lessons for other eradication efforts, or would smallpox remain a unique achievement in the history of absolute eradication, as some people thought?

Two answers stand out from the official and other accounts – political will, and a new strategy that came to be known as 'surveillance-containment'. The first, political will, is a difficult thing to measure and account for, whether at the level of WHO's inner workings, or, just as importantly, at the level of the many governments that were involved. Certainly, Henderson and his consultants showed great determination, in the face of considerable scepticism, to achieve the results asked of them. Henderson was tenacious in putting together the numerous bilateral agreements needed between WHO and national governments to get national vaccination campaigns organized. He was a skillful negotiator, determined, but also tactful enough to overcome the resistance, even at times the opposition, of many public health officials who had reasons, many of them sound from a public health point of view, not to give smallpox eradication the priority demanded by the WHO in Geneva. But political will and determination were attributes of many more people than Henderson and his experts – unsung and unnamed people who participated in their thousands to make smallpox eradication finally work in their own countries. It also characterized many national governments, who put their own money into smallpox eradication, and who, in the end, mustered the political commitment to the cause, because they did not want to disassociate themselves from what had become a worldwide, technical project associated symbolically with the ideas of modernity and progress. As several commentators have pointed out, how could a country that could explode an atomic bomb, as India did in 1974, not get rid of smallpox?

The second factor in smallpox's successful eradication identified in the official accounts is more technical. It refers to a new method introduced in the smallpox campaign in the late 1960s, a method that Henderson and many others came to consider as the key to success in smallpox eradication. Surveillance-containment (S-C) as it came to be called, was first seen as a supplement to, and then eventually a replacement for, mass vaccination. As a technique, it is closely associated with the work of Dr William H. Foege, a CDC consultant who had been working in Nigeria as a medical missionary when he joined the CDC-USAID smallpox project.[97] In December 1966, when an epidemic of smallpox broke out in Ogoja, Nigeria, Foege found himself with insufficient supplies of smallpox vaccine to undertake mass vaccination, and this led him to concentrate on vaccinating people at the site of the epidemic – all those who had had contacts with smallpox; within a short period he found the epidemic had ended. On the basis of this experience, in 1968 Foege proposed that, since smallpox in rural areas spread slowly, and tended to cluster in particular places, vaccinators should concentrate their work on places where outbreaks occur, vaccinating only those people who had had direct contact with smallpox victims. This meant all the victims had to be quickly identified and if possible isolated in their own homes; then each and every person who had been in contact with them had to be tracked down so they could be vaccinated, even after exposure. Using his knowledge of the seasonal fluctuations that occur in smallpox transmission, Foege then generalized the method to propose that, in the future, vaccinators concentrate their efforts on containing outbreaks of smallpox during smallpox's seasonal low-point, when its incidence was lowest; at this time, any outbreaks of smallpox were more obvious and visible, and also easier to manage. In this fashion, smallpox transmission could in effect be 'stamped out'. The undertaking required careful surveillance and reporting methods, but it meant vaccinating a far smaller percentage of the population than mass vaccination techniques.

Foege first presented the new strategy to smallpox staff in Abidjan, Nigeria, in May 1968.[98] As Ogden notes, some people thought it simply 'another crackpot headquarters scheme'. But Dr Donald R. Hopkins, a medical officer in Sierra Leone, one of the most smallpox-infected countries in West Africa, and a country where only 66 per cent of the population was vaccinated, decided to give it a try; he reached zero cases in nine months. In May 1970, smallpox ended in West Africa.[99]

At first, S-C was seen as something to be used as a supplement to mass vaccination – as a method to be followed when vaccine supplies ran short. But many on the CDC and WHO staff began to speak of the S-C method as the entire solution to eradication, giving it priority *over* mass vaccination. The official account of the SEP acknowledges that the suggestion by some officials that mass vaccination was not necessary, in any circumstances, was actually misleading, and simplistic; and when some people became doctrinaire on the matter, going so far as argue that it was against policy to carry out mass vaccination campaigns, the matter became contentious. Mass vaccination was, after all, the method that WHO and its Expert Committee on Smallpox had been recommending for years; it was understandable that many of the people involved in running mass vaccination campaigns resisted shifting gear. Having finally managed to get their governments and populations behind the idea, the officials were reluctant to give it up, especially for something that called for greater resources, in terms of surveillance and reporting staff, than they often felt that they could afford. Many directors of vaccination campaigns, in their determination to meet their targets for mass vaccination, as a result simply turned a deaf ear to the new request by WHO.

So how important was S-C to the last inch in eradication? In some places it certainly was; in others its role is less clear. Even in Africa, where Foege first developed the method, surveillance-containment was not totally adopted; in Upper Volta, where the French served as advisors to the eradication campaign, there was no change in strategy from mass vaccination, and yet smallpox was extinguished.

Another example is Brazil. Brazil was the most smallpox-endemic of the countries in the PAHO region of the Western Hemisphere; sharing borders with every nation in South America except Chile and Ecuador, it was the source of constant re-importations of smallpox into its increasingly smallpox-free neighbours. At the start of the intensified smallpox campaign, Brazil was rightly judged to be the key place if eradication of smallpox in the Western Hemisphere was to be achieved. But its smallpox eradication efforts were viewed very critically by Henderson; his recent book pulls no punches, calling the intensified stage of the smallpox eradication campaign in Brazil 'a regrettable saga', even though eradication was achieved in only four years.[100] Understandably perhaps, Brazilians do not see the story in quite the same way.[101]

Brazil is a big country, geographically and in population size. It was at the time also poor, and racially stratified; it had a cumbersome federal system, with health programmes organized at the state level, with many diseases and programmes competing for attention. At the national level, the country had only launched its national malaria eradication programme a few years before, and this absorbed a large number of health personnel and resources. There were probably fewer than 10,000 cases of smallpox a year (even accounting for under-reporting), all of them of the *Variola minor* kind. Smallpox was simply not the country's highest health priority. None of these factors figure in the accounts of the 'insiders' running smallpox eradication at the centre; they were in fact outsiders to the national and local settings in which health policies were being carried out. Even the fact that Brazil was operating under military rule when the intensified programme started is not mentioned in the semi-official account, a situation that resulted in many dismissals of health officials for essentially political reasons, and considerable turnover of personnel.

As Amrith says, the situation on the ground was messy, and messy in each country in its own way.

The Brazilian Ministry of Health had in fact started mass vaccination against smallpox in 1958, but progress was very slow; by 1961 only 600,000 people had been vaccinated in 18 of the 20 states; further efforts were made in 1962–6 but coverage rates remained low, reaching less than 10 per cent in some southern states, and just over 40 per cent in more northern ones. Finally responding to international pressure, as WHO voted to launch the Intensified Smallpox Eradication Programme, the Brazilian government established its National Campaign to Eradicate Smallpox in 1966. Supervised and co-ordinated by the federal authorities (by then based in the new capital, Brasília), and organized and run at the state and local level, the aim was to conduct a three-year campaign during which more than 90 per cent of Brazil's 95.8 million people would be vaccinated – an impossibly high figure (as noted, the United States had got rid of smallpox with a vaccination rate of barely 40 per cent).

The launch of the campaign overlapped with, and was indeed the project of, the military dictatorship, which had staged a military coup in March of 1964 against the then elected civilian President; the period of military rule extended to 1985 (democracy being fully re-established only in 1989).[102] The coup resulted in the immediate closure of Congress, the banning of all political parties, and the imprisonment (and in some cases the torture and disappearance) of many civilians. The intensely nationalistic generals ran the country in authoritarian fashion and this gave a certain impetus to the international project of eradication (rather as Vargas had ruled from the centre in the 1930s and early 1940s). The regime signed up to malaria eradication in 1965, and it followed a year later, in 1966, with smallpox eradication, which it viewed as a programme that fitted in with its nationalistic desire to show technical competence, improve its image abroad, and associate the government with a US-supported, international project.

Nevertheless, the smallpox eradication campaign got off to a slow start, suffering from constant changes in administration and staff, and unpredictability in its funding. The national vaccination service had five directors in the five years between 1967 and 1971. The money was not enough, and though WHO had identified Brazil as the only country left in the Western hemisphere with endemic smallpox, the money from PAHO, little though it was, was for political reasons of equity, distributed by Horwitz to many countries, instead of largely to Brazil.[103] Mass vaccination began in 1967, aiming to get 30 million people vaccinated that year, but in the event only six million were (and even this figure was questioned).

Surveillance-containment methods were introduced slowly, but unevenly, and only towards the very end of the campaign. Geneva's presence in Brazil was in fact quite minimal; according to Henderson, the programme directors were quite touchy about outside help. A crucial appointment was Dr Leo Morris, a statistician and epidemiologist who had been Henderson's right-hand man at the CDC and who was sent by the WHO to Brazil in March 1967 to work on improving the country's system of smallpox surveillance and reporting (this was the same Dr Leo Morris who had tested the jet injector in the Amazon in 1965). The new system of surveillance Morris introduced promptly revealed some serious problems with the procedure for reporting smallpox cases, as it invariably did. In one incident, in July 1967, the town of Branquinhas, in the state of Bahia, reported an outbreak of smallpox where vaccinators had supposedly already completed mass vaccination. Investigation showed they had in fact reported vaccinating a larger number of people than actually lived in the town; the reports were in fact falsified. This pointed to the need to inspect the work of the vaccinators – Soper's method.

By 1969, surveillance methods were in place in four of the country's 26 states (plus the federal district); but at the end of the year the main surveillance officers were dismissed and the director of the national programme resigned.[104] The highest priority of the Brazilian officials was to get mass vaccination done. By 1969, the Brazilian programme had at least 1,000 staff involved in the field, the number of people being vaccinated each month was about 1.3 million, and the number of smallpox cases being reported each year was less than 5,000. But mass vaccination had not yet started in several large states, and rigorous surveillance was still not the norm; any time it was used, there were found to be many more cases of smallpox than had been reported, sometimes as many as 50 times more. In 1969, for instance, in a town called Ittinga, Bahia, an investigation by a surveillance unit of a single case revealed an epidemic unnoticed by the authorities, in which 618 people got smallpox out of a population of 9,277.

In a letter to the deputy director of PAHO in February 1970, Henderson reported that 'surveillance, such as it is, is collapsing along with a good many other things'. But he went on to say: 'Candidly, I'm afraid that WHO is in no small way at fault. Despite Brazil having been recognized as the No. 1 problem ... Money has been directed to smallpox projects in any number of countries (most recently Venezuela!) when, in fact, the real need is Brazil.'[105]

Finally, in 1970–71, the USAID provided some bilateral assistance, covering 30 per cent of the programme's costs, and the Brazilian government allocated more funds; by this time, epidemiological surveillance units were in place in every state and over 6,000 reporting posts had been set up throughout the country. The last outbreak of smallpox in Brazil occurred in Rio de Janeiro in 1971, the cases being identified by house-to-house searches. The outbreak was stamped out by tracing and vaccinating all contacts; the very last case was recorded on the 19 April 1971.

By chance both Candau, the Director-General of WHO, and Horwitz, the Director of PAHO, were in Brazil at the time, and were there to witness what turned out to be the end of smallpox in Brazil. In all it had taken an expenditure of only $4,506,369 by the Brazilian government, $1,763,780 by PAHO and $892,195 from the US government, between 1967 and 1971, to achieve this end (these figures do not include the considerable contributions made by the state governments within Brazil).

As WHO's official record conceded, the final success of smallpox eradication in Brazil was 'testament to a generally well-managed, systematic vaccination campaign and vaccine standards that tolerated a substantial margin of error', as much as to the systematic use of S-C procedures. Officials in Geneva considered the Brazilian officials recalcitrant, but as they said, the system worked – at least in the Brazilian case.

Surveillance-containment was of great importance, however, to India, where it was not clear that mass vaccination by itself could have done the job. Reaching 100 per cent of the population was not possible; identifying and tracing every case, and so stamping out smallpox wherever it appeared, was.

Surveillance was also essential to the eradication certification process, in Brazil as in all the other places. The idea of issuing certificates that would serve as a guarantee that eradication had really been achieved had originated with Soper in relation to the eradication of the *Aedes aegypti* mosquito, and then adopted in malaria eradication. Since the pay-off in eradication was that, once the disease had disappeared, all routine vaccinations could be given up, it was essential that countries were confident that smallpox had really been extinguished. The definition of smallpox eradication established by WHO was the elapse of two years without any cases following the last recorded case in a country or region. An International Commission for the Certification of Eradication was set up, which laid out the guidelines as to how to carry out the process of evaluation. In 1973, the PAHO Region of WHO became the first region in the world to be certified as free of smallpox. The last case of indigenous smallpox was reported in Somalia in 1977; a further two years of anxious monitoring by independent teams of experts passed before WHO was able to certify that the entire world was actually free of smallpox.

After Smallpox: To Destroy or Not to Destroy the Virus?

Unfortunately, the end of smallpox as a human disease did not end the story of smallpox. Many questions remained. Should research be continued on the smallpox virus? This immediately connected to the larger question: what should be done with remaining stocks of smallpox virus? Should they be deliberately destroyed too, on grounds of safety? When eradication was achieved, stocks of variola virus were scattered across the world, in many laboratories, many of them forgotten, obscure, or not safe. The danger of smallpox virus escaping from unsecured labs was demonstrated in 1978, when virus escaped from a smallpox research lab in Birmingham, in the UK, where it infected a woman working in an office above it. Belatedly diagnosed as having *Variola major*, she died one month later. The head of the laboratory committed suicide. Some 341 contacts were traced and vaccinated.[106]

It was clear there were good arguments for requiring most laboratories to destroy their stocks. By 1981, countries with samples were down to five (China, Britain, South Africa, the United States and the Soviet Union). By 1984, only two laboratories were authorized by WHO to keep them, the CDC in Atlanta, Georgia, and the USSR at a laboratory in Moscow. But whether or not to take the next and ultimate step, and destroy the very last laboratory samples was a matter that divided the public health and scientific community. By 1984, all countries had given up routine smallpox vaccination, so from then on, immunity in populations steadily declined (though some countries continued for several years to vaccinate their military personnel).

The story of the debate between the 'destructionists' and the 'anti-destructionists' over the fate of the smallpox virus has been focus of several recent accounts. The prolonged struggle over the matter within WHO was intensified by the revelation in the mid-1990s that the USSR (and perhaps other countries) had been engaged in a clandestine programme of weaponizing the virus.[107] The news upset the entire calculation about the destruction of the virus, and led to the decision at WHO being repeatedly postponed; after a destruction date was set for 1995, supported by many countries such as India, several other countries, including the UK, Russia and the United States, argued for a policy of retention, so that further research on new tools to fight the disease could be developed. Within the United States, the Department of Defense was the most resistant to destroying the last samples. The end-date of the virus samples for this reason kept on being put off; as of the time of writing, the decision has still not been made.

Henderson's position on this issue is, as usual, very interesting. He has long been a destructionist when it comes to the smallpox virus, its destruction logically marking the absolute end to smallpox as an organism. But Henderson has also been increasingly concerned about bioterrorism, growing more and more worried as time has passed about what the release of smallpox as a weapon would do to civilian populations that are almost all without any immunity. In 1998, Henderson established a Center for Civilian Biodefense Studies at Johns Hopkins University, Baltimore. Then came the events of 9/11, followed a few days later by the deliberate release of anthrax spores. Fears of bioterrorism moved from WHO and expert circles out into the wider world. Almost 30 years had passed since the US had given up routine smallpox vaccination. Smallpox vaccine was put in production, and in 2002 President Bush planned a massive vaccination campaign, first aimed at vaccinating ten million Americans, then modified to vaccinate 450,000 hospital and medical staff, with 'first responders' such as the police and firefighters to follow afterwards, for a total of about ten million people. Henderson did not think this a wise plan; he considered that the risks of vaccination complications outweighed the risk of a bioterrorist smallpox attack, and knew from experience that, in the event of an attack, the best way to stop the epidemic was by immediately ring-fencing it via contact-tracing, isolation and vaccination. He was right, and the vaccination programme was, in Henderson's words, 'an abject failure'. Fewer than 40,000 people agreed to be vaccinated.[108]

This is a very big and unfinished story; but the events have added an unexpected twist to the eradication equation. If President Bush's original plan had been followed, the US would have vaccinated millions of people after the events of 9/11. If so, it would have undone one of the key promises of eradication, namely, that once eradication is achieved, all the costs of keeping stocks of viable vaccine, and all the risks of vaccination, can be given up forever.

In 1980, the events and challenges just described were not foreseen. Instead, quite other factors put a question mark over eradication. The smallpox success was universally applauded as a great accomplishment, as it indeed was. But where to go from there – that was the issue. What would smallpox eradication signify, beyond the relief anyone would feel that a truly horrible, often fatal, and disfiguring human disease was gone forever. Would the smallpox campaign herald a new era of disease eradication efforts? Did it teach new lessons? Was eradication after all a satisfactory method of public health intervention, or not? These are the issues I take up in the final chapter of this book.

7 Controversies: Eradication Today

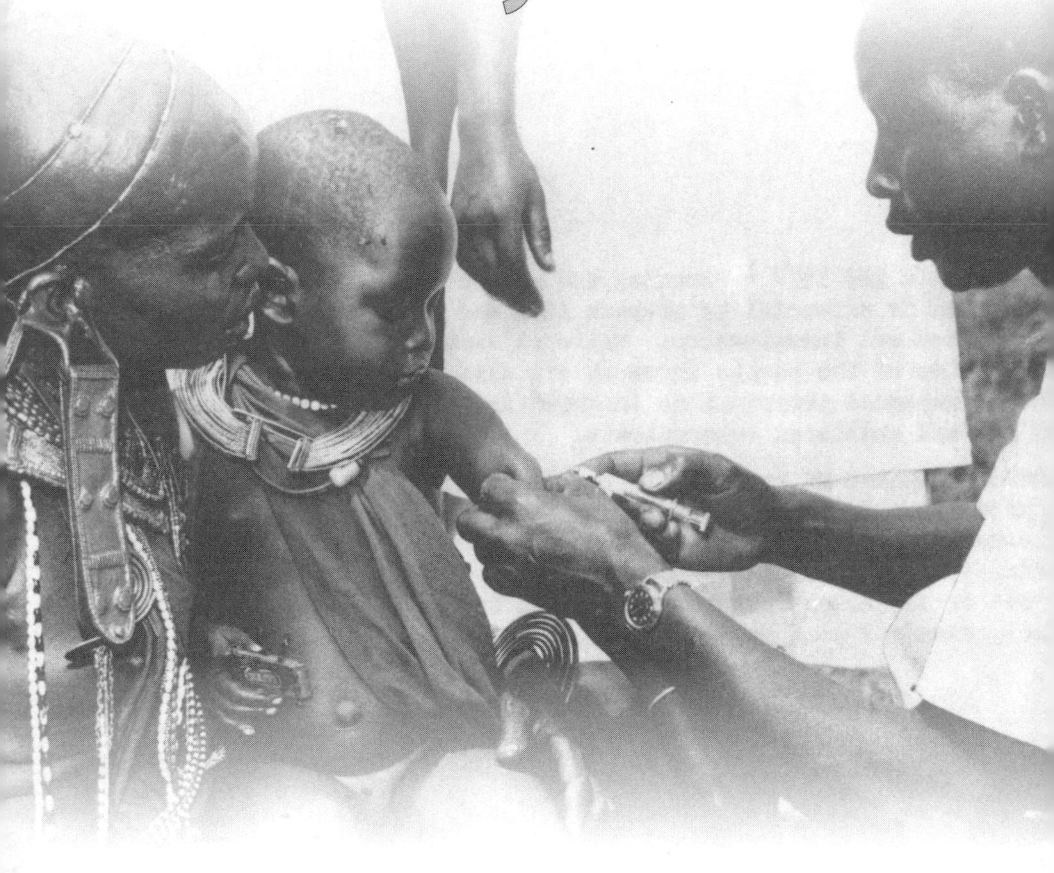

Soper died in 1977 before any of the eradication campaigns he had championed had succeeded. True to form, he kept his faith in eradication to the end. He blamed the failures on poor administration, faulty methods, lack of understanding – but never the concept itself. He stood firm by his absolutist dictums. At his 80th birthday celebrations, tributes poured in from his disciples and admirers – testimonials to a brilliant general on the battlefield of public health.[1]

After his death, Soper's faith in disease eradication as a goal in international health appeared to be vindicated, not just by the eradication of smallpox, but also by the launching of two new worldwide eradication campaigns, both supported by WHO and other international health organizations. Were Soper alive now, he would no doubt be pleased to know it was his office, PAHO, which led the way by announcing in 1985 a campaign to eradicate polio in the entire Western Hemisphere in five years. In 1988 the other regional offices of WHO followed suit, setting the year 2000 as the completion date for worldwide eradication. In 1991, the WHO endorsed yet another global eradication project, against Guinea Worm Disease (GWD; medical name, dracunculiasis), a disease which at the time afflicted millions but which many people had never even heard of. In addition, several regional eradication efforts were begun (for example, against measles in the Americas).

Soper would also certainly be gratified to know that the definition of disease eradication being used today is his: it stands for an absolute disappearance. Even the moral and economic language used to justify eradication echoes Soper's. Eradication, it is said, 'brings health equity and social justice and frees scarce resources for other purposes'.[2] It represents 'the ultimate achievement in public health', or 'the ultimate in sustainability and social justice'.[3]

Eradication campaigns, it seems, are here to stay.

Primary Health Care and the Challenge to Eradication

Or are they? I ask this question because one of the legacies from the past is the ambivalence, or even outright hostility, many people in the international health community feel towards eradication as a strategy. Eradication campaigns are expensive; they channel too many funds and energy into single diseases, when people suffer from many infections and have multiple needs; they set global priorities against local ones; they often operate independently of the health services of the countries involved; and they are very difficult to do.

People ask: do they, or can they, work? Thus far the polio eradication campaign has repeatedly failed to meet its deadline. Eradication fatigue is setting in as, after billions of dollars have been spent, the campaign confronts the classic problem of the final inch. Some of polio eradication's original advocates have even changed their minds; they think that the world should give up the quest, and settle instead for a policy of continuous and effective polio control.[4]

In regard to these issues, Donald A. Henderson stands as an emblematic figure, because of the ambivalence he has consistently expressed about eradication – as well as about some of its alternatives. Despite the decade he had dedicated to smallpox eradication, Henderson did not become a great proponent of disease eradication more generally. He has drawn attention repeatedly to the fact that smallpox eradication was in doubt until the very last case. Moreover, by the time smallpox eradication was in fact achieved, Henderson points out, eradication was being more or less written off the international public health agenda. At the very moment that the World Health Assembly (WHA) convened its 150 delegates in a formal ceremony in Geneva in May 1980, to sign the document announcing success, the smallpox eradication effort, said Henderson, was being 'critically maligned by traditional international health planners'. To these critics, 'the smallpox campaign epitomized the worst of what they characterized as anachronistic, authoritarian, "top down" programmes which they saw as anathema to the new "health for all" primary health care initiative'.[5]

Henderson was here referring to the major reorientation in outlook that had taken place within WHO in the late 1960s and into the 1970s, away from disease eradication and towards a much greater emphasis on the development of Primary Health Care (PHC). The right to basic health care had been part of WHO's charter from its founding; but the emphasis on PHC, well represented by Dr Brock Chisholm, the first Director-General of WHO, had been marginalized by WHO's post-war concentration on controlling and/or eradicating communicable diseases. Starting in the 1960s, as many more post-colonial, newly independent countries joined WHO, there was a revived interest in the social bases of ill health. There was a growing concern about the absence in most developing countries of even the most elementary of health services outside the main urban centres; about the huge disparities in life-chances between the rich and poor nations, and between rich and poor people within nations; and about the absorption of so much of WHO's resources in eradication campaigns that were apparently unable to meet their goals. The failure of the malaria eradication campaign in the late 1960s made an especially strong impression. Was it right that one disease should absorb at the height of its campaign almost two thirds of the WHO's regular budget? Was it not better to concentrate first on putting in place some basic health services in countries where they were woefully lacking, and where most people had no access to modern medical care? Had not eradication campaigns also fared best in those places where some basic health services already existed?

The new Director-General of WHO, the Danish physician Halfdan T. Mahler, who took over from his predecessor Marcelino Candau in 1973, thought so, redirecting the energies and policies of WHO towards PHC. Mahler had the missionary zeal of a Soper, but for a different cause – 'Health for All by the Year 2000'. This was the short-hand slogan Mahler used to draw attention to the idea that what people most needed was not the complete elimination of one or two targeted diseases, but the provision of basic, continuous, health care services – to emphasize that the chief causes of ill-health were multiple, not single, and above all, social and economic, and not just a matter of bacteria or insects.

There were many developments within international public health that converged in the late 1960s and early 1970s to downplay the importance of single-disease eradication campaigns and to open up the field to broader currents of ideas about health in relation to economics and politics. This is the period in which Thomas McKeown's ideas about the socio-economic determinants of the nineteenth-century health transition began to have an influence beyond the UK example. Then there was the more radical figure of Ivan Illich, who criticized the medical, technically driven and essentially urban approach to disease that predominated in the rich, industrialized countries, arguing that Western medicine was the cause of ill health, not the solution to it. René Dubos's ecological approach to disease represented yet another strand in the debate, drawing attention to the ways in which humans and disease pathogens have co-evolved, and to the need to find methods to control diseases, rather than extirpate wholesale pathogens or vectors. In the US, John H. Bryant's study of the huge disparities in health and health services in developing countries, *Health and the Developing World* (1969) was another influential source of ideas about health and poverty.[6]

Political events also shaped the debate. The Cuban Revolution in 1959 presented an alternative model for providing basic health in a socialist setting, making access and equity fundamental to achieving health for all. China (which finally joined the WHO in 1972, replacing Taiwan), presented yet another approach, with its cadres of the so-called barefoot doctors (now referred to as paramedics), made up of peasants who, after a few months training, fanned out into rural areas to bring basic preventive health care services and health education to the masses.[7]

These new ideas were not universally admired within the WHO. The US opposed anything and everything that smacked of what it called socialized medicine (and it stretched the definition of 'socialized' to include pretty much every and any health delivery system that departed from its own privatized, highly individualistic, curative model). Its Cold War rival, the USSR, had its own reasons for objecting to the barefoot doctor model, which they saw as the antithesis of their own medically oriented, scientific and modern system of health care (the Soviet Union being at the time, of course, the bitter rival of China within the Communist world). To the Soviets, primary health care sounded too like primitive health care, a second-best health system for the poor.[8] They preferred their own model of a highly centralized system of health services based on the most modern scientific medicine.

Many people in public health, however, were very supportive of the new emphasis on primary health care services. The model of expensive, single-disease eradication campaigns was felt to be exhausted. Field experience had shown that technically driven health initiatives in the developing world often foundered because of the absence of even the most elementary infrastructure in basic health care. Instead of eradication sowing the seeds of basic services, as the eradicationists had hoped, the relationship seemed to go in the other direction – it was the pre-existence of basic health care services that allowed eradication to succeed. As we have seen in chapter Five on the Malaria Eradication Programme, consideration of this fact had led the WHO in the mid-1960s to propose that eradication campaigns against specific diseases be integrated with general health services wherever possible, and to recommend that the poorest of the developing countries spend a pre-eradication year putting some basic health infrastructures in place, before starting the attack phase of a malaria eradication campaign.[9]

When, then, the idea of 'Health for All by the Year 2000' was put forward by Halfdan Mahler in 1976, it caught on, giving rise to wide-ranging discussions and debates. The culminating point of the shift in attitudes was the International Conference on Primary Health Care, organized by WHO and UNICEF and held from 6–12 September in 1978 in Alma-Ata (the capital of the eastern Soviet Republic of Kazakhstan, a location the USSR had insisted on, paying for the conference with a contribution of $2 million so as to forestall the conference going to a city in China). Attended by some 3,000 delegates from 134 countries and 67 UN agencies, as well as many national organizations and well-known political figures (for example, Senator Edward M. Kennedy), Alma-Ata was a huge jamboree in the middle of the Cold War. The final *Declaration of Alma-Ata* that emerged was approved by acclamation; endorsed the next year by the World Health Assembly, it remains to this day a touchstone of WHO's philosophy (reiterated by the current Director-General of WHO, Dr Margaret Chan, in *The World Health Report* for 2008, which had the title *Primary Health Care [Now More Important Than Ever]*).

But if PHC was easy to vote for, it was not so easy to make a reality. One reason, in fact, that the Alma-Ata Declaration could be so readily approved by so many different countries, with completely different political outlooks and agendas, was that the Declaration was so general in scope. The Declaration called for a return to WHO's original definition of health as a 'state of complete physical, mental and social wellbeing'; it committed the world to a 'New International Economic Order' that would guarantee health for all; it emphasized the fundamental human right to health and universal provision of services; it made participation and solidarity keys to health services, as well as social justice and the need for equity; and it emphasized Primary Health Care as the necessary and integral cornerstone of every country's health system.[10]

Who could vote against any of these fine ideals? But also, how could such ideals be translated into concrete action (especially when no special budget was allocated for such ends)? Where to start? With malnutrition, the health of mothers and children, with local health units, or the development of rural health?

In fact, the decades after Alma-Ata were decades of disappointment and setbacks in regard to the PHC initiative. In the 1980s, political support for the post-war welfare state was already beginning to fall apart in many countries, to be replaced by aggressive economic liberalization and privatization promoted especially by the United States as the supposed path to economic development. Developing countries were buffeted by neo-liberal ideology, the so-called 'Washington consensus' (meaning an emphasis on investment in finance and industry, a concentration on fighting inflation, and the slashing of social spending), the market 'reforms' of the Chicago school of economists; many had to deal with massive government debt, IMF-dictated 'restructuring', falling revenues, and often, political instability. The emphasis everywhere was on cost-benefit analyses, short-termism, and 'hard headed practicality' (meaning under-investment in long-term public health and/or health care infrastructure). In many countries, the secular improvements in morbidity and mortality that had characterized the period roughly between 1950 and 1975 slowed down, or were even reversed. The trend was away from building up inclusive and equitable health services and towards the privatization of health care and even, in many places, the more or less complete collapse of whatever had passed for public health services.[11]

In addition, and perhaps in response to the shifting ideological ground, several public health experts, who had been trained to think of health in terms of medical advances and technical tools, wanted to operationalize Alma-Ata, by turning the broad idea of PHC into Selective Primary Health Care (SPHC) – something very different.[12] Following a meeting organized by the Rockefeller Foundation in Bellagio, Italy in 1979, and attended by representatives from the World Bank, the Ford Foundation and USAID (all increasingly players in international health, and with the money to set the agenda), SPHC was presented as an interim but practicable set of objectives, four in all, and known by the acronym GOBI. This stood for Growth monitoring, Oral rehydration, Breast feeding and Immunization. Behind these four objectives lay the demand for clear and measurable targets and measurable results.[13]

Many people in the public health field reacted very negatively to the idea of SPHC, seeing it as a sly way of returning to vertically organized, technically driven programmes, of introducing business methods (and perhaps corporate interests) into health care, and of generally perverting PHC's original purpose of putting in place comprehensive health care systems.[14] Debate, much of it acrimonious, lasted for years. The priorities within SPHC were also criticized; oral rehydration, for instance, worked as an emergency, technical solution to the immediate threat of death in children, but it did not touch the fundamental causes of the diarrhoeas that cause life-threatening dehydration in the first place, such as unclean water and poor sanitation.

Of the selective goals, immunization had the strongest rationale and probably the greatest impact. The intensified smallpox programme that started in 1967 was strengthening the capacity of many countries to deliver vaccines at a time when several new vaccines were appearing, notably those for polio and measles. In general, vaccination against numerous childhood diseases was becoming routine in the Western world, and there was a growing feeling that these benefits to children's health could and should be extended to the poorest children of the world. In recognition of these trends, in 1974 the World Health Assembly voted to set up an Expanded Program on Immunization (EPI), initially targeting six vaccine-preventable communicable diseases – tuberculosis, diphtheria, measles, tetanus, pertussis (whooping cough) and polio – with the goal of immunizing 80 per cent of the world's infants by 1990.[15] The EPI represented a set of disease-specific, technical interventions; though not eradication campaigns, they had much in common with them. Immunization was something the WHO could help organize, and organize well. And the results were initially very promising. When the EPI got launched in 1977, less than 5 per cent of the world's children had been immunized against the diseases.[16] After a slow start, with coverage rates in the mid-1980s of little more than 20 per cent, and little change therefore in disease incidence (for example, tetanus, polio and measles), the figure for all six diseases reached about 80 per cent by 1994 (as high a coverage rate in some developing countries as in the rich, western countries). Success had depended on overcoming many obstacles in order to train immunizers, secure a cold chain (meaning a chain of refrigeration facilities to keep the vaccine viable in its passage from a laboratory or manufacturer to its point of use in the field), and set up systems of delivery and surveillance.

Many people attribute the large decrease in mortality rates in children under the age of five in the period from roughly from 1970 to 1995, when the GDP in several developing countries actually declined or stagnated, to immunization.[17] The high rates were not achieved everywhere, nor were they always maintained; as a service, immunization in developing countries had, according to one account, 'a very fragile organizational structure', and could hardly serve as a primary health care service. Nevertheless, at the time, it seemed to many people that the EPI represented the most significant international public health initiative in the developing world.[18]

In regard to these trends and debates in international public health, Henderson found himself in the middle. In general he agreed with the critics that too often eradication campaigns had been run in a hierarchical and inflexible manner that doomed them to failure. The malaria eradication campaign especially, he said, had been organized from the centre down, as an independent, autonomous service with no community involvement. All the national MEPs , he said, 'had to adhere rigidly to a highly detailed, standard manual of operations', and were 'conceived and executed as a military operation to be conducted in an identical manner whatever the battlefield'.[19]

But when the same criticisms were directed at the smallpox eradication campaign, Henderson bristled. He maintained that the SEP was modest, not rich, in resources and personnel, and in this respect a far cry from the malaria eradication campaign; that the SEP was situated in communities, not outside, or above them; that it relied on the support and participation of thousands of local people; and that it was flexible and adaptable, not rigid and military-like in character.

Beyond this, however, he was not ready to go. He did not think other eradication campaigns should follow smallpox. As a result of making his views known, says Henderson, he was dropped from many of the workshops and international meetings held on eradication in the two decades after smallpox eradication was announced in 1980.[20]

But neither did the 'Health for All' alternative recommend itself to Henderson. 'I have no idea what "health for all by the year 2000" means', he said in 1980, 'and I know of no-one who expects to achieve it'. The key idea seemed to be 'horizontal programmes' in place of eradication's 'vertical programmes'. But like many people who had worked in very poor countries, Henderson believed effective public health interventions needed to be specific, otherwise the efforts were often wasted. To Henderson, a vertical programme was one that had clear objectives, proper disease surveillance mechanisms in place, and assessments to monitor progress, while the horizontal models of primary health care that he had seen, he said, 'best describe the sleeping position of the workers'. He concluded: 'Regrettably, I feel we are now working in a fog of slogans, of hazy ill-defined objectives, and of philosophy rather than of definite programs.'[21]

Eradication Redux

Other people, though, continued to see eradication as a viable option. As early as 1976, Dr Donald R. Hopkins, whose experience working on the smallpox eradication campaign in West Africa had left him much more positively inclined towards eradication than Henderson, was already asking, 'After Smallpox Eradication: Yaws?'[22] When the yaws idea did not seem to catch on, he and his colleague, William H. Foege (who, in 1977, became the director of the US Centers for Disease Control) proposed instead the eradication of Guinea Worm Disease (GWD).[23]

Eradication was also finding new sponsors. Between 1980 and 2000, in fact, numerous conferences and workshops were held on the topic, starting with a meeting in Washington organized by the National Institutes of Health (NIH) in 1980 within months of the formal declaration of smallpox eradication.[24] In 1988, The Carter Center in Atlanta, inspired by smallpox eradication, set up an International Task Force for Disease Eradication (ITFDE); meeting six times between 1989 and 1992 (with a final report appearing in 1993), the members evaluated 90 diseases and conditions for their potential eradicability, concluding there were five good candidates – polio, GWD, mumps, rubella and cysticercosis (pork tape worm disease). In 1997 an important workshop at Dalhem, Germany, examined past failures in eradication and the criteria to be used in disease selection.[25]

Oddly enough, given the tremendous effort and money that had been put into eradication campaigns in the past, the criteria had rarely been examined at all systematically.[26] All that could really be said about the 'first generation' of eradication campaigns (pre-1980) was that the choices had been essentially circumstantial, historical and contingent. Would this also be the case for future eradication efforts? The hope was that it would not – that lessons drawn from the many past failures to eradicate, and the one success, would point the way towards a set of rational criteria that could be applied in the future.[27]

The need for clarity on these matters was evident to the experts at the National Institutes of Health in the US, meeting in 1980, when they found there was little agreement even about the most basic of terms used in discussing disease eradication. The first order of business was therefore to settle on some definitions. After some preliminary discussions, it was decided that Soper had got it right, that eradication had henceforth to represent the most absolute standard possible in public health and mean that an infection has disappeared completely from all countries in the world because transmission of the causative organism has ceased completely. With eradication posited as a reduction to zero, and an irreversible effect, disease 'control' was situated at the other end of the spectrum, and stood for the mere reduction of a disease in prevalence. This seemed to leave a space in the middle for a third term that would signify something less than worldwide eradication, but more than mere control. 'Regional eradication', appeared to do the job, but since the term eradication had to stand for an absolute, whereas regional eradication left open the possibility of re-infection of eradicated areas, a regional eradication seemed to be a contradiction in terms. It was decided instead to introduce the word 'elimination' for regional eradication.[28] In its own review of the terms and meaning of eradication, the Carter taskforce (ITFDE) came to the same conclusions and seconded these definitions.

But the terms nonetheless remained slippery. For example, did eradication imply that a disease agent itself had been removed entirely from nature, as well as from laboratories (where the remaining stocks of smallpox virus were kept after 1980)? At Dahlem, a new word, 'extinction', meaning that the pathogen had been destroyed forever, was added to clarify this point. Could eradication refer to the complete disappearance of the worst clinical symptoms of a disease, but not the pathogen itself – if, for example, the blindness caused by onchocerciasis (river blindness) were to be eradicated, even though the microfilariae were not? Or would this latter situation be covered best by the term 'elimination'? Could elimination be stretched to mean simply the reduction of a disease by a certain amount, as when the WHO adopted neonatal tetanus in 1989 for 'elimination', meaning its reduction to less than one case per district by 1996? What was meant by 'district'? And what about leprosy, which in 1991 WHO voted to eliminate, defining elimination in this case to mean the reduction of leprosy cases to less than one person per 10,000? A press release from the WHO in March 1997 only added to the terminological confusion by announcing that lymphatic filiariasis, river blindness, leprosy and Chagas disease could all be 'eliminated as public health problems within ten years' – in effect meaning they could be 'controlled'.

The conferees at the Dahlem workshop pointed out that none of these WHO usages were consistent with the definitions adopted previously by the ITFDE and other expert groups.[29] But getting consistency has proved difficult.[30] The WHO's current elimination projects against leprosy, vitamin A deficiency, congenital syphilis and blindness from trachoma continue to rely on many different definitions of 'elimination'. Eradicationists want definitional absolutes, in keeping with their absolute goals; public health advocates often prefer terms that are more ambiguous, perhaps because of their rhetorical possibilities. Hopkins, at any rate, has suggested this is the reason 'disease elimination' is so widely used at WHO and elsewhere; it has a ring to it, the hint of a promise of something close to eradication, and this may serve to bring in the support of politicians and outside funds for projects that really have no intention, or perhaps the possibility, of achieving even a 'regional eradication'.[31]

The criteria suggested for disease selection are equally open-ended and hard to pin down. They are generally divided into three categories: the biological/technical; the economic and the socio-political. Biological/technical criteria seem the most straightforward. The factors here concern a disease's basic characteristics. Does its pathogen have any other host than humans? If it does – if it has an animal reservoir, as yellow fever does – then it cannot in principle be eradicated. Is the disease easy to diagnose? If not, then eradication is difficult. Technically, is there a proven intervention, such as a vaccine, or a drug? Also important is the assessment of a disease's epidemiological characteristics, especially how infectious it is.[32]

Economic criteria, given a prominent place in the deliberations at Dahlem, relate to the economic burden of a disease places on a population *per capita*; the availability or otherwise of funds to carry out an eradication campaign; and cost-benefit calculations as to the whether the up-front expenditures would be less than the costs of continued control. Political criteria refer to the political visibility of a disease, and political will to support eradication: How stable, politically, is a country where eradication is supposed to take place? How committed are governments or agencies to eradication? What about the means of transport (of vaccines, technical staff), and communications?

These criteria are all sensible. But each set of criteria opens up a host of often quite intangible or difficult-to-ascertain matters. Even the idea of an effective intervention, seemingly one of the most unambiguous of the biological criteria, is not as straightforward as it first appears; a vaccine that works in, say, the Americas, for epidemiological or socio-economic reasons might not work as well in a very different area and population (for example, the oral polio vaccine in India). What about 'field-proven strategies'?[33] How big does the field have to be before it is proven adequate for an eradication campaign? As E. H. Hinman had said years before, we can only know for certain that eradication is technically feasible once eradication is achieved (and so far it has been achieved only once).[34]

On the economic side, the cost-benefit example of smallpox eradication seems compelling, but this is a retrospective view of a long process that had ticked along for years without adequate commitment, funding or organization.[35] After eradication, too, the potential threat of rogue or bioterrorist release of smallpox virus has altered the cost-benefit calculation. With other eradicable diseases, the cost-benefit calculation may be very different than with smallpox – for example, the eradication of Neglected Tropical Diseases (NTDs). This group of diseases, of which GWD is one, finally began to get some attention at the WHO in the 1990s; largely rural, the eradication of NTDs would bring at best only indirect economic benefits to the world at large, perhaps by improving the agricultural productivity of the infected populations. The real benefit will be to the infected populations themselves. To eradicate NTDs would be to remove some of the most socially excluding, debilitating, often disfiguring and economically burdensome afflictions known to mankind, from some of the most marginalized and impoverished people in the world; the control or eradication of such diseases will, then, certainly require external sources of funding and has to be done on the grounds that health is a benefit, in and of itself, to those freed from infection.[36]

The political criteria were recognized at Dahlem as usually the most critical to success in eradication, but also the most open-ended. Since eradication depends on the participation of all the countries where the disease is endemic, an eradication campaign requires cooperation and collaboration on a scale that is very unusual in international affairs and difficult to bring about politically. How are we to measure in advance, or create, the political commitment or social support needed (two of the criteria listed by the IFTDE)?

Despite these ambiguities in the eradication agenda, by the time the WHO co-sponsored a large conference on the topic in Atlanta, Georgia in February 1998, with over 200 conferees representing some 81 organizations, eradication seemed to be fully back on the international agenda.[37] By this point both the global polio and GWD eradication campaigns had been going on for several years (and regional eradication of polio in the Americas had already been achieved, with the last case occurring in Peru in 1991). The expectation was that new campaigns would be added to the list in the future.

A final factor affecting the improved status of eradication concerned Primary Health Care. While PHC remained a fundamental ideal at WHO, the two decades since Alma-Ata had yielded few tangible results. It had proven difficult to shift WHO's limited resources away from disease-specific projects to supporting more basic services. Deciding how to help improve such services in impoverished countries, each with its own political agenda, governance, resources and health needs, was not an easy matter. The potential tension between time-limited, disease-specific eradication campaigns, and long-term, sustainable, basic health programmes was widely recognized; the debate about top-down versus bottom-up programmes was not about to go away. Nonetheless, it appeared that more people in international public health were open to the idea of disease eradication than they had been in the 1970s.

One of them was Dr Halfdan Mahler, the Director-General of WHO who for years had 'carried the WHO banner in opposition to vertical public health programs'. He now changed his mind. He was persuaded that vertical programs, such as those of immunization, 'could serve as "messenger DNA" for the insertion of effective, and equitable, measures into the vector of Primary Health Care'. In May 1988, Mahler placed polio eradication on the agenda for the meeting of the WHA (his last as D-G).[38]

Thus it was once again hoped that, at least in some cases, eradication, if done well, could greatly benefit the development of basic health services, as Soper had once argued. Of course, the old 'Soperian' model of eradication, with its para-military style, its top-down authoritarian structure and its organizational autonomy was no longer seen as valid. But was it possible that a new model of eradication could be found that would overcome some of the limitations of the first generation of eradication campaigns? More generally, how would eradication fit within the rapidly changing field of international health in the twenty-first century?

New Models of Disease Eradication? Polio and Guinea Worm Disease

The two ongoing worldwide eradication campaigns against polio and GWD disease provide information that takes us part way to answering the first of these questions. Both campaigns have achieved dramatic reductions in disease incidence, but after more than two decades of effort neither has reached the magical number of zero incidence; both have had to reset repeatedly their target dates for completion.

The question that interests me here is whether the campaigns represent more than a dramatic reduction in the incidence of a single disease, commendable though such a result surely is. Do they also represent broader contributions to overall public health in poor countries?

I start with polio eradication, the better known of the two campaigns because of polio's fearsome reputation as a childhood disease that can cause severe paralysis and a lifetime of disability.[39] Polio had peaked in the United States in the 1950s, with severe epidemics occurring in 1952 and 1953, with 58,000 and 35,000 cases respectively. Competition to find a polio vaccine had been fierce, resulting in the production of two, Salk's inactivated polio vaccine (IPV), introduced in 1955, and Sabin's live virus oral polio vaccine (OPV), licensed in 1962. Their widespread use in Western, industrialized countries brought down polio incidence quickly and were central elements in the new immunization era in health.[40]

From a biological/technical point of view, polio seemed quite like smallpox and appeared to meet the newly laid-out criteria for eradication. It was a viral disease that was spread by oral-fecal contamination. The disease was fairly easily diagnosed (from the appearance of flaccid muscle paralyses). There was no apparent animal reservoir of the virus. And it was vaccine-preventable. Sabin, the inventor of the oral polio vaccine, proposed in the 1960s that mass immunization could eradicate polio worldwide; but with the exception of Castro's Cuba, which, beginning in 1962, used mass immunization 'days' to wipe out polio, the idea was not taken up. WHO was in no mood to contemplate a worldwide effort, being fully engaged in malaria eradication. Once PHC came to the forefront in WHO deliberations, even the Expanded Programme on Immunization was viewed by many people as a vertical initiative unsuited to the needs of basic health care, as we have seen.

However, PAHO's director, the Brazilian Dr Carlyle Guerra de Macedo, who took office in 1983, was a strong proponent of childhood immunizations, as was the Chief of the Expanded Programme on Immunization at PAHO, another Brazilian, Dr Ciro de Quadros.[41] De Quadros thought a vertical programme of immunization would strengthen, not weaken, health systems, especially by improving capacity in disease surveillance, laboratory analysis and the delivery of vaccine services to the populations that needed them. Brazil's success in this regard was an important example of what could be done. In 1980, after many years of poorly coordinated polio immunization campaigns, Brazil had begun a programme of National Immunization Days (NIDs); organized twice a year, with two months' interval between them, the programme aimed to vaccinate all children under five, regardless of their previous polio vaccination history. The number of polio cases at the time was not great, but the cases were widely scattered across the large country, so a nationwide, mass immunization campaign was called for; once it was launched, the numbers of polio cases fell rapidly, with only 45 cases being reported in 1983, and the last case being registered in March 1989.[42] In May 1985, the 37 members of PAHO announced a plan to eradicate polio in the Americas in five years.[43] The WHA followed suit in 1988 with an announcement of the goal of eradicating polio worldwide.[44] Despite Halfdan Mahler's endorsement of the project, the officials at WHO were not initially enthusiastic about it; the budget set aside was tiny, just enough to support a single staff person in Geneva.[45] In the circumstances, the enthusiasm, financial aid and organizational support of Rotary International, especially its network of volunteers, were crucial to the launch (and continued functioning) of the polio eradication effort.[46]

At the time the global effort started, paralytic polio was still endemic in 125 countries in five continents, and there were an estimated 350,000 cases a year worldwide – although, as usual, the data were not reliable (there was considerable under-reporting). On the plus side, the majority of cases were clustered in a few highly endemic countries. On the negative side, polio was more difficult to eradicate than smallpox. While all smallpox infections produce some symptoms (a rash), many cases of polio are symptomless, which makes them hard to identify. For every person whose polio infection results in paralysis, in fact, somewhere between 200 and 1,000 people will be infected who will show only mild, flu-like symptoms that are easy to overlook. These people with inapparent infections can continue to infect other people with the virus for several weeks. Another difficulty is that acute flaccid paralysis (AFP) can be caused by infections other than polio. To diagnose polio cases with certainty requires a laboratory stool test, a large demand on a poor country's health infrastructure. By the time such tests are carried out, many other children may have become infected.

The oral polio vaccine (OPV) was selected over the inactivated vaccine for eradication in developing countries because it is cheap, effective, and can easily be delivered by volunteers. But both the Sabin and the Salk polio vaccines require multiple doses, not the single application needed in smallpox. With the OPV, for example, children have to be brought back two and sometimes three or even more times, at intervals separated by only a few months; in the most stubborn areas up to fifteen doses may be needed. The oral vaccine also requires a cold chain to keep it viable. The vaccine therefore has certain limitations.[47]

The principal policies for getting rid of polio had been worked out in the PAHO countries. There were four elements: improved routine immunization; supplementing routine polio vaccination with mass immunization campaigns; putting in place a system of poliovirus surveillance (linked to prompt and accurate systems of reporting, and a network of laboratories); and ensuring a prompt response to outbreaks.[48]

Sabin had argued the case for basing polio eradication on supplemental immunization in developing countries, because such countries tended to have low levels of routine immunization, too low to interrupt transmission.[49] Even in those places where the EPI had, exceptionally, reached 80 per cent polio vaccination coverage, these rates were not enough to stop polio in places where transmission was year-round, the climate was hot, population densities were very high and there were very poor levels of sanitation. Rather than relying on existing health services for the delivery of polio vaccine, the supplemental vaccination usually took the form of special 'National Immunization Days' (NIDs) – days set aside for mass immunizations. This was the method Cuba used in 1962 to eliminate wild poliovirus (and which it has continued to rely on), as had Brazil; it was also a familiar method in many other countries, NIDs having been used in the previous smallpox eradication campaign.

In the 1980s very good results were achieved by these methods in Mexico, Costa Rica and other Latin American countries. China, after experiencing a number of bad epidemics in 1989–90, which left some 10,000 children paralysed, launched its NIDs in 1993, and success there spurred the eradication programme of the entire Western Pacific Region of WHO.

However, the scale of polio immunization required to keep up the momentum for eradication is quite staggering. In 2003, a WHO report indicated that over 20 million volunteers were involved in polio eradication in middle-income and low-income countries.[50] According to the medical doctor and writer Atul Gawande, 'in one week in 1997, some 250 million children were vaccinated simultaneously in China, India, Bhutan, Pakistan, Bangladesh, Thailand, Vietnam, and Burma. National immunization days have reached as many as half a billion children at one time – almost a tenth of the world's population.'[51]

As is to be expected of so huge an undertaking, there have been setbacks along the way. In 2003–6 there was a serious resurgence of polio. Stephen Cochi, the director of the CDC's Global Immunization Division, has summarized the main causes. First was the reduction of NIDs and supplementary immunizations in India in 2001–2 (largely for financial reasons). Then in 2003–4, rumours that the polio vaccine caused women to become sterile, or was unsafe, led several Muslim states in northern Nigeria to stop immunizing children. Combined, these events resulted in the spread of polio between 2003 and 2006 to 27 previously polio-free countries. It took a huge effort, revised tactics, and $500 million to get polio back under control (and not before 5,000 additional paralyses from polio had occurred in Nigeria). The year 2007 was a turning point, a 'do-or-die' moment, as Cochi puts it, when the polio eradication effort had to be rapidly stepped up to stop outbreaks.[52] By June 2008, polio was again endemic in only four countries: Pakistan, India, Nigeria and Afghanistan. The total count of polio cases for 2008 was 1,654 cases worldwide, for 2009, 1,604, and for 2010, 1,292 cases.[53]

Given the enormous scale of the global polio eradication undertaking, it is right that we ask what impact such determined pursuit of a single disease to the very last case has had on health infrastructures more generally, especially in the poorest countries where polio has long been endemic. Immunization against childhood infections certainly counts as one of the 'greatest benefits of mankind', and the reduction of polio incidence to a miniscule fraction of the numbers that once existed, along with the reduction of measles or yellow fever (vaccines against which are often combined with polio immunizations, depending on the epidemiology in the countries concerned) represents a very important contribution to the improvement of the health of poor children. But how should these benefits be delivered? Through eradication campaigns, or some other way?

In 1988, these questions were very much on the minds of the delegates to the World Health Assembly when polio eradication was being considered.

This was at the height of the PHC movement, so when the WHA voted to endorse a global polio eradication campaign, it stipulated that the eradication initiative had also to strengthen basic health infrastructures.

Proponents of polio eradication tend to say that polio eradication has done so. In the PAHO countries, they argue that it has produced a cadre of trained epidemiologists, created a network of virology laboratories, helped improve countries' capabilities in health planning, increased regional cooperation and the development of information systems concerning vaccination coverage, and led to the most comprehensive surveillance system for human health that has ever existed in the hemisphere, with the participation of over 20,000 health units reporting weekly on the presence or absence of acute flaccid paralyses. More generally, they believe polio eradication has added prestige to the health sector, by encouraging a 'culture of prevention'.[54]

This is an impressive list that understandably underscores its contributions in improving immunization services. But not all would agree that the results have been equally good everywhere. The Taylor Commission, which was set up in 1995 specifically to evaluate the impact of the EPI initiative and polio eradication in PAHO countries in the ten years since the campaign had started, agreed there were indeed several positive outcomes, but found some less favourable ones as well. The Commission reported, for instance, that the pay-offs from polio eradication were not as great in the poorest countries of the Americas as they were in the middle-income countries, which tended to have adequate health infrastructures already in place.[55] Taylor noted that donors tend to have great influence on health programmes (in some countries in sub-Sahara Africa, 40 per cent or more of health expenditures come from external [foreign] sources); and with a large campaign like polio eradication, there tends to be an excessive focus of effort on one disease, at the expense of a broader approach to ill health.

Taylor and his colleagues also raised some of the ethical issues that surround eradication more generally.[56] Polio eradication, for instance, sets a global priority ahead of local priorities, with the result that poor countries may find their own health planning distorted. In many countries, polio was not the most urgent of their public health problems when the eradication effort began; a survey in Ghana in 1984, for instance, found that polio was ranked only 33rd in priority, out of 48 diseases (malaria and measles ranked at the top).[57] Finally, there is the problem that polio eradication sets up a separate, parallel and unsustainable system of financing, vaccine supply and transport. This was, Taylor said, 'top-down mobilization, not bottom-up'. Once polio is almost (but not quite vanquished), would some of the money be made available for other public health needs, or would it all be expended on pursuing the elusive target of absolute eradication?

From a cost-benefit point of view, also, the calculations need to be re-examined. The benefit of eradication is usually calculated in terms of the health savings to be expected once eradication is achieved; one estimate by WHO put predicted savings (from cessation of vaccination and care of the paralysed) at $1 billion a year. But to whom would these savings accrue? Taylor pointed out that such benefits accrue less to poor countries than rich ones, because paralysed children in most poor countries do not get any such care or rehabilitation anyway. And although the amount of money pouring into Africa or India for polio eradication over the last 21 years has been huge (an estimated $3 billion worldwide between 1988 and 2007), the recipient countries have also had to spend a lot of their own resources merely to participate in the eradication effort. It is estimated, in fact, that 80 per cent of the costs of polio eradication are borne by individual countries.

Taylor's overall conclusion? That the promise of building a health infrastructure through polio eradication has not always been fulfilled.[58] Polio eradication thus represents an effort that, while from one point of view is utterly worthy of praise, from another can be seen as a Western, technical 'fix' that will not in fact produce solutions to the long-term health problems of poor populations. 'If the campaign succeeds, it may be mankind's single most ambitious accomplishment', says Gawande. 'But this is a big if.' He adds: 'International organizations are fond of grand-sounding pledges to rid the planet of this or that menace. They nearly always fail, however. The world is too vast and various to submit to dictates from on high.'[59]

Guinea Worm Eradication: A Different Model

GWD eradication tells a rather different story. This is a disease for which there is neither a drug nor a vaccine. Prevention (by means other than a vaccine) is therefore the only means of interrupting transmission. This basic fact about GWD has altered the way in which eradicating the infection has been carried out, bringing it much closer to the PHC model than other eradication efforts. In these regards I view the GWD story as a very interesting experiment – a potentially important alternative model or case study of a public health intervention.[60]

GWD was an obscure infection to most people in the west when it was proposed for eradication– one of those conditions known, if at all, for being, indeed, neglected.[61] Since almost no surveys of GWD had ever been carried out, it was very difficult to get a clear picture of incidence. In 1981, when Hopkins and Foege first suggested GWD eradication, they cited estimates of between ten and 48 million people being infected annually.[62] A later estimate in 1986 put the figure at a large but more manageable 3.2 million in twenty countries. Most cases of GWD were never reported; it was something poor rural people simply suffered.

Yet it is a very old disease whose symptoms had been recorded over the centuries, and whose parasitic origins were uncovered in the 1880s. The infection is transmitted to humans in one way only, through drinking water that is contaminated by minute arthropods called Cyclops, which harbour the larvae of the Guinea worm (*Dracunculus medinensis*). When someone drinks dirty contaminated water from a well or a pond, the larvae enter the human body, reproduce and, after an incubation period of a year, eventually a female worm, laden with new larvae, makes its way to the surface skin of the infected individual, through which it proceeds to emerge, often from a lower limb but also from other locations. The slow emergence of a worm up to 70–80 cm (28–31 in) in length is extremely painful and incapacitating, preventing walking (if it emerges from a limb) and working for weeks at a time. The affected individual often uses a stick to roll the worm around to help slowly pull it out. Seeking relief from the irritation and pain, infected people often immerse themselves in a cooling source of water; this provides the opportunity for the female worm to release its larvae, thereby contaminating the water, and starting the cycle again.

GWD met the biological and technical criteria for eradication: its diagnosis was unambiguous (the emergence of a worm); there was no other animal reservoir than the Cyclops; the latter, the transmitting agent, was not a mobile insect; and preventive interventions existed. In their letter, Hopkins and Foege linked the choice of GWD eradication to the launch of the UN's International Drinking Water and Sanitation Decade, which had set a target of providing clean water for all by the year 1990 (one of many such grand but unfulfilled targets).[63] Why not use some of the $20 to $30 billion expected expenditures to give priority to areas where GWD was endemic? Hopkins and Foege pointed out that GWD was the only disease that could be completely eradicated by substituting clean drinking water for dirty, since no other mode of transmission existed, and human beings were the only hosts for the worm. In principle, since the incubation period was a year, recurring infections could be stopped within a year of introducing clean water, as long as no larvae were allowed to re-enter the new water supply. GWD also had the advantage of being relatively confined in its distribution to certain places and/or countries in the Middle East, Asia, Latin America and, above all, Africa. Expectations for success in eradication were based on earlier programmes that had managed to eliminate GWD from many large areas and/or countries of the world (for example, the Soviet Union had eradicated GWD in Central Asia between 1925 and 1931).

From an economic point of view, the benefits of eradication (as opposed to mere control) were considered to be great, and accrued almost entirely to the affected populations. In 1986, The Carter Center set up its global Dracunculiasis Eradication Program (Hopkins moved to The Center as Vice President for Health Programs the next year).[64] In 1991, the WHO added its own resolution supporting worldwide eradication, the deadline for completion being set, much too optimistically, for 1995.[65] The financial aid of multiple international donors (various national governments of the countries with endemic GWD, UNICEF, The World Bank and eventually the Bill and Melinda Gates Foundation) has been essential, though the money has never been quite enough (between 1987 and 2007, external funds amounted to $147 million, a fraction of the costs of polio eradication).

Starting slowly, the GWD eradication effort gathered momentum, the concentrated focus on tackling a specific disease bringing about remarkable and rapid declines in the disease's incidence. To take one particularly striking case, in 1991, Uganda, with a budget of approximately $5.6 million, and the third-highest number of cases (125,000) reported from any endemic country, eradicated GWD in twelve years.[66] India's eradication effort took longer, starting in the 1980s and achieving zero cases by 1997. Worldwide, the approximately 3.5 million cases in twenty countries in Africa and Asia had by 1986 been reduced to 25,000-odd. Ten years of further effort brought the worldwide figure down to 4,600 (registered in December 2008), to 3,190 (by the end of 2009), and to less than 2,000 in 2010.[67] This is an extraordinary reduction of a long-standing disease of poverty.

What merits special attention is the distinctive mode of operations that the project has developed. The original plan had been to concentrate on building new water wells designed in such a way as to prevent the infection of the water by the worm's larvae. This fitted in with the intentions of the international 'water' decade; providing clean water has long been the *sine qua non* of modern health, preventing all sorts of water-transmitted infections. But building wells in rural areas proved costly and not always effective; the wells were not always deep enough, or placed near enough to where people lived in their villages; they were hard to maintain, and people often reverted to using their familiar, nearby watering holes and ponds.[68] The migration of populations was another problem. Chemical treatment of water to kill the Cyclops was a method that had been used successfully in India and elsewhere in the 1980s, but it took a long time, and was considered not to be always practicable.

Instead what proved most effective was to approach the problem of infected water differently, using preventive measures based on changing human behaviour – often considered to be the hardest thing to change of all. In many poor countries, local filters were already used to get clean water; the

GWD eradication project extended this idea to get rid of a specific infection. As spelled out by Hopkins and Ernesto Ruiz-Tiben in 1991, based on the experiences of GWD eradication in Pakistan, Ghana and Nigeria, the preventive programme needed the following elements: First, under a national plan of action involving the national government and the Ministry of Health, a baseline survey was carried out to identify and register all the endemic villages in the country. The next step was to identify each and every active case; here the campaign moved to the village level, relying on village-based health care workers, or if they did not exist or could not be found, on volunteers from each village.[69] They were given basic training on how to find and register or report every person with a worm.

The fundamental element was health education – instructing everyone in three basic messages: guinea worms come from drinking contaminated water; people with emerging worms must not contaminate sources of drinking water; and people can protect themselves from future infections by filtering their water, or only drinking from safe sources.[70] Education about GWD was the crucial element: most people did not connect drinking dirty water with worms that emerged from their bodies a year later. Filtering mud from a glass of water, and showing people the tiny Cyclops, was a direct demonstration. Filters, both on wells and for individual use at the end of drinking straws, were experimented with, until satisfactory types were found and widely distributed.

The key to GWD eradication has been the intense mobilization and above all, participation, of people at the village or community level – a different model from that used in most eradication campaigns before. As the numbers of GWD cases declined, active surveillance and containment became ever more important; the same was the case with keeping careful records. Starting in 1991, most national programmes began setting up 'case containment centres' – special huts set aside for infected individuals to live in while the worm emerges, in order to ensure that the worm has no chance of entering the drinking water supply. Incentives are offered, such as topical medical treatment of wounds, and help with food and water, until the worm exits and dies. Other elements that have helped push national programmes towards success have been the use of well-known figures such as President Carter himself, and prominent African politicians and other celebrities, to publicize the campaigns.[71]

This is not the place to give a complete account of all the details, ups and downs, successes and setbacks, country by country, of GWD eradication. My purpose here is to try to assess the GWD eradication campaign's contributions to public health in the countries concerned; to find out whether the project manages to combine the potential strengths of a specific-disease effort, with the broad concerns for public health equity and the delivery of basic health services that are needed.

Certainly, Hopkins and Ruiz-Tiben see the GWD eradication programme in these terms. They cite the improved agricultural productivity that comes from the elimination of GWD, as well as improved school attendance and infant care. They also believe that the mobilization of communities around public health, and especially the creation of a network of volunteers across rural areas of Africa, is a significant contribution. Moreover, in some places the network is being used to expand health services, by 'piggy-backing' new elimination and/or control projects directed against other NTDs, such as onchocerciasis, lymphatic filariasis, schistosomiasis and trachoma. The Carter Center has already helped distribute 20 per cent of the 530 million doses of the drug ivermectin that are being used to prevent river blindness (onchocerciasis). In two Nigerian states, the network originally recruited for river blindness control is now also delivering drugs and health education for lymphatic filariasis and schistosomiasis, Vitamin A supplements, and insecticide-treated bed nets for malaria control.[72] Many diseases are of course co-endemic (for example, malaria and trachoma in Ethiopia), so combining health interventions makes sense.

The expansion of the networks to include more diseases and more interventions raises the question of 'integration', the new watchword in international public health. Usually, integration in public health means merging a specific disease effort with the regular health services of a country. To the GWD eradicationists, though, integration means basing the eradication effort in a local community, with corresponding high levels of community participation and/or direction, and adding to a community-based network a new disease-specific effort. They generally resist merging GWD work with basic health services.[73] Two reasons for this are given; first is the general absence of such basic services in rural Africa, and second is the argument that, even where they do exist, such services tend to be largely passive, not active, and disconnected from the rural villages where so much disease is found.

There is also great reluctance to disband the volunteer health networks prematurely, before eradication is achieved. Hopkins and others see that as a recipe for failure. The idea, instead, is that the eradication network itself should become the organization through which to extend basic health services to the poorest and remotest places. 'I would prefer an excellent vertical programme to a mediocre integrated programme any day', Hopkins has remarked.[74]

This is an argument most eradicationists wind up making in one form or another. In defending eradication as a method of providing a legitimate model of health care, its proponents often refer to the specificity of the training that eradication demands, the perfection in execution it requires, the importance of maintaining systematic surveillance and containment, of setting measurable goals, undertaking continuous assessment, and keeping careful records (Soper would recognize all these points). Those involved in GWD eradication fear that the village-based networks and skills that have been built up around a specific disease over many years (sometimes decades) might get lost, or overwhelmed, in a general and fragmented system of basic health care.

The people leading GWD eradication are especially positive about what it shows can be done with health education and simple preventive measures. Hopkins argues that most people have a rational interest in their own health, and are willing to take action, but are wary of being told what to do by strangers, or foreigners. Thus a system that is specific, but based on simple methods, and organized by volunteers in villages, commends itself because it works.

Finally, Hopkins and those at The Carter Center like GWD eradication because, when all is said and done, they think it a great equalizer; to eradicate, Hopkins says, you have to go to all the places where the diseased population lives, to their villages – whether the population with GWD is small (as it was in Cameroon), or large (as it was in Nigeria). Eradication needs international financing behind it, he maintains, because in a country like Cameroon, with its small incidence, getting rid of every case of GWD is simply not the highest public health priority. Yet unless its few remaining cases are identified and dealt with, eradication cannot succeed. This is, again, close to Soper's own view of the inherent equity in eradication. Taking the example of tuberculosis as an eradicable disease, Soper commented 'Eradication cannot sacrifice the minority under the blanket classification – "no longer of public health importance"', meaning by this that when the goal is mere 'control', public health can settle for overall low incidence per capita, and disregard the rights of people who live in remote areas or places difficult to reach. To work, eradication has to cover everybody, so 'protection of all the population becomes the only acceptable professional public health standard'.[75] It is a rather different idea of health equity than is usual, when equity is used to refer to the methods needed to address unjust disparities in health outcomes between groups; to the distribution of resources to those most in need of them – the disadvantaged, the disempowered, the poorest, the least educated. In eradication, equity means that, for it to work, every single person with an infection has to be identified and treated if the goal of zero transmission is to be met, whatever their economic or medical situation. It is a definition that derives from that of eradication itself.

In other respects, the GWD eradication programme is un-Soperian, in being participatory and organized from the village-level up. It suffers from the some of the limitations of other disease-specific projects in that, being focused largely on a single disease, it cannot have a holistic approach; the young woman who has by preventive measures been protected from GWD infection also needs pre-natal and maternal care, and better nutrition. These latter needs the GWD eradication project by itself cannot meet. It is therefore a question of priorities; in the absence of the primary health care that remains the ideal in health circles, GWD eradication proponents feel they have nonetheless achieved a lot, and perhaps have laid a potentially fruitful building block towards the more sustainable and comprehensive health care that is really needed.

Is Eradication Feasible or Even Necessary?

Judged as a project of concentrated single-disease control, then, the GWD campaign can be called a brilliant success. Judged as a project of community-based health care, it has a great deal to recommend it.

Judged as an eradication campaign, however, as it must be (since it has always been advertised and run as such), it has been, as Hopkins acknowledges, 'unexpectedly long and difficult'.[76] The original target date of 1995 has come and gone, and so has the new deadline of 2009. Nonetheless, the determination to complete the job is there, and the end seems almost in sight. It may well be that GWD will become only the second human disease ever to be eradicated. President Carter has by now been involved with GWD eradication for 24 years; at 85 (in 2010) he says he is determined to outlive the guinea worm.[77]

Polio eradication appears more elusive. Though the number of polio cases has fallen to the merest fraction of what it once was, the remaining pockets of infection are proving difficult to eliminate, and the overall number of cases reported worldwide of about 1,500 per year has remained roughly the same since 2000. In August 2009 the WHO issued a warning that polio was still was spreading in Nigeria; by the middle of the month, 124 Nigerian children had already been paralysed. In addition to Nigeria, polio is still occurring in other countries – in Chad, Angola and Sudan, probably as a result of importation. Most worrying to WHO officials is that some of the paralyses are the result of a mutation in the live virus used in polio immunization itself. Furthermore, even if polio eradication were to be achieved, there are real questions about the hidden circulation of new polio virus variants, especially the most virulent type-1 variant; and about how, or even whether, polio immunization might be given up – a key rationale for the eradication project.[78]

The costs of pursuing eradication at this point are enormous. In August 2009, India set aside $657 million in its budget for polio eradication in

2010–11 alone (and the WHO noted that this followed similar commitments in past years). Gawande puts these sums into perspective by calculating (in 2007) that the cost per polio case detected worldwide is $600, while the entire health budget of India amounts to only $4 per person per year. 'Even if the campaign succeeds in the eradication of polio', he says, 'it is entirely possible that more lives would be saved in the future if the money were spent on, say, building proper sewage systems or improving basic health services'.[79]

Proponents argue that eradication is nevertheless a *bona fide* solution to relevant public health problems; that pushing to absolute zero is worthwhile in its own right, as well as from an economic point of view; and that the financial gains from the removal of polio will be calculated in billions of dollars (one estimate predicted $3 billion of savings in world expenditures by 2015 if eradication were to be achieved). They reject the view that, as eradication becomes focused on the remaining few cases in the world, the cost per every case detected becomes impossibly high, arguing that this is to overlook the huge savings in ill health, suffering and economic costs made by all the cases the campaign has already prevented. The main point is, to press on to the last case. Everything, they maintain, about an eradication campaign is dictated by this end purpose. If it were merely a control effort, the operation would not take the form it has, and the post-eradication benefit would of course not be gained, namely the giving up of all controls for that disease, for ever and ever. To them, the costs of giving up are greater than pursuing eradication to its logical conclusion. The end is in sight; giving up at this point would be a disaster.

But would it? What if eradication is not feasible, or necessary?[80] Why not settle for what has been achieved already?

D. A. Henderson's scepticism about eradication is well-known; he has not been, as he says, a 'bold eradicator'.[81] He praises Hopkins for being a 'brilliant and persuasive advocate and strategist' for GWD eradication, and for approaching GWD in the right way, with community involvement, proper surveillance and political commitment. Initiatives like this he thinks capable of being 'key steps in revolutionizing and revitalizing public health', because they set measurable goals, and are willing to look at alternatives for achieving them, 'without assuming, as we so often have, that every intervention, every vaccine, every drug, must somehow be directed or dispensed by some sort of primary health care'. Not being a fan of PHC or horizontal structures in health *per se*, Henderson is quick to insist on specificity and clear, measurable objectives in health work.

But Henderson is quite consistent in also thinking that in most cases setting eradication as the end-point of public health in the international sphere is a mistake. Eradication is too difficult to achieve, too costly and results in the constant adjustment of target dates and constant disappointment, with the consequent loss of morale of health workers. His advice? That we should not be blinded to a range of new public health programmes 'by staring too fixedly at the blinding beacon of a few eradication dreams'.[82]

Many others agree; they say that eradication is not worth it, medically, politically, economically or ethically. The criticisms of health professionals, especially those who once favoured eradication, probably sting the most.[83] In 2006, for instance, Dr Isao Arita, a WHO health official who had worked on smallpox eradication and had served on the technical advisory committee to the Expanded Programme on Immunization and Poliomyelitis Eradication, created a storm of controversy and disappointment among polio eradication advocates when he announced that he had changed his mind about polio. 'Is Polio Eradication Realistic?', he asked. His answer was: 'no'.[84]

He and his co-authors pointed out that between 1988 and 2006, $4 billion of international financial aid had been spent on polio eradication, and a further $1.2 billion would be needed to complete the task, assuming it could be done. They pointed, as well, to the failure of the campaign to meet the original target date of 2000. In that year, polio still existed in 23 countries, and in 2005 in sixteen. The figures on costs did not include the resources spent by the recipient countries in mobilizing to absorb polio eradication programmes. They reminded their readers that the world's population was now much larger than it had been when polio eradication had started (growing from four billion people in 1988 to 6.2 billion in 2006), with nearly all the increase occurring in the poorest areas of the world. In addition, the National Immunization Days used in polio eradication tend not to leave a legacy in health infrastructure, and it is not clear that polio vaccination can ever be given up. In short, the cost-benefit analysis of polio eradication for poor countries is quite different from that of smallpox.

Arita's recommendation is that, in the circumstances, the global strategy should shift from eradication to 'effective control'. Effective control does not mean giving up the extraordinary gains made against polio; it means pressing ahead until the annual number of cases of polio is less than 500 and the number of nations with polio less than ten. All global eradication programmes at that point should become part of WHO's Global Immunization, Vision, and Strategy (2005); oral polio vaccine (OPV) should be stockpiled, and continued OPV vaccination should be part of routine services in developing countries, so that the benefits gained thus far would be sustained. Understandably, those involved in polio eradication feel as people did when giving up on malaria eradication was proposed: that it is intolerable to think of losing all that had been gained in the near-elimination of polio over decades of effort. The picture has become even more confused and charged by the recent announcement by the previously sceptical Henderson that he has changed his mind: polio, he now thinks, is eradicable, given the resources, new methods and determination being brought to bear on the task by the Bill and Melinda Gates Foundation.[85]

Public Health in a Globalized World: A Changed Terrain

Arita and others are right to place eradication in the broader context of the health conditions that exist today, above all that of the gross deterioration we see in the state of health in the poorest countries of the world. The period roughly between 1945 and 1975 was one of the developing world's health transitions, meaning generally reduced levels of mortality and morbidity and improved longevity. But post-1975 we entered a new era of economic globalization, based on market fundamentalism and the 'free' flow of capital across the world, with its economic booms and its many busts. This has resulted in growing inequality, both within and between societies. It is estimated that, while the global economy has grown seven-fold since 1950, the disparity between the richest twenty countries and the poorest twenty more than doubled between 1960 and 1995. Today, almost half of the world's population lives on less than $2 a day. In Sub-Saharan Africa, mortality rates for children under five are between 100–200/1,000 (compared to eight in the USA and four in Japan); routine immunizations against childhood diseases like measles (a great killer) cover 50 per cent of children at best; and AIDS and malaria place intolerable burdens on populations and compete for attention and the limited resources of impoverished economies.

These economic realities bring into sharp focus the old argument about the economic determinants of health; economic and other social inequalities translate into inequalities in health. The virtual collapse of public health in post-Soviet Russia is just one example of how fragile many public health systems are, and how easily buffeted by the shock of naked and unregulated market forces. Male life expectancy actually fell in Russia for the first time in decades. The poorest countries in the world, many of them in Africa, have experienced even worse results; they had anyway seen much more modest gains in health than those in Asia and Latin America in the post-war period, only to have these gains virtually reversed from the 1980s on by economic setbacks, failures in governance, war, conflict over resources and global trade policies that have greatly disadvantaged their domestic economies. There has also been a huge resurgence in many places of diseases such as malaria and tuberculosis, as well as devastating new infections, notably HIV/AIDS. The response to HIV/AIDS, the major pandemic of our times, has been completely inadequate at the international level, often for ideological reasons (for example, the refusal by the US under President George W. Bush to support condom use to prevent infection), with the result that millions of people have now acquired the infection, with very large numbers dying, leaving huge numbers of orphaned children in the poorest countries, above all in Africa.

Globalization has also affected the institutions that govern health policies. Brown, Cueto and Fee have recently traced the history of the substitution of the word 'global' for the earlier term 'international' at the WHO; the word became fashionable at the organization in the 1990s, they say, and was directly tied to the recognition of the impact on societies of the global interdependence of capital, goods, people, ideas, information and technology, of the degradation of the environment, the inequalities in the distribution of health services, and the spread of infectious diseases.[86] Microbes, it is often said, know no borders; today, the compressed time/space character of globalization has intensified the potential for the spread of diseases, whether resurgent 'old' ones, or new and 'emerging' ones. Improving selected aspects of health in poor countries that might threaten rich countries with diseases has always been a feature of the latters' foreign policies, but the globalized and inter-connected world of today gives a special edge to global health policies as 'an investment in self-protection'.[87]

This investment takes many forms, from bilateral, government-to-government health programmes, to massive injections of money from private philanthropies. In 2000, in response to the growing disparities between rich and poor populations, 147 heads of state signed up to the UN's Millenium Development Goals (MDGs), eight in all, aimed at reducing poverty and inequalities in education, health, and gender. The MDGs were greatly influenced by the economist, Jeffrey Sachs, who had moved from advising 'shock' policies in Bolivia and post-1989 Poland, to health economics, arguing in his book, *The End of Poverty* (2005), that poverty and disease are major barriers to economic growth in the poorest countries, and that both could be eradicated through massive foreign aid (he proposed $195 billion a year by 2015), and fairly quickly (for example, in twenty years in Africa).[88] Gallup and Sachs argue that, controlling for factors such as tropical location, intensely malarial countries have lowered income levels compared to countries without malaria (on average, 1.3 per cent less per person growth per year). Lowering malaria would therefore, Sachs argues, increase economic growth. This is, of course, an old argument in public health. Given the uncertainties that surround what mix of factors creates economic improvement in the lives of poor people, however, it may be better to argue that bad health and high mortality, especially infant and child mortality, is something to be tackled in and by itself. Health should be treated as a fundamental human right, as WHO says.

Between 2002 and 2006, Sachs served as Director of the MDGs, whose purpose is to set definite targets and deadlines (rather as eradication campaigns do). For example, MDG 1, to eradicate extreme poverty and hunger, sets the target of halving by 2015 the proportion of people whose income is less than $1 a day. MDG 6 is directed at combatting HIV/AIDS, malaria and tuberculosis, indicating that for malaria it aims to halt and reverse the incidence by 2015. These are laudable goals, though many people argue that, like so many such grand goals before them, they are too grand and too vague to be met.[89]

Private philanthropy is very much part of this new global economy of health – more privately sourced money is pouring in to deal with disease than probably at any time before in human history. Health philanthropy has as a result become a very crowded field, with foundations, private-public partnerships and a huge number of non-governmental organizations (NGOs) engaged in a bewildering and overlapping array of health initiatives across the world.[90]

Today, in fact, the philanthro-capitalists (as they have been dubbed) call the tune in international health, with the WHO displaced from the leadership role it had commanded between 1948 and the late 1970s, and becoming instead a supplicant for resources and attention.[91] In 1982, the WHO's budget was frozen (by a vote of its members). Further depletions of the resources of the only legitimate representative global organization in health came from ideological attacks on the UN system as a whole. In 1985, the US Republican administration under President Ronald Reagan expressed its hostility to the UN by paying only 20 per cent of its assessed contributions to the UN agencies; it withheld entirely its contribution to WHO's regular budget because of its opposition to WHO's Generic Drug Programme, which predictably, the US pharmaceutical companies lobbied hard against (the budget has since been restored by the Obama administration). It is a sign of WHO's impoverished and reduced status that today only 9 per cent of the costs of the WHO-led polio eradication campaign is paid for by WHO funds.[92] Though supplemental donations have long been a part of how WHO operates, today outside money dwarfs the WHO's own regular budget. The World Bank, especially, has since the 1980s taken on a new role by giving large loans for health programmes as part of its development strategies.

The most striking example of the power and influence of philanthrocapitalism is The Bill and Melinda Gates Foundation (GF). Founded by Bill Gates in 1999 with stocks from his company Microsoft, today the foundation has at its disposal an estimated $31 billion of Gates's own money, as well as an additional $37 billion in stocks in Bershire Hathaway Inc., the hedge fund run by Warren Buffet (given in 2006). Its annual expenditures on health rose from $1.5 billion in 2001 to $7.7 billion in 2009.[93]

The GF is, if you like, the Rockefeller Foundation of the global era. It shares with the RF a science-based, technology-driven idea of how to solve the problems of global health. The emphasis is on new research breakthroughs and technological inventions. As Bishop and Green say, the new venture capitalists use the language of business and aim to harness the profit-motive to achieving a social good. Add to the mix the role of rock stars like Bono, or well-known public figures like President Bill Clinton (who has his own foundation), celebrities who speak out about the dire poverty and disease-ridden condition of the poorest countries, especially those in Africa, and we see that the profile of global health has been raised to levels hitherto never reached. But what will be the outcome? There is a fervent belief that solutions to the problems of disease and ill health in the world will be found. But what kind of solutions?

The trouble with these private initiatives is that, however dedicated to their aims and wise in their choices of goals and methods, they tend to each have their own favourite disease, or diseases, which become the focus of their activities. The foundations also answer largely to themselves and their technical staff; they channel their money into programmes selected by themselves, or their panels of expert advisors, rather than those chosen by the recipients of their financial and technical aid; and they almost inevitably divert people with much-needed technical, nursing and medical skills away from whatever basic health services may exist in poor countries, into the better paid foreign-funded health projects.

Of course, many initiatives, especially those working in partnership with the WHO, achieve beneficial outcomes – we would certainly put GWD eradication in this category. Pressure on the pharmaceutical companies from the Gates Foundation, the Clinton Foundation and the Global Fund to Fight AIDS, Tuberculosis and Malaria also led to a huge reduction in the price of AZT and other anti-AIDS drugs. Even William Easterly, the development economist who is most critical of the entire foreign aid business, argues that health is an area where foreign aid has probably had its greatest success.[94] At the same time, however, many philanthropic efforts represent schemes that are worked out at a distance, geographically and culturally, from the places where the schemes are to be applied. As in the MEP, there is often a gap between such projects and the realities on the ground. There is no doubt, too, that many private foundations tend to rely too much on new technical and medical innovations when considering health aid.

In a trenchant critique of the Bill and Melinda Gates Foundation's 'Grand Challenges' initiative, which the foundation launched in 2003, soliciting scientists from around the world for innovative research proposals on diseases that plague the poorest countries, such as malaria, Anne-Emmanuelle

Birn points out that the foundation explicitly excluded from consideration any proposals that focused on the social and economic determinants of disease and ill-health. This was so even when including a social dimension to their proposed interventions would greatly increase the possibility that the Gates Foundation's help would improve the overall health of populations.[95] Moreover, as Birn says, two thirds of children's deaths and four-fifths of all deaths are preventable through *existing* measures, whether technical (for example, vaccinations) or social (for example, improving clean water supplies or sewage disposal). 'The frustration in international circles is how effective measures remain unused', she comments.[96] The greatest challenge to the Gates Foundation, and others like it, is to realize that the social, political, economic and local factors cannot be separated from the biological and medical when considering the determinants of disease and its solutions.

Another problem concerns the medicalization of public health, such as over-reliance on mass distribution of antibiotics and anti-malaria drugs, without being sure the drugs reach those who most need them, and without being certain they will not result in the development of microbe and insect resistance. New drugs are necessary, both for old diseases like malaria, but also for the many NTDs that are only now being given the attention they are due. But history shows us that an over-dependence on drugs and chemicals can have unforeseen and negative consequences. (Already, for instance, plasmodium resistance has developed to artemisinin, the most recent 'wonder' anti-malarial drug.)

Finally, we need to recognize that however well-intentioned, generous and technically sophisticated the activities of philanthropic institutions are, and however many partnerships they forge (for example, between the Bill and Melinda Gates Foundation and several WHO-led efforts at disease control), their activities are often uncoordinated; are often so disease-specific that they cannot address the public health needs of impoverished countries in any consistent way (according to Garrett, there are more than 60,000 HIV/AIDS-related non-governmental organizations alone); and cannot, by themselves, provide an overall general, regulatory and policy framework for 'global' health. This is what, historically, the WHO once provided.[97] The mandate of WHO needs to be strengthened, not weakened, otherwise we run the risk that private capital and interests will determine how the bulk of health aid is spent.

Battle-Ground Malaria: Eradication, Once Again?

Among the many initiatives and programmes of health aid in the recent past, perhaps none has made more news or been more surprising than Bill and Melinda Gates' announcement in October, 2007 that their foundation's goal in malaria was complete eradication. This was no casual use of a word but a considered decision to set an absolutist end-point. Whatever the Gates Foundation does, it means large sums of money, incentives, a pulling of people and ideas into the Gates Foundation's orbit.

Malaria, and especially malaria in Africa, is at the centre of current debates about poverty, development and ill health. After a period of steep declines before 1980, malaria has made a comeback, with by now an estimated 300–500 million malaria cases a year, and one million deaths (90 per cent of which are in Africa). HIV/AIDS joined with malaria appears to make things worse.[98] The large sums of money going to malaria have already led to questions about how to spend it. Debates often pit experts in Western think-tanks or research institutions, looking for technical solutions, against those who work in the field and who think of malaria in terms of sustainable and long term control – a reprise, in some ways, of the debate between eradicationists and colonial malaria experts in Kampala in 1950.

When the GF announced they saw the endgame of malaria control as eradication, they were apparently taken by surprise at the largely negative reaction. They did not intend to signal by their statement an all-out, short-term and immediate global eradication campaign like the MEP, as some people seemed to think. Their timeframe is much longer; but since eradication is in principle achievable, they decided to announce this as the ultimate goal.[99] Their view is that reductions in malaria from the deliberate interventions of the MEP were remarkable, were curtailed by a much too short timeframe, and are today generally overlooked or dismissed by critics of eradication. Looking to the future, they see a new era in malaria investigations being made possible by well-selected and well-funded scientific investigations.[100] These could well result in the next two to three decades in new anti-malaria drugs to replace those to which the plasmodia have become resistant.[101]

The foundation has also set its sights on an anti-malaria vaccine. Such a vaccine has long been a dream of malaria research – but an unfulfilled dream. A vaccine is often seen as the ideal intervention to achieve eradication, but the barriers to discovering one in the case of malaria are extraordinarily high, the plasmodium and the anopheline mosquitoes being extremely wily, adaptive and capable of high reproductive rates. Despite the difficulties, many avenues are being pursued (though field trials of potential vaccines have proved disappointing).[102] But many people remain unconvinced; they continue to maintain that no vaccine alone will be able in the next decade or two to eradicate malaria – that multiple strategies, adapted to different human circumstances and vectors, will be needed.

The GF's bold declaration of eradication as their goal is, of course, very much in keeping with its general science-based outlook towards disease, and reflects as well the power of a single foundation to set policy targets for the rest of the world. It is a striking example of the idea that 'eradication is the venture capital of public health' – of the notion that 'the risks are huge but so are the results'.[103]

And yet, in all the discussions among public health officials and scientists about eradication that had taken place since smallpox eradication was announced in 1980, malaria had never been selected as a possible candidate. The past failure weighed too heavily for that. From that failure, people had rediscovered the complexity of the biological, ecological, social and economic determinants of the disease; there was little appetite for a one-size-fits-all, technical fix, and an appreciation of the need to link anti-malaria work to basic or primary health care. The best that could be aimed for was prevention and control, which would require an integrated strategy involving multiple social, political and medical components. These lessons are partially reflected in the Roll Back Malaria (RBM) programme, WHO's first large-scale project on malaria since the end of malaria eradication; starting in 1998, the RBM aimed to reduce by 2010 malaria morbidity and mortality by 50 per cent and 75 per cent, respectively, of the levels that existed in 2000. Basing its work largely on the distribution of Insecticide Treated Bed Nets (ITNs), malaria incidence has been reduced steadily in some countries (for example, Ethiopia, Rwanda and Zambia), but diagnosis and treatment is lagging behind nearly everywhere else. As usual, the RBM's goals were 'nominal' targets that could not be met completely.[104]

In the circumstances, most malaria specialists believe that eradication is either not achievable, or unrealistic.[105] Yet to many people's further surprise, Dr Margaret Chan, the current Director-General of WHO, immediately applauded the idea of malaria eradication, seeing it as a long-term, not a short-term, project that might take 'multiple decades' (as Gates told reporters), but one that would have an immediate and large influence, owing to the power and pull of the Gates Foundation.

Some Soperian Moments?

So where does eradication now stand in our current globalized economy? Since this book began with Soper, perhaps it should end with him too. The context is the return of many diseases that were once greatly reduced in incidence – tuberculosis, yaws, yellow fever and malaria. Especially alarming, dengue fever is on the rise, especially the often-fatal variant, dengue haemorrhagic fever (DHF).

These developments have produced some 'Soperian' moments – moments when public health experts reconsider Soper's methods, while acknowledging the quite different political circumstances in which they must be employed. For instance, Soper's achievement in eradicating *Anopheles gambiae* in Brazil has led to the proposal that his larviciding techniques be added to current malaria control methods in Africa.[106]

Soper's anti-vector methods are especially relevant to the control of dengue fever. Dengue is a human infection caused by an arbovirus; like yellow fever it is transmitted largely by the urban *Aedes aegypti* mosquito, of Soper fame; but unlike yellow fever today, dengue thus far has no vaccine.[107]

As noted in chapter Four, when Soperian vigilance against the *Aedes aegypti* was given up in the 1970s, owing to the availability of a yellow fever vaccine, no one was thinking about dengue fever, which at the time caused only sporadic epidemics in the Americas. Today, however, dengue is a very serious public health problem, spreading rapidly in both Asia and the Americas, and causing ever more serious epidemics. Altogether, there are probably 50–100 million cases of dengue infection worldwide a year, roughly 400,000 of them dengue haemorrhagic fever (DHF), the most fatal variant of the four dengue fever virus variants (resulting in the deaths of 5 per cent of those infected). Another alarming trend is that a growing number of the DHF infections are found in children under fifteen. The best that can be done for dengue patients is hospitalization and prompt rehydration.[108]

Pending the development of a vaccine (and there are several under trial), there is nothing for it but to return to the methods of Soper – meaning mosquito surveillance and vigilant larviciding. In 1996, PAHO's Directing Council passed a resolution – yet again – urging member countries to develop national plans to reduce *Aedes aegypti* as a matter of urgency. But in every other respect there was no going back to Soper's day. The original goal of eradicating the mosquito had to be given up; history showed that every time a country certified complete eradication of the vector, it was negated by the mosquito's return within a few years. The new aim was instead control – meaning permanent systems of epidemiological surveillance, laboratory testing of the virus and its variants and identification and treatment (usually with insecticides) of the breeding spaces of the mosquitoes. Physically, the density of human urban settlement is far greater today than it was in the 1940s and '50s; many cities in the developing world now have populations of twelve, fifteen or even twenty million people; slums, with their inadequate housing, and their lack of piped water and proper garbage removal, have proliferated – creating perfect breeding conditions for the *Aedes aegypti* mosquito.

Politically, too, the Soperian era has passed. Militant top-down programmes are simply not acceptable short of severe emergencies (or extremely authoritarian polities).

Instead, Soper's methods have to be adapted to new political norms of public health, meaning a respect for human rights and community participation. To take an example, I have looked at Brazil, where by far the greatest number of cases of dengue in the Americas occur (about 70 per cent of the total). In 2002, the city of Rio had a massive epidemic, with 280,000 cases of infection and 91 deaths. The epidemic of 2007–8 was smaller, but still resulted in 75,000 cases. The military had to be called in to fumigate houses and to set up temporary tent hospitals (actually large metal structures like containers) to take in the thousands of patients who overwhelmed the city hospitals.

To move from this kind of reactive, short-term response, to a much more proactive, long-term sustainable programme of dengue control, the public health officials I interviewed are searching for a new political and cultural model – one that is Soperian in being disease-specific and vigilant about identifying and destroying *Aedes aegypti* larvae, but quite different in its social organization.[109] When Soper used a vertical approach and relied on teams of insecticiders and inspectors, his ideas about vector eradication were not absorbed or accepted necessarily by the local populations, but imposed on them. Today's approach aims to be much more bottom-up, organized in local communities, and based on collaboration, cooperation and modern communications (such as mobile phones). Like Soper, the officials rely on careful mapping of risk areas; but their eyes in the local communities are largely those of resident volunteers, who are recruited and trained in the job of reporting abandoned and neglected sites where mosquitoes are breeding (today thousands of such community health workers are involved across the cities and municipalities of Brazil). The health officials I met believe their most innovative contribution is to approach dengue control as a fundamentally social problem, and not just a problem of mosquitoes, whose solution will depend on the involvement of people from all sectors of society – the local community and mayor's office at the municipal level, the health authorities at the level of the state, and finally, the federal government, which serves as the national coordinator of the effort.[110]

As a final example of a 'Soperian' moment, we might cite the programme to control American trypanosomiasis (otherwise known as Chagas disease after the Brazilian physician Carlos Chagas, who discovered the parasite, the insect vector and the clinical symptoms of a hitherto unknown human infection in 1909). This is a very strange, essentially chronic disease; it is transmitted by a large insect called a triatoma that lives in houses that are poorly constructed, with cracked walls in which the insects can hide, and from which they emerge at night to feed on the sleeping inhabitants. Infection starts with an acute feverish stage, usually in childhood, and then is followed, many years later, in a percentage of the infected population, by a chronic phase involving odd digestive disturbances and heart arrhythmias (which can cause sudden death in young adults). Chagas disease currently infects millions of people in Latin America, and globalization (meaning in this case, migration) is bringing it into new areas of North America and Europe. It is one of the many neglected diseases left out of the picture in the current 'flurry of global health advocacy and resource mobilization'.[111] Celebrity medical philanthropy has passed it by.

Soper never got involved in Chagas disease control in Brazil, but the methods being used to deal with it today have their Soperian aspects, in being almost entirely focused, as with dengue, in getting rid of insects, Soper's speciality.[112] Starting in 1991, the 'Southern Cone Initiative' (involving Argentina, Bolivia, Brazil, Chile, Paraguay and Uruguay) was organized, in a major and cooperative public health effort focused on stopping transmission by attacking with insecticides the main insect vector of the disease in the region, the *Triatoma infestans* (and to a lesser extent, by improving rural houses so as to prevent their infestation by the vector). Transmission was declared eliminated in Uruguay in 1997, in Chile in 1999, and in Brazil in 2006. This is an important milestone. The challenge now is to keep up surveillance, and to get treatment and care to the many people who were infected in the past and now bear the burden of the chronic condition, for which there are few if any effective drugs.[113]

Note that the elimination aimed for thus far is regional, and is aimed at eliminating only one of several triatome vectors responsible for Chagas transmission in the Americas. As such, the campaign operates, like dengue control, in a very different fashion from the vertical campaigns of Soper's day. It is more modest in ambition, and when it uses the word 'eradication', it uses it in a loose rather than a technically absolutist fashion.[114] In many ways we might think of it as a new paradigm (no doubt with its own paradoxes and problems). First, the project is in effect 'owned' (planned, directed, organized, staffed) by the participating countries themselves. Second, as with dengue control, community participation (volunteers trained to report on housing infestations) and local support (via health education) are assumed to be essential. Third, research forms a critical component of the campaigns (it is understood that epidemiological and other knowledge of the disease is incomplete).[115] The watchwords are 'multi-pronged' or 'integrated' approaches, and 'adaptation to local realities'. The model is political, rather than purely biomedical; it is participatory and more democratic in intention, without giving up the commitment to disease specificity in its technical methods.

Those involved in such disease-specific efforts know that the programmes alone cannot provide health to populations, as WHO has defined health; primary or basic health care systems are fundamental and must work in concert with targeted efforts, whether for measles vaccination, Chagas disease control, dengue mosquito reduction or other initiatives. Indeed, building primary care services is more important than ever, a point made by Dr Margaret Chan, the Director-General of WHO in her 2008 World Report.[116] Poorer countries struggle to get such combined services, but there are examples. In Brazil, for instance, in the 1980s public health doctors, galvanized by their opposition to military rule, and by the crisis of HIV/AIDS, managed to organize specific, targeted health policies for those infected with the retrovirus (including, crucially, free treatment with retrovirals for all those who are HIV-positive); they also managed to draw on, and put to use, the new commitment to human rights that had developed as part of the resistance to military rule, and thereby make the right to health a fundamental element in the new Constitution that was drawn up in 1988, after the military had finally stepped down and full constitutional government was restored.[117]

Concomitant with the response to HIV/AIDS, the other necessary element to improving health in Brazil was to put in place the *Sistema Único de Saúde* (known as SUS, and standing for 'Unified Health Service'), also in 1988. This is the first, universal, publicly funded health care system to be established in the country, one that guarantees every Brazilian citizen free access to healthcare.[118] It is still far from perfect; SUS is not organized around primary care doctors, but is largely dependent on specialist care, and as a result is curative rather than preventive in orientation, and too hospital-based. As a system, SUS also has to compete against numerous private insurance schemes in the country which have long dominated the health sector, and which together in effect divide Brazil's health services into a first-class system for the rich, and a second-class system for the poor. Brazil has still a long way to go in overcoming economic and racial inequalities in one of the most unequal countries in the world, inequalities that translate into inequalities in health and access to good quality health care which are felt across regions, states, ethnicity and class.[119]

Nevertheless, SUS is a very important development, providing health care that previously was simply not available to the majority of Brazil's citizens. As Kunitz, Szreter and others have argued, deliberate social and public health policies by the state, broadly defined to include such things as sickness insurance, access to medical care and routine vaccinations, delivered universally and as a right, are crucial factors in overcoming the disruptive and unequal impact of economic growth.

As we have seen, the GWD eradication campaign in Africa also provides a new model of public health action in very poor countries that lack the infrastructure and political commitment necessary for the development of the kinds of primary health care services that are found in a middle income country like Brazil. But the GWD model can be emulated in other places *without the commitment to absolute eradication*. Better by far to have a sustainable project, disease-focused, but with an ever-widening public health agenda, such as we see is possible with the GWD initiative. Eradication campaigns organized around a single disease absorb a great deal of a country's financial and other resources in the pursuit of a single goal; when the goal proves elusive, very often the gains are not sustained, because the project is not linked to other health projects or health care systems.

Eradication will no doubt continue to keep a place in the arsenal of possible public health interventions but, in my view, eradication campaigns should be exceptional and rare.

References

Introduction

1 F. Fenner et al., 'What is Eradication?', in *The Eradication of Infectious Diseases*, ed. W. R. Dowdle and D. R. Hopkins (New York, 1998), p. 11, quoting the definition given by the US Centers for Disease Control (CDC).

2 For example, malaria disappeared in Britain by the end of the nineteenth century, as a result of ecological changes and alterations in patterns of human settlement, but without any particular measures directed against it. See Mary J. Dobson, *The Contours of Death and Disease in Early Modern England* (Cambridge, 1997).

3 Incidentally, only one animal disease, rinderpest, a highly contagious disease of cattle, has been completely eradicated worldwide by deliberate efforts. A decades-long global campaign, based on animal vaccination, ended in success, with the official UN announcement made on 28 June 2011. This book is about the eradication of human diseases, not animal diseases, but there are parallels in their histories. The eradication of diseases in animals is potentially more straightforward than the eradication of diseases in human beings, because fewer ethical constraints apply: we can cull animal herds if we have to, and indeed as we have done since the eighteenth century. Many diseases, such as foot-and-mouth disease, have been eradicated locally or regionally, but not globally. Culling and other methods of 'stamping out' diseases has in practice been very difficult to achieve, in part because of the intense commercial interests that are involved in saving herds from severe culling, even in the face of epidemics (or, in the case of foot-and-mouth disease in the UK, resistance, also for commercial reasons, to a rational plan of animal vaccination).

4 World Health Organization, *The Global Eradication of Smallpox: Final Report of the Global Commission for the Certification of Smallpox Eradication* (Geneva, 1980). Three further deaths were connected to the accidental release of smallpox virus from a laboratory in Birmingham, England, in 1978; one death occurred from smallpox, one by suicide (of the laboratory's director) and the third was the smallpox victim's father, who died of a heart attack.

5 In addition to the deaths, seventeen other people were infected, but recovered. Over the years, suspicion was directed at several individuals, all in the United States; in 2008, the FBI accused Dr Bruce Ivins, a microbiologist and researcher at the US Army Medical Research Institute of Infectious Diseases, who was working on improving a vaccine for anthrax, of being responsible. Ivins committed suicide on 29 July 2008, before federal officials could charge him. Considerable scepticism remains about the conclusions of the official investigation.

6 The discussions and events concerning smallpox bioterrorism are well described by Jonathan B. Tucker, in his book, *Scourge: The Once and Future Threat of Smallpox* (New York, 2001), especially chap. 11. The original WHO-decision that all stocks of smallpox virus be destroyed had been put on hold earlier, when a defector from the USSR to the United States in the 1980s revealed that the Soviet Union had weaponized large quantities of smallpox, in contravention of the Biological Weapons Convention.

7 President George W. Bush announced in December 2002 a new plan to vaccinate ten million Americans against smallpox, starting with mandatory vaccinations for members of the armed forces, to be followed by voluntary vaccinations for 'first responders' in an emergency, such as firefighters, the police and health workers. Complications, including some deaths, from smallpox vaccination led to a temporary suspension of the programme and to growing resistance. Most health workers argued that the risks of vaccination, to themselves, but also to the unvaccinated patients they treated in hospitals and clinics, far outweighed the benefits of vaccination. By December 2003, less than 40,000 had been vaccinated. See D. A. Henderson, *Smallpox – The Death of a Disease. The Inside Story of Eradicating a Worldwide Killer* (Amherst, NY, 2009), pp. 292–7.

8 Letter to the Editor by Dr Timothy Baker, 'Malaria Eradication in India: A Failure?', *Science*, 319 (5870) (21 March 2008), p. 1616. WHO's figures have recently been challenged as a very serious undercount of death rates in rural areas, which take place outside of health care facilities and out-of-sight of reporting systems; see Neeraj Dhingra, et al., 'Adult and Child Malaria Mortality in India: A Nationally Representative Mortality Survey,' published online at www.thelancet.com (21 October 2010) DOI:10.1016/S0140-6736(10)60831-8. The authors' estimates, based on 'verbal autopsies' (house-based comments on recent deaths in families and communities) suggest low-to-high estimates of 125,000 to 277,000 malaria deaths per year.

9 Leslie Roberts and Martin Enserink, 'Did They Really Say ... Eradication?', *Science*, 318 (5856) (7 December 2007), pp. 1544–5.

10 *The Eradication of Infectious Diseases*, p. 20, Table 3.1.

11 For example, John Farley, *To Cast Out Disease: A History of the International Health Division of the Rockefeller Foundation (1913–1951)* (Oxford and New York, 2004).

12 An excellent account of the Rockefeller Foundation's activities in Mexico is given by Anne-Emmanuelle

Birn, in *Marriage of Convenience: Rockefeller International Health and Revolutionary Mexico* (Rochester, NY, 2006). For a re-conceptualization of the history of hookworm infection, labour and the 'new science', see Steven Palmer, 'Migrant Clinics and Hookworm Science: Peripheral Origins of International Health, 1840–1920', *Bull. Hist. Med.*, 83 (4) (2009), pp. 676–709.

13 Randall M. Packard, *The Making of a Tropical Disease: A Short History of Malaria* (Baltimore, MD, 2007); Marcos Cueto, *Cold War, Deadly Fevers: Malaria Eradication in Mexico, 1955–1975* (Baltimore, MD, 2007).

14 Two older books, written at the height of the post-war eradication fervour, are E. E. Harold Hinman's *World Eradication of Infectious Diseases* (Springfield, IL, 1966), and Greer William's *The Plague Killers* (New York, 1969). Neither are critical accounts, nor could the authors anticipate what would happen with malaria, smallpox and later eradication efforts. A more recent book, still breezy and anecdotal in style, but useful in covering the post-war campaigns against malaria, smallpox and polio, is by Cynthia A. Needham and Richard Canning, *Global Disease Eradication: The Race for the Last Child* (Washington, DC, 2003).

15 Soper lacks a modern biography. His autobiographical *Ventures in Health: The Memoirs of Fred Lowe Soper*, ed. John Duffy (Washington, DC, 1977), is an important resource, though curiously impersonal. A collection of his published articles appeared as *Building the Health Bridge: Selections from the Works of Fred L. Soper, M.D.*, ed. J. Austin Kerr (Bloomington, IN, and London, 1970). Soper left a large archive of his diaries, letters and papers to the National Library of Medicine (NLM) in Washington; the library has made selected documents drawn from the collection available online. See 'The Fred L. Soper Papers', Profiles in Science, National Library of Medicine (http://profiles.nlm.nih.gov/VV/). His unpublished papers are found at NLM, Collection Number Ms C 359, The Fred Lowe Soper Papers, and consist of 74 boxes of manuscripts and case items, and 114 volumes of documents (consisting mainly of Soper's collection of reprints of articles).

16 'The Reminiscences of Dr Alan Gregg' (1958), p. 135, in The Alan Gregg Papers, NLM, Profiles of Science, at http://profiles.nlm.nih.gov/FS/.

17 Quoted in Farley, *To Cast Out Disease*, p. 16.

18 NLM, Ms C 359, Soper Papers, Box 2. Candau in a cable.

19 Quote from Marcos Cueto, *The Value of Health: A History of the Pan American Health Organization* (Washington, DC, 2007), p. 91.

20 See Fred L. Soper, 'Meaning of Eradication – Revolutionary Concept', in NLM, Ms C 359, Soper Papers, Box 30, Daily Files, 1964, Folder: October–December 1964 (dated 15 December 1964).

21 Editorial Introduction to Fred L. Soper lecture, 'Rehabilitation of the Eradication Concept in Prevention of Communicable Diseases', *Public Health Reports*, 80 (10) (1965), pp. 855–69, Introduction on p. 854.

22 John Duffy, Editor's Note, in Soper, *Ventures in World Health*, pp. xiii–xiv.

23 NLM, Ms C 359, Soper Papers, Box 14, from a review in 1970 by Bruce-Chwatt of *Building the Health Bridge*.

24 Today the member countries are grouped into six regions, each with its own regional office; these are Africa (Brazzaville, Congo), Americas (Washington, USA), South East Asia (New Delhi, India), Europe (Copenhagen, Denmark), Eastern Mediterranean (Cairo, Egypt) and Western Pacific (Manila, The Philippines).

25 NLM, Ms C 359, Soper Papers, Box 12, Soper notes on 'Conversation with Dr John Hume', New Delhi, India (5 December 1955), p. 5 of document.

26 Ilana Löwy, 'Epidemiology, Immunology, and Yellow Fever: The Rockefeller Foundation in Brazil, 1923–1939', *J. Hist. Biology*, 30 (1997), pp. 397–417.

27 *Yellow Fever*, ed. George Strode (New York, 1951). With an effective vaccination in hand, the Foundation believed that mosquito control and vaccination were adequate to control yellow fever. Farley, *To Cast Out Disease*, p. 16, says Soper left the foundation under a cloud, though he provides no direct evidence.

28 Malcolm Gladwell, Annals of Public Health, 'The Mosquito Killer', *New Yorker* (2 July 2001), pp. 42–51.

29 NLM, Ms C 359, Soper Papers, Box 12, Document, 'Conversation with Dr John Hume', New Delhi, p. 5.

30 Fred L. Soper, 'Problems to be Solved if the Eradication of Tuberculosis is to be Realized', *Amer. J. Pub. Health*, 52 (5) (1962), pp. 734–48, here p. 735.

31 Geoffrey M. Jeffery, 'Malaria Control in the Twentieth Century', *Amer. J. Tropical Med. and Hyg.*, 25 (3) (1976), pp. 361–71, here: p. 367.

32 Rene Dubos, *Man Adapting*, with a new introduction by the author (New Haven, CT, 1980), p. 379.

1 Eradication and Public Health

1 See Stephen J. Kunitz, *The Health of Populations: General Theories and Particular Realities* (Oxford, 2007), pp. 9–26, where he discusses the two revolutions.

2 Figure from Jeffrey Sachs, *The End of Poverty: How We Can Make it Happen in our Lifetime* (New York and London, 2005), p. 194.

3 James C. Riley, *Rising Life Expectancy: A Global History* (Cambridge and New York, 2001), p. 1. Mortality and life expectancy are useful measures for purposes of country-to-country comparisons, but do not reveal considerable variations within countries across class, geography and other lines of social division.

4 See Michael Worboys, *Spreading Germs: Diseases, Theories, and Medical Practice in Britain, 1865–1900* (Cambridge, 2000), especially chap. 7, where he examines the multiple meanings that were attached to bacteriology and its slow penetration into medical practice. Fumigation designed to remove poisonous miasms in the pre-bacteriological era was used in the post-bacteriological era to remove insect vectors.

5 Kunitz, *The Health of Populations*, p. 11.

6 Lester S. King, 'Dr Koch's Postulates', *J. Hist. Med. Allied Sci.*, 7 (4) (1952), pp. 350–61, points out that Koch himself did not emphasize these logical principles, but Koch's work exemplified them so clearly and originally that the postulates are called after him. Koch's postulates set out the necessary conditions for infectious disease, but not the sufficient conditions; people could test positive for the presence of the diphtheria bacillus, for example, yet show no signs of the disease. Other factors, such as previous infections, help determine the susceptibility or immunity of individuals.

7 The Culicidiae family of mosquitoes includes the genus of Anopheles, Culex (transmitting West Nile fever, filariasis, and St Louis encephalitis, among other viral infections), and *Aedes aegypti* (originally called *Stegomyia fasciata*, the vector of urban yellow fever and dengue). African and American trypanosomiasis (sleeping sickness, and Chagas disease) were also shown by the end of the first decade of the twentieth century to be conveyed to human beings by tsetse flies and triatoma bugs respectively.

8 Quote from Kunitz, *The Health of Populations*, p. 12. This book gives a lucid account of the epistemological changes associated with the 'new public health' in the United States in the early years of the twentieth century, showing how the rise of the profession of public health was particularly closely associated with bacteriology, the establishment of bacteriological laboratories, and the introduction of new techniques of disease control.

9 A similar analysis could be made with yellow fever. Its immediate cause is a viral infection transmitted by the bite by an infected mosquito. Yellow fever vaccination can prevent infection, as can strict mosquito control. But yellow fever also has social and economic determinants, such as the unsanitary rubbish, abandoned rubber tires, tin cans and soda bottles that litter the urban slums of cities in regions such as Latin America; the water that collects in such receptacles provides the perfect breeding place for the *Aedes* mosquito that transmits urban yellow fever (and dengue). Regular rubbish collection and the provision of clean piped water would be perhaps more expensive than mosquito-clearing and killing, but also would provide more long-lasting, social improvements that would reduce the risk of yellow fever as well as water-borne infections.

10 For example, in 1909, the Brazilian researcher, Dr Carlos Chagas, discovered the parasite, insect vector and clinical symptoms of a hitherto unrecognized human disease, *American trypanosomiasis* (commonly called Chagas disease).

11 Brazil is generally considered to have had one of the best responses to HIV/AIDS, while the South African government, under President Mbeki, was notorious in public health and AIDS-activist circles for rejecting the retroviral theory of AIDS infection. This position has begun to be reversed under President Zuma. On Brazil, see Herbert Daniel and Richard G. Parker, *Sexuality, Politics, and AIDS in Brazil: In Another World* (London and Washington, DC, 1993).

12 Politically, McKeown's thesis was originally associated with the political left; but in the 1980s it was taken up by the political right and interpreted as validating neo-liberal market approaches to health. Right-wing appropriation of the McKeown thesis is perhaps one reason for the efforts by historians and social scientists to re-instate the importance of social, political and public health, intentional interventions if health for all is to be reached. James Colgrove, in his article, 'The McKeown Thesis: A Historical Controversy and its Enduring Influence', *Amer. J. Pub. Health*, 92 (5) (May 2002), pp. 725–9, suggests that McKeown's battles against the over-medicalization of health in Britain's National Health Service (NHS) may have led McKeown to downplay the part played by medicine and public health in lowering mortality and morbidity.

13 Figures from Simon Szreter and Graham Mooney, 'Urbanization, Mortality, and the New Standard of Living Debate: New Estimates of the Expectation of Life at Birth in Nineteenth-Century Cities', *Econ. Hist. Rev.*, 51 (1) (1998), pp. 84–112, here: p. 88.

14 It is well known that malnutrition is correlated with reduced immunity to disease, and good nutrition to disease resistance. For McKeown's publications, see Thomas McKeown and R. G. Record, 'Reasons for the Decline in Mortality in England and Wales During the Nineteenth Century', *Population Studies*, 16 (2) (1962), pp. 94–122; Thomas McKeown, R. G. Record and R. D. Turner, 'An Interpretation of the Decline of Mortality in England and Wales during the Twentieth Century', *Population Studies*, 29 (3) (1975), pp. 391–422; Thomas McKeown, *The Modern Rise of Population* (New York, 1976); and his *The Role of Medicine: Dream, Mirage, or Nemesis?* (London, 1976). The term 'optimistic' to describe the McKeown thesis is used by Kunitz, in *The Health of Populations*, pp. 22–3. Others have called it a 'nihilist' theory; see Amy L. Fairchild and Gerry M. Oppenheimer, 'Public Health Nihilism vs Pragmatism: History, Politics, and the Control of Tuberculosis', *Amer. J. Pub. Health*, 88 (7) (1998), pp. 1105–17.

15 Colgrove, 'The McKeown Thesis', gives an excellent review.

16 Szreter and Mooney, 'Urbanization, Mortality, and the New Standard of Living Debate', pp. 84–112. The reference to Hobsbawm is E. J. Hobsbawm,

'The British Standard of Living, 1780–1850', in *The Standard of Living Debate in the Industrial Revolution*, ed. A. J. Taylor (London, 1975), pp. 82–92.

17 See Simon R. Szreter, 'The Importance of Social Intervention in Britain's Mortality Decline *c.* 1850–1914: A Re-interpretation of the Role of Public Health', *Social History of Medicine*, 1 (1) (1988), pp. 1–38. Along somewhat the same lines as Szreter, see Anne Hardy, *The Epidemic Streets: Infectious Disease and the Rise of Preventive Medicine, 1866–1900* (Oxford, 1993). The interventions referred to by Szreter concern improving water standards and sewage disposal.

18 See Colin Leys, 'Health, Health Care and Capitalism', in *Morbid Symptoms: Health Under Capitalism*, ed. Leo Panitch and Colin Leys, *Socialist Register 2010* (London, 2009), pp. 1–28.

19 Simon Szreter, *Health and Wealth: Studies in History and Policy* (Rochester, NY, 2005).

20 Kunitz, *The Health of Populations*, especially pp. 45–56. The quote is from p. 76. The literature on McKeown is now enormous. In 2002, the *American Journal of Public Health* devoted an issue to the McKeown thesis. See especially for references and analysis, Colgrove, 'The McKeown Thesis'; Simon Szreter, 'Rethinking McKeown: The Relationship between Public Health and Social Change', *Amer. J. Pub. Health*, 92 (5) (May 2002), pp. 722–5; and Bruce G. Link and Jo C. Phelan, 'McKeown and the Idea that Social Conditions are Fundamental Causes of Disease', *Amer. J. Pub. Health*, 92 (5) (May 2002), pp. 730–32.

21 Riley, *Rising Life Expectancy*, chap. 1; on the control of water-borne diseases in Japan without the aid of sewage systems, see p. 76.

22 Data from Cueto, *The Value of Health*, p. 93.

23 Tim Dyson, 'India's Population – the Past', in *Twenty-First Century India: Population, Economy, Human Development, and the Environment*, ed. Tim Dyson, Robert Cassen and Leela Visaria (Oxford, 2005), p. 26.

24 Sunil Amrith, *Decolonizing International Health: India and Southeast Asia, 1930–1965* (Basingstoke, Hampshire, 2006), p. 100.

25 Dyson, 'India's Population', p. 26.

26 Leela Visaria, 'Mortality Trends and the Health Transition', in *Twenty-First Century India*, pp. 32–56, here: p. 33.

27 A recent report suggests that malaria infections may increase the amount of HIV in a person's blood tenfold. Thus the reduction of one disease may result in a reduction in the other. See *The Guardian* (Friday, 8 December 2006), p. 17.

28 To this day, much of Africa lacks adequate and clean water and sewage systems. Of the 10.5 million children who are estimated to have died throughout the world in 2001 before they reached the age of five, 99 per cent of whom were in low income countries and more than 40 per cent in sub-Saharan Africa, the primary causes of their deaths were under-nutrition and poor access to safe drinking water and sanitation. Data from Anthony C. Gatrell and Susan J. Elliott, *Geographies of Health: An Introduction*, 2nd edn (Chichester, West Sussex, 2009), p. 88.

29 Amrith, *Decolonizing International Health*, p. 179.

30 John Luke Gallup and Jeffrey D. Sachs, 'The Economic Burden of Malaria', *Amer. J. Pub. Health*, 64 (1, 2) (2001), pp. 85–96.

31 Anne-Emannuelle Birn, 'Gates's Grandest Challenge: Transcending Technology as Public Health Ideology', *The Lancet*, 366 (9484) (6–12 August 2005), pp. 514–19.

32 The demographer, Samuel Preston, disagrees that disentangling the various contributions of different factors is impossible. He concludes that 1) the greatest mortality declines after the Second World War were in developing countries, where infectious diseases still predominated; 2) international health programmes were focused in the developing world, precisely where the greatest potential for mortality reduction existed; 3) by the mid-1960s, there was a significant slowing of mortality decline, as diseases more closely tied to standards of living came to predominate in poor countries, for example, diarrhoeal diseases. By this time, too, support for vertical campaigns was already declining. See Samuel H. Preston, 'The Changing Relation between Mortality and Level of Economic Development', *Population Studies*, 29 (2) (July 1975), pp. 231–48.

33 The social welfare provisions put in place after the war in Europe continued to widen the state's commitment to everyday security against unemployment and sickness, and add to health services, sometimes, as in the UK, in a universal system, thereby greatly improving the health of populations.

34 John C. Caldwell, 'Routes to Low Mortality in Poor Countries', *Population and Development Review*, 12 (2) (June 1986), pp. 171–220; and 'Health Transition: The Cultural, Social and Behavioural Determinants of Health in the Third World', *Social Science and Medicine*, 36 (2) (1993), pp. 125–35.

35 Richard G. Wilkinson, *Unhealthy Societies: The Afflictions of Inequality* (London and New York, 1996); the analysis is widened to social dysfunctions more generally (for example, alcoholism, obesity, violence and crime) in Wilkinson and Kate Pickett, *The Spirit Level: Why More Equal Societies Almost Always do Better* (London and New York, 2009). For a recent review of the Wilkinson thesis, see David Runciman, 'How Messy it All Is', *The London Review of Books*, 31 (20) (22 October 2009), pp. 3, 5–6. The mechanisms by which social inequality is translated into health inequality even in rich countries with universal health services, such as the UK, are unclear. Wilkinson points to bio-psychosocial mechanisms involving status anxiety in hierarchical societies; critics of this explanation point to neo-

materialist factors.

36 Matthew Gandy, 'Deadly Alliances: Death, Disease, and the Global Politics of Public Health', *PLoS Med.*, 2 (1): e4 (doi:10.1371/journal.pmed.0020004).

37 Andreas Rinaldi, 'The Global Campaign to Eliminate Leprosy', *PLoS Med.*, 2 (12): e341 (doi: 10.1371/journal.pmed.0020341).

38 Ralph H. Henderson, 'Primary Health Care as a Practical Means for Measles Control', *Reviews of Infect. Diseases*, 5 (3) (May–June 1983), pp. 592–5.

2 Imperial Origins

1 *Yellow Fever*, ed. George Strode (New York, 1951), p. 12.

2 The International Health Division (IHD) of the Rockefeller Foundation was first called the International Health Commission (1913–1916); then the International Health Board (1916–1927); and finally the International Health Division (1927–1951). For simplicity, I refer to it throughout this book as the IHD.

3 Fred L. Soper, *Ventures in World Health: The Memoirs of Fred Lowe Soper*, ed. John Duffy (Washington, DC, 1977), p. 13.

4 As quoted in *Building the Health Bridge: Selections from the Works of Fred L. Soper*, ed. J. Austin Kerr (Bloomington, IN, 1970), p. xiv.

5 Sunil Amrith, *Decolonizing International Health: India and Southeast Asia, 1930–1965* (Basingstoke, Hampshire, 2006).

6 Nancy Leys Stepan, 'Tropical Medicine and Public Health in Latin America: Essay Review', *Med. Hist.*, 42 (1) (January 1998), pp. 104–12.

7 James D. Goodyear, 'The Sugar Connection: A New Perspective on the History of Yellow Fever', *Bull. Hist. Med.*, 52 (1) (1978), pp. 5–21. Among urban epidemics, the epidemic of 1793 in Philadelphia has received the most attention from historians. See J. Worth Estes and Billy G. Smith, eds, *A Melancholy Scene of Devastation: The Public Response to the 1793 Philadelphia Epidemic* (Philadelphia, PA, 1997).

8 See Margaret Humphries, *Yellow Fever and the South* (Baltimore, MD, 1992), p. 41.

9 Khaled J. Bloom, *The Mississippi Valley's Great Yellow Fever Epidemic of 1878* (Baton Rouge, LA, 1993).

10 A black regiment was sent to Cuba by the US army in 1898 in order to aid white military victims of yellow fever. Of course, the black soldiers died too, and the regiment had to be sent back to the United States. The view that black people have innate resistance is still put forward by some historians, despite the lack of evidence of specific genetic mechanisms. The case of yellow fever is very different from malaria, where known genetic immunities have been identified, but they are associated with populations and not races in the old-fashioned sense of the term 'race'. See Nancy Leys Stepan, *The Idea of Race in Science: Great Britain, 1800–1960* (London, 1982), pp. 172–81, for a discussion. Among those claiming, on the basis of historical evidence, that black people have an innate racial immunity to yellow fever, see Kenneth F. Kiple and V. H. Kiple, 'Black Yellow Fever Immunities, Innate and Acquired, as Revealed in the American South', *Social Science History*, 1 (4) (1977), pp. 419–36, and Kiple's book, *The Caribbean Slave: A Biological History* (Cambridge, 1984), pp. 177–8. For a reply to Kiple, see Sheldon Watts, in 'Yellow Fever Immunities in West Africa and the Americas in the Age of Slavery and Beyond', *Journal of Social History*, 34 (4) (2001), pp. 955–67, and Kiple's 'Response to Sheldon Watts', *Journal of Social History*, 34 (4) (2001), pp. 969–74.

11 Humphries, *Yellow Fever and the South*, pp. 114–147. The US Marine Hospital Service became the Public Health and Marine Hospital Service in 1902, and the United States Public Health Service in 1912.

12 Andrew Cliff, Peter Haggett and Matthew Smallman-Raynor, *Deciphering Global Epidemics: Analytical Approaches to the Disease Record of World Cities, 1888–1912* (Cambridge, 1998), p. 49.

13 Louis A. Pérez Jr, *Cuba and the United States: Ties of Singular Intimacy*, 3rd edn (Athens and London, 2003), p. 97.

14 John B. Judis, *The Folly of Empire: What George W. Bush Could Learn from Theodore Roosevelt and Woodrow Wilson* (New York, 2004), p. 11.

15 Niall Ferguson, *Colossus: The Rise and Fall of the American Empire* (New York, 2004), p. 13.

16 For example, the US added huge chunks of territory (what eventually became the states of Texas, New Mexico, Arizona and California), which it wrested from Mexico by warfare. See Judis, *The Folly of Empire*, pp. 22–7.

17 Ferguson notes that the only democracy in Central America by 1939 was Costa Rica, the only country in the region where the US had never intervened. Ferguson, *Colossus*, p. 58.

18 The Panama Canal Zone was part of what had previously belonged to Colombia; the US navy was used to support Panamanian separatists in their quest to establish Panama as an independent state, in return for the territory in which it would build the Panama Canal. See Ferguson, *Colossus*, p. 54.

19 Quoted in Lisa Appignanesi, *Simone de Beauvoir* (London, 2005), from de Beauvoir's book, p. 104. This book was based on de Beauvoir's travels through the United States in 1947 just after the end of the Second World War and during the first stirrings of the Cold War.

20 See William Coleman, *Yellow Fever in the North: The Methods of Early Epidemiology* (Madison, WI, 1987). Between 1900 and 1925 there were several investigations of yellow fever in West Africa; Sir Rubert W. Boyce, from the Liverpool School of Tropical Medicine, studied yellow fever in West Africa,

British Honduras and the West Indies; he concluded West Africa had never been free of yellow fever, yet many disputed this. See A. F. Mahaffey, 'Progress in the Conquest of Yellow Fever During the Period 1905–1930', in *Yellow Fever: A Symposium in Commemoration of Juan Carlos Finlay*, The Jefferson Medical College of Philadelphia, 22–23 September 1955 (Philadelphia, PA, 1956), p. 157.

21 Nancy Stepan, 'The Interplay between Socio-Economic Factors and Medical Science: Yellow Fever Research, Cuba, and the United States', *Social Studies of Science*, 8 (4) (1978), pp. 397–423; this gives due emphasis to the Cuban side of the story. For a good re-telling of the 1898 war from the perspective of the US and military medicine, see Vincent J. Cirollo, *Bullets and Bacilli: The Spanish–American War and Military Medicine* (New Brunswick, NJ, 2004); for a recent book emphasizing the effects on Cuban independence in public health, see Mariola Espinosa, *Epidemic Invasions: Yellow Fever and the Limits of Cuban Independence, 1898–1930* (Chicago, IL, 2009).

22 And a near military disaster as well. See especially Louis A. Pérez Jr, *The War of 1898: The United States and Cuba in History and Historiography* (Chapel Hill, NC, and London, 1998), pp. 90–94.

23 Letter from Reed to Dr William C. Gorgas, Chief Sanitary Officer for Havana, on 29 July 1901, in NLM, Ms C 359, Fred L. Soper Papers, Box 51.

24 Cirollo, *Bullets and Bacilli*, pp. 28–33, says only 100 of the total complement of 192 army doctors were available for field service, and even so, he estimates that twice that number was really needed.

25 The biggest killer in the camps was typhoid fever; ibid., p. 33.

26 Cirollo, *Bullets and Bacilli*, p. 125, judges the typhoid board to be the most significant, because it resulted in the US army eventually (in 1911) introducing mandatory anti-typhoid inoculation for its troops, the first army in the world to do so. The Reed Board's yellow fever work is, however, far better known.

27 'Report of Maj. W. C. Gorgas, Medical Corps, United States Army (July 12, 1902)', in *Yellow Fever; A Compilation of Various Publications. Results of the Work of Maj. Walter Reed, Medical Corps, United States Army, and the Yellow Fever Commission* (Washington, DC, 1911), pp. 234–38.

28 H. R. Carter, 'A Note on the Interval Between Infecting and Secondary Cases of Yellow Fever from the Records of Yellow Fever at Orwood and Taylor, Mississippi, in 1898', *New Orleans Medical and Surgical Journal*, 52 (1900), pp. 617–36.

29 François Delaporte's *The History of Yellow Fever: An Essay on the Birth of Tropical Medicine* (Cambridge, MA, 1991) focuses exclusively on this question, and argues that a visit to Havana by two doctors from the Liverpool School of Tropical Medicine in mid-July, 1900, led the Reed Commission to turn their attention to the mosquito hypothesis, on a direct analogy with malaria mosquito transmission. The evidence for this, however, is thin.

30 Stepan, 'The Interplay between Socio-Economic Factors and Medical Science', deals with these events.

31 There were several reasons for his failure to convince others; the main problem was that Finlay inoculated individuals with infected mosquitoes too soon after the mosquitoes had fed first on yellow fever victims. Thus he – like the Reed Board initially – failed to grasp the issue of extrinsic incubation. In Finlay's defence, one might add that his main aim was to vaccinate people – to give non-immune people a light and not fatal infection, so they would thereafter be immune, something he felt possible if a mosquito bit an individual soon after being infected with the yellow fever germ itself.

32 They failed precisely because the infected mosquitoes were allowed to bite the non-immune volunteers too soon, before the mosquitoes were infective.

33 Stepan, 'The Interplay Between Socio-Economic Factors and Medical Science', p. 411.

34 To this day we really don't know the sequence of events, guesses and transferral of knowledge that led to the success of the Reed Commission; there are many speculations. What is clear is that the mosquito theory of yellow fever was backed by Carter in principle. Espinosa quotes a note Carter sent to Lazear in June 1900, in which Carter expressed his support of the mosquito theory, which Lazear was the first to test; however, Lazear's actual mosquito inoculations took place some weeks after the letter and were not carried out in such a way as to indicate that Lazear had fully grasped Carter's understanding of extrinsic incubation.

35 W. Reed, J. C. Carroll, A. Agramonte and J. Lazear, 'Yellow Fever: A Preliminary Note', *Public Health Papers and Reports*, 26 (1900), pp. 37–53.

36 By this time only Reed remained non-immune among the original four members of the Board (one of whom had died); it was decided it was not sensible for Reed to risk dying from further experiments, so Reed was himself never a subject of inoculation (though he is often portrayed in historical accounts as though he were). The first volunteers (other than the members of the Reed Board themselves and then US army recruits) were Spanish immigrants; they were paid, and signed consent forms, which absolved the US government of all potential claims against it, making this historically the first time, apparently, that a consent protocol of some kind was used in medical research. Agramonte commented later that the written consent was used 'so that our moral responsibility was to a certain extent lessened'. See A. Agramonte, 'The Inside History of a Great Medical Discovery', *The Scientific Monthly*, 1 (3) (December 1915), pp. 209–37, here: p. 234.

37 W. Reed, J. C. Carroll and A. Agramonte, 'The

Eteiology of Yellow Fever: An Additional Note', *J. Amer. Med. Assn*, 36 (7) (16 February 1901), pp. 431–440. For a general account, see *Yellow Fever: A Symposium in Commemoration of Carlos Juan Finlay*. The Jefferson Medical College of Philadelphia, 22–23 September 1955.

38 Juan Guiteras, 'Experimental Yellow Fever at the Inoculation Station of the Sanitary Department of Havana with a View to Producing Immunization', *American Medicine*, 2 (1901), pp. 809–17. Carroll also experimented with transmitting yellow fever to non-immune individuals using blood, producing three cases, but following the deaths from Guiteras's work, Carroll was ordered by Reed to stop. The lack of deaths in the Reed Board's last set of inoculation experiments may have been due to the lucky fact that the particular strain of yellow fever virus involved was not lethal; in Guiteras's cases, all three people who died had been bitten by mosquitoes infected by the same patient.

39 The pathogenic agent of yellow fever is a filterable virus. Carroll established the ultramicroscopic size of the agent following a suggestion that it had parallels with the disease agent in foot-and-mouth disease, which Loeffler and Frosch had shown in 1898 was so small it could pass through a fine porcelain sieve.

40 *Yellow Fever*, ed. Strode, pp. 303–304. H. W. Thomas managed to infect a chimpanzee in 1907 by inoculation, and show that after it recovered, it was immune to further attacks of yellow fever, but his work did not lead to further investigations.

41 Many other questions existed. In the case of the yellow fever mosquito, though many doctors swore it only fed at night, so that people were safe from its bite in the daytime, others disagreed. The range the *Aedes aegypti* mosquito could fly, how long it could live, whether once infected by the yellow fever virus the mosquito remained infected for the rest of its life and whether an infected female mosquito transmitted the infection to its progeny, were all unsettled matters.

42 Members of a Pasteur Mission sent to Rio de Janeiro (1901–1905) to study yellow fever in the wake of the Reed Board's work, had negative results in testing other mosquitoes.

43 Henry Carter, *Yellow Fever: Its Epidemiology, Prevention, and Control* (Lectures Delivered at the United States Public Health Service School of Instruction by H. R. Carter, Senior Surgeon United States Public Health Service), suppl. n. 19 to the *Public Health Reports*, 11 September 1914 (Washington, DC, 1914), p. 4.

44 The investigations into yellow fever carried out immediately after the Reed Commission, by various groups of physicians in Mexico, Cuba and Brazil confirmed the Reed Board's conclusions but did not add much that was new to them. For the experiments by Brazilians that preceded the control work in Rio de Janeiro, see Nancy Stepan, *Beginnings of Brazilian Science: Oswaldo Cruz, Medical Research and Policy, 1890–1920* (New York, 1976), p. 144. A French mission also confirmed the mosquito theory over several years of work in Brazil; see Ilana Löwy, *Virus, Moustiques et Modernité: La Fièvre Jaune au Brésil entre Science et Politique* (Paris, 2001), pp. 68–83.

45 Finlay had proposed such methods in his paper, 'Mosquitoes Considered as Transmitters of Yellow Fever and Malaria', *New York Medical Record* (27 May 1899), p. 379, and re-published in his *Obras Completas* (Havana, Cuba, 1965), vol. II, pp. 254–259, where he mentioned isolation of yellow fever patients in hospitals, mosquito 'blinds' for windows, and attacking mosquito larvae sources with chemicals.

46 New mosquito-based quarantines were put in place that were more selective than the old quarantines; for instance, if a ship had been at sea for more than 20 days, without yellow fever cases, it was thought it was unlikely to harbour any mosquitoes infected with yellow fever, so there was no need for the detention of passengers.

47 Gorgas had the advantage of being immune to yellow fever, having recovered from the disease as a young army medical officer. Working with yellow fever carried risks. Six of the Rockefeller Foundation's yellow fever researchers died in the course of various yellow fever experimental investigations: *Yellow Fever*, ed. Strode, pp. vii and 633.

48 W. C. Gorgas, 'Results in Havana During the Year 1901 of Disinfection for Yellow Fever, Under the Hypothesis that the Stegomyia Mosquito is the Only Means of Transmitting the Disease', *The Lancet*, 160 (4123) (6 September 1902), pp. 667–70, here: p. 670.

49 For an account of the campaign (one among many), see Hugh H. Smith, 'Controlling Yellow Fever', in *Yellow Fever*, ed. Strode, pp. 546–628.

50 Gorgas later concluded that, given the difficulty of identifying everyone with yellow fever and isolating them, either at their own home or in hospitals, the easiest method was to concentrate on destroying the larvae of mosquitoes in their breeding sites of water nearby where people lived. See Socrates Litsios, 'William Crawford Gorgas (1854–1920)', *Perspectives in Biology and Medicine*, 44 (3) (2001), pp. 368–78. Gorgas advocated relying only on anti-larval methods at the First Pan American Sanitary Conference in 1908.

51 William C. Gorgas, 'A Few General Directions with Regard to Destroying Mosquitoes, Particularly the Yellow Fever Mosquito', in *Yellow Fever: A Compilation of Various Publications*, pp. 239–50. Gorgas's account dates from 1904.

52 In 1901, when the town of Santiago de las Vegas, situated twelve miles outside of Havana became infected, the same methods were applied and within six weeks yellow fever had disappeared.

53 Smallpox vaccination was also made compulsory

in Cuba under the US authorities. See chapter Six of this book.

54 Espinosa, *Epidemic Invasions*, p. 90.

55 Humphries, *Yellow Fever in the South*, p. 163.

56 Sir Rubert Boyce, *Yellow Fever Prophylaxis in New Orleans, 1905*, Liverpool School of Tropical Medicine Memoir 19 (Liverpool, 1906).

57 Stepan, *Beginnings of Brazilian Science*, especially pp. 85–91. The campaign to enforce compulsory smallpox vaccination failed, however, and Rio suffered a major epidemic in 1908. The first to apply the mosquito theory in Brazil was actually Dr Emilio Ribas, in towns in the interior of the state of São Paulo in 1901 and 1903.

58 Julie Greene, *The Canal Builders: Making America's Empire at the Panama Canal* (New York, 2009), focuses on the cost paid by the workmen in America's most important imperial project.

59 The actual management of the project was in the hands of a Panama Canal Commission.

60 The recent dissertation by Abernathy gives a detailed history, emphasizing the narrow geographical territory involved. See David Ray Abernathy, *Bound to Succeed: Territoriality and the Emergence of Disease Eradication in the Panama Canal Zone*, unpublished PhD, University of Washington, Department of Geography (2000). On the artificial character of the main towns involved in the canal work, see Sharon Phillips Collazos, 'The Cities of Panama: Sixty Years of Development', in *Cities of Hope: People, Protests and Progress in Urbanizing Latin America*, ed. Ronn Pineo and James A. Baer (Boulder, CO, 2000), pp. 240–57.

61 Since Colon and Panama City were situated outside the Canal Zone itself, they were formally the responsibility of the local Panamanian health authorities, but Gorgas took charge of the isolation and anti-mosquito measures, since they were places where many non-immune US and Caribbean workers lived and congregated.

62 Litsios, 'William Crawford Gorgas', p. 373.

63 Gordon Harrison, *Mosquitoes, Malaria and Man: A History of the Hostilities Since 1880* (London, 1978), p. 165.

64 William C. Gorgas, *Sanitation in Panama* (New York, 1918), pp. 182–205.

65 The number of workers admitted to hospital fell from 821/1,000 in 1906, to 76/1,000 in 1913. The overall death rates fell from 15.3/1,000 in 1905 to 6/1,000 in 1914. Sir Malcolm Watson was very impressed with the work of the Sanitary Department on malaria, but was nonetheless uncertain as to how the different sanitary methods contributed to the overall result. For instance, he remarked that he found almost no screening in Colon, and said that figures showed that by 1912, only 15 per cent of the total Panama Canal Zone population lived in screened houses. The infection rate for malaria among black workers was considerably higher than that of white labourers, as was their rates of pneumonia; see Sir Malcolm Watson, *Rural Sanitation in the Tropics* (New York, 1915), chap. 7.

66 One of Gorgas's admirers was Sir Ronald Ross, who included two chapters by Gorgas (and Le Prince, Gorgas's right-hand man) in his influential book, *Prevention of Malaria* (New York, 1910). Ross met Gorgas personally on board a ship in New York harbour when Ross arrived in the USA, on his way to an international congress in St Louis.

67 William C. Gorgas, 'Sanitation in the Canal Zone', *J. Amer. Med. Assn*, 49 (1) (6 July 1907), pp. 6–8.

68 Watson, *Rural Sanitation in the Tropics*, p. 2.

69 Greene, *The Canal Builders*, pp. 130–40.

70 Watson, *Rural Sanitation in the Tropics*, p. 1.

71 Quotes from the interesting analysis by Scott L. Montgomery, *The Scientific Voice* (New York and London, 1996), pp. 142–3, and p. 183.

72 Ronald Ross, *Report on the Prevention of Malaria in Mauritius* (London, 1909), p. 92.

73 Geoffrey M. Jeffery, 'Malaria Control in the Twentieth Century', *Amer. J. Tropical Med. and Hyg.*, 25 (3) (1976), p. 365.

74 Nancy Leys Stepan, 'Race and Gender: The Role of Analogy in Science', *in Science, Race and Ethnicity: Readings from Isis and Osiris*, ed. John P. Jackson Jr (Chicago, IL, 2002), pp. 5–21.

75 Montgomery, *The Scientific Voice*, pp. 140–41.

76 David Arnold, 'Disease, Medicine and Empire', in *Imperial Medicine and Indigenous Societies*, ed. David Arnold (Manchester, 1988), p. 19.

77 See chapter Five.

78 Edmund Russell, *War and Nature: Fighting Humans and Insects with Chemicals from World War I to Silent Spring* (Cambridge and New York, 2001), pp. 3–4. The historian, Paul Weindling, in *Epidemics and Genocide in Eastern Europe, 1890–1945* (Oxford, 2000), goes much further, asking whether there is an eradicationist or exterminatory core essential to modern bacteriology; he links the draconian aspects of public health, especially in war, to the concept of disease eradication. He points out that coercive routines were common in public health in Germany, as was the use of chemicals (including poison gas) to get rid of germs and vectors; there was furthermore a close connection between the military and the new bacteriology. Ultimately, however, Weindling's own analysis shows that the connections between the efforts to control or exterminate disease pests (for example, of typhus) by chemical means, and the rise of German racism and especially the extermination of the Jews by the Nazis in the Holocaust, have to be understood as the historically contingent and specific outcomes of Nazi ideology and Nazi power, rather than inherent products of bacteriology itself.

79 Greer Williams, *The Plague Killers* (New York, 1969), p. 197.

80 Amy Fairchild, et al., 'The Exodus of Public Health: What History Can Tell us about the Future', *Amer.*

J. Pub. Health, 100 (1) (January 2010), pp. 54–63. The authors argue that ever since the loss of the broader social and reform agenda, public health in the United States has struggled to define itself, and has been in effect marginalized within the biomedical system of health care.

81 William C. Gorgas, 'Sanitation in the Tropics with Special Reference to Malaria and Yellow Fever', *J. Amer. Med. Assn*, 52 (4) (3 April 1909), pp. 1075–7.

82 Ronald Ross, *Mosquito Brigades and How to Organize Them* (New York, 1902).

83 These events are described in chapter Four of this book.

84 Gorgas, 'Sanitation in the Tropics, with Special Reference to Malaria and Yellow Fever'.

85 Humphries, *Yellow Fever in the South*, p. 160.

86 Boyce, *Yellow Fever Prophylaxis in New Orleans*, p. 16.

87 Quote from F. Haskin, *The Panama Canal* (New York, 1914), as cited in Abernathy, *Bound to Succeed*, p. 149.

88 The original scientific paper which claimed a causal connection between MMR vaccination and autism was first published in the Lancet 1998; it was later withdrawn by the editors, on the grounds that subsequent studies did not show the expected association; there were also ethical questions surrounding the treatment of the children and conflicts of interest. For the retraction see *The Lancet*, 375 (9713) (6 February 2010), p. 445. The lead author, A. J. Wakefield, was also struck off the UK's Medical Register for unethical behaviour towards children who were his medical patients.

89 Sir Ronald Ross, on the other hand, bowing to the realities of the lack of enthusiasm among the colonial authorities for spending any money beyond what was absolutely necessary on colonial public health, and the general lack of confidence in his anti-mosquito measures in dealing with malaria, settled for purely voluntarily organized (and voluntarily funded) mosquito brigades. See Ross, *Mosquito Brigades and How to Organize Them*.

90 Ross, *Report on the Prevention of Malaria in Mauritius*, p. 89 gives this figure.

91 Ross, *Mosquito Brigades and How to Organize Them*, p. 34.

92 See, for instance, the defence of the continued use of DDT in the control of malaria by Donald R. Roberts, Penny Masuoka and Andrew Y. Au, 'Determinants of Malaria in the Americas', in *The Contextual Determinants of Malaria*, ed., Elizabeth A. Casman and Hadi Dowlatabadi (Washington, DC, 2002), pp. 35–58.

93 Humphries, *Yellow Fever in the South*, p. 172. Another very important factor was the absence of jungle or sylvan yellow fever in the USA; the significance of the jungle cycle of for yellow fever eradication was not grasped until the early 1930s. See chapter Three of this book.

94 *Yellow Fever*, ed. Strode, p. 12.

95 William C. Gorgas, 'A Few General Directions with regard to Destroying Mosquitoes, Particularly the Yellow Fever Mosquito', in *Yellow Fever: A Compilation of Various Publications*, pp. 239–50, from a piece dated 1904.

96 James Carroll, 'Yellow Fever: A Popular Lecture', in *Yellow Fever: A Compilation of Various Publications*, p. 215, from a lecture delivered in 1905.

97 Carter, *Yellow Fever: Its Epidemiology, Prevention, and Control*, p. 10. The title of the book on anti-mosquito work in Panama by Joseph Le Prince, Gorgas's chief sanitary inspector and right-hand man, made the shift from control to eradication clear: *Mosquito Control in Panama: The Eradication of Malaria and Yellow Fever in Cuba and Panama* (New York and London, 1916).

98 Carroll in 'Yellow Fever: A Popular Lecture', in *Yellow Fever: A Compilation of Various Publications*, p. 215.

99 Quotation and figures from Ross, *Report on the Prevention of Malaria in Mauritius*, pp. 89–90.

100 Soper, *Ventures in World Health*, p. 10.

3 Paradoxes: The Rockefeller Era

1 I refer here to the title of E. Richard Brown's book, *Rockefeller Medicine Men: Medicine and Capitalism in America* (Berkeley, LA, and London, 1979).

2 John Farley, *To Cast Out Disease: A History of the International Health Division of the Rockefeller Foundation (1913–1951)* (Oxford and New York, 2004), p. 16, names Soper as one of the field officers to merit this title.

3 See note 2 for chapter Two of this book.

4 Fred Lowe Soper, *Ventures in World Health: The Memoirs of Fred L. Soper*, ed. John Duffy (Washington, DC, 1977), p. 92.

5 Soper, *Ventures in World Health*, p. 93.

6 Soper, *Ventures in World Health*, p. 153.

7 Altogether, in Rio alone there were 738 registered cases and 478 deaths (many of them foreigners or immigrants). Data from Fred L. Soper, *Proposal for the Continental Eradication of Aedes aegypti*. (1942), in *Building the Health Bridge: Selections from the Works of Fred L. Soper, M.D.*, ed. J. Austin Kerr (Bloomington, IN, 1970), p. 44. See also Fred L. Soper, 'The Rehabilitation of the Eradication Concept in the Prevention of Communicable Diseases', *Public Health Reports*, 80 (10) (October 1965), pp. 855–69.

8 Greer Williams, *The Plague Killers* (New York, 1969), p. 264.

9 The Rockefeller Foundation was endowed with 72,000 shares of the Standard Oil Company, worth (by Farley's calculation) more than 700 million in 1990 dollars; see Farley, *To Cast Out Disease*, p. 3.

10 Farley, *To Cast Out Disease*, p. 5.

11 Anne Marie Moulin, 'The Pasteur Institutes between the two World Wars: The Transformation of the International Sanitary Order', in *International Health Organizations and Movements, 1918–1939*, ed. Paul Weindling (Cambridge, 1995), p. 253.

12 Paul Weindling, 'Philanthropy and World Health: The Rockefeller Foundation and the League of Nations Health Organization', *Minerva*, 35 (1997), pp. 269–81.

13 Darwin H. Stapleton, 'Lessons of History? Anti-Malaria Strategies of the International Health Board and the Rockefeller Foundation from the 1920s to the Era of DDT', *Public Health Reports*, 119 (March–April 2004), pp. 206–15, here: p. 208.

14 One result of the technocratic orientation and detailed recordkeeping of the RF is its remarkable archive, now housed in the Rockefeller Archive Center in Sleepy Hollow, New York. For information about the archive and for online search tools, see: www.rockarch.org

15 *Yellow Fever*, ed. George Strode (New York, 1951), pp. 631–33.

16 Farley, *To Cast Out Disease*. The historical literature on the RF is now very large. A first wave of studies tended to be semi-official and generally uncritical; a second wave highly critical and tended to reduce the RF little more than a tool of US imperialism and capitalism. A third (present wave) is less reductive and more nuanced. As examples of the first, see Raymond B. Fosdick, *The Story of the Rockefeller Foundation* (New York, 1952), and Robert Shaplen, *Toward the Well-Being of Mankind* (New York, 1964). Among the anti-imperialist critiques, see Brown, *The Rockefeller Medicine Men*, and Saúl Franco Agudela, 'The Rockefeller Foundation's Antimalarial Program in Latin America: Donating or Dominating?', *International Journal of Health Services*, 13 (1) (1983), pp. 51–67. Examples of the third wave include Steven Palmer, 'Central American Encounters with Rockefeller Public Health, 1914–1921', in *Close Encounters with Empire: Writing the Cultural History of US–Latin American Relations*, ed. Gilbert A. Joseph, Catherine C. LeGrand and Ricardo D. Salvatore (Durham, NC, 1998), pp. 311–32, and his *Launching Global Health: The Caribbean Odyssey of the Rockefeller Foundation* (Ann Arbor, MI, 2010); and *Missionaries of Science: The Rockefeller Foundation in Latin America*, ed. Marcos Cueto (Bloomington, IN, 1994). For a discussion of recent historiography of the RF, see Nancy Leys Stepan, 'The National and the International in Public Health: Carlos Chagas and the Rockefeller Foundation in Brazil, 1916–1930s', *Hispanic American Historical Review*, 91 (3) (2011), pp. 469–502.

17 Palmer, *Launching Global Health*.

18 Weindling, 'Philanthropy and World Health'. The United States was not a member of the League of Nations.

19 Peter J. Hotez, *Forgotten People, Forgotten Diseases: The Neglected Tropical Diseases and Their Impact on Global Health and Development* (Washington, DC, 2008), p. 14.

20 See Steven Palmer, 'Migrant Clinics and Hookworm Science: Peripheral Origins of International Health, 1840–1920', *Bull. Hist. Med.*, 83(4) (2009), pp. 676–709, for a brilliant new interpretation.

21 Quoted in Farley, *To Cast Out Disease*, p. 4.

22 Farley, *To Cast Out Disease*, chaps 2, 4 and 5, and Palmer, *Launching Global Health*. The side effects of oil of chenopodium could in certain circumstances be even more dangerous. See Steven Palmer, 'Toward Responsibility in International Health: Deaths Following Treatment in Rockefeller Hookworm Campaigns', *Med. Hist.*, 54 (2) (2010), pp. 149–70.

23 For a recent, comparative account, see Palmer, *Launching Global Health*.

24 Quoted in Palmer, *Launching Global Health*, p. 67; see H. H. Howard, *The Eradication of Ankylostomiasis* (Washington, DC, 1915).

25 Quoted in Soper, *Ventures in World Health*, p. 37.

26 See Palmer, *Launching Global Health*, pp. 67–76, for a description.

27 Soper, *Ventures in World Health*, p. 9.

28 'The Reminiscences of Dr Alan Gregg' (1958), pp. 112 and 116, The Alan Gregg Papers, at Profiles in Science, the National Library of Medicine Profiles in Science: http://profiles.nlm.nih.gov/fs/b/b/n/v.

29 Christian Brannstrom, 'Polluted Soil, Polluted Souls: The Rockefeller Hookworm Eradication Campaign in São Paulo, Brazil, 1917–1926', *J. Hist. Geog.*, 25 (1997), pp. 25–45; and Ilana Löwy, '"Intervenir et représenter": Campagnes sanitaires et élaboration des cartographies de l'ankylostomiase', *History and Philosophy of the Life Sciences*, 25 (2003), pp. 337–362.

30 Soper, *Ventures in World Health*, pp. 53–54.

31 Eventually a total of 424,128 people out of a population of 646,416 were treated for hookworms in Paraguay between 1924 and 1928. Many people got a second treatment, boosting the figures of those treated further (with further numbers treated by the Paraguayan government). Figures from Soper, *Ventures World Health*, pp. 66–7.

32 Lewis W. Hackett, 'Presidential Address', *Amer. J. Tropical Med. and Hyg.*, 9 (2) (March 1960), pp. 105–15.

33 Farley, *To Cast Out Disease*, p. 37. These assessments involved counting the number of people who attended public health lectures, or the number of privies in a region.

34 The reduction in hookworm that did occur in the USA in the decades before the Second World War was due to a mix of such factors, including public health education and treatment, economic growth and the massive movement of people from the poorer southern to the richer and more urban northern states.

35 'The Reminiscences of Dr Alan Gregg', NLM Profiles in Science, p. 118.

36 According to Soper, the RF in Brazil had abstained from enforcing sanitary regulations, such as requirements to build latrines, because it did not want to get involved with sanctions against the public for non-compliance. But he thought that the RF ran a greater risk in treating people with dangerous drugs, which at times caused 'severe intoxication', than in enforcing sanitary regulations. Soper always insisted successful public health interventions had to be backed up by the law.

37 Soper, *Ventures in World Health*, p. 67.

38 Farley, *To Cast out Disease*, p. 44. In fact, the IHD became involved in TB work, in Canada, Jamaica and Mexico.

39 Farley, *To Cast out Disease*, p. 55.

40 Soper, *Ventures in World Health*, p. 67.

41 The reasons for the absence of yellow fever in places like India, where the *Aedes aegypti* mosquitoes are common, are not entirely settled to this day. It is possible that dengue fever, transmitted by the same mosquito, gives immunity to people against the yellow fever virus. The possibility of introducing yellow fever to completely non-immune Asian populations remained a concern of Soper's until the end of his life.

42 Rose wrote a memo, 'Yellow Fever: Feasibility of its Eradication', on 27 October 1914. See Williams, *The Plague Killers*, p. 210.

43 Gorgas was elected chairman of the Medical Section of the Congress, which then proposed the eradication of yellow fever in the Americas. The proposal urged 'the American Republics in which yellow fever prevails or is suspected of prevailing enact such laws for its eradication as will best accomplish that result'; to which was added that 'Inasmuch as yellow fever exists in some of the European colonies in America, they be invited to adopt measures for its elimination'. *Pan American Resolution: Second Pan American Scientific Congress, the Final Act and Interpretive Commentary Thereon*. Prepared by James Brown Scott, Reporter General of the Congress (Washington, DC, 1916), p. 38, Article 40.

44 Fosdick, *The Story of the Rockefeller Foundation*, p. 59.

45 Farley, *To Cast Out Disease*, p. 88.

46 Heather Bell, *The Frontiers of Medicine in the Anglo-Egyptian Sudan, 1889–1940* (New York, 1999), p. 165.

47 Farley, *To Cast Out Disease*, pp. 90 and 92.

48 Marcos Cueto's term in 'Sanitation from Above: Yellow Fever and Foreign Intervention in Peru, 1919–1922', *Hispanic American Historical Review*, 72 (1) (1992), pp. 1–22.

49 Marcos Cueto, *The Return of the Epidemics: Health and Society in Peru During the Twentieth Century* (Aldershot, 2001), chap. 2, here: p. 39.

50 Figures from *Yellow Fever*, ed. Strode, pp. 556–65. For a detailed account, see Anne-Emmanuelle Birn, *Marriage of Convenience: Rockefeller International Health and Revolutionary Mexico* (Rochester, NY, 2006), pp. 47–60.

51 See Nancy Leys Stepan, *Beginnings of Brazilian Science: The Oswaldo Cruz Institute, Medical Research and Policy, 1890–1920* (New York, 1981), pp. 84–91, 114, for an account of the campaigns. On the discovery of rural ill-health by Brazilian doctors, see Nisia Trindade Lima, 'Public Health and Social Ideas in Modern Brazil', *Amer. J. Pub. Health*, 97 (7) (July 2007), pp. 1168–77.

52 Soper, *Ventures in World Health*, pp. 27 and 33. A visit to the state of Alagoas, however, dented their optimism; they came to doubt that other states would be as efficient as Pernambuco.

53 Noguchi arrived in the USA in 1900, ostensibly on the invitation of Dr Simon Flexner at the University of Pennsylvania, whom he had met when Flexner visited Japan. After three years, Noguchi moved with Flexner to the Rockefeller Institute in New York.

54 Noguchi's unusual life, from humble beginnings in Japan to well-known Rockefeller scientist, is described in Gustav Eckstein, *Noguchi* (New York, 1930), and Isabel R. Plesset, *Noguchi and His Patrons* (London, 1980).

55 His first announcement appeared in Hideyo Noguchi, 'Contribution to the Etiology of Yellow Fever', *J. Amer. Med. Assn*, 72 (3) (1919), pp. 187–8. At the time, spirochetes were very much in the news, having been implicated in several other diseases, including syphilis (on which Noguchi had worked previously), and there was considerable uncertainty about the distinctions that existed between the different spirochete species that caused jaundice-like diseases. This goes part way to explaining why Noguchi seized on the spirochete, but only part way. Weil's disease is a rather rare infection of human beings and animals.

56 His papers were published in the *Journal of Experimental Medicine*, edited by Dr Simon Flexner, a chief mentor of Noguchi's at the Rockefeller Institute.

57 According to Farley, *To Cast Out Disease*, p. 93, in October 1918, in Peru, Noguchi vaccinated 325 members of families of a non-immune battalion and another 102 individuals, making a total of 427, only five of whom Noguchi claimed came down with yellow fever, while in the population at large, in contrast, he said there had been 386 natural cases, of which 217 died. By the end of 1925, some 20,000 individuals in Ecuador, Brazil, Mexico, Peru and other places, had been vaccinated with Noguchi's vaccine.

58 This is an incomplete list of the problems with Noguchi's work. For instance, Noguchi was able to inoculate animals with supposed yellow fever with blood drawn from a yellow fever patient six days after infection, whereas the Reed Board clearly

demonstrated that human blood drawn from a victim was only infective in the first one or two days following infection.

59 Paul Franklin Clark, 'Hideyo Noguchi, 1876–1928', *Bull. Hist. Med.*, 33 (1) (January–February 1959), pp. 1–20.

60 Juan Guiteras, 'Observations on Yellow Fever, in a Recent Visit to Africa', *The Archives of Diagnosis*, 14 (1) (1921), pp. 1–14; and Aristides Agramonte, 'Some Observations Upon Yellow Fever Prophylaxis', *Proceedings of the International Conference on Health Problems of Tropical America* (Kingston, Jamaica, 1923), pp. 201–27. There were many other critics.

61 Max Theiler and A. W. Sellards, 'The Relationship of *L. icterohaemorrhagiae* and *L. icteroides* as Determined by the Pfeiffer Phenomenon in Guinea Pigs', *Amer. J. Trop. Med.*, 6 (6) (1926), pp. 383–402. Theiler was a South African born, UK-trained doctor who joined the department of tropical medicine at Harvard in 1922. From 1930–1964 Theiler worked at the Rockefeller Institute for Medical Research in New York City, where he and several other scientists developed the 17D vaccine.

62 Max Theiler and Hugh H. Smith, 'The Use of Yellow Fever Virus Modified by In Vitro Cultivation for Human Immunization', *J. Exptl. Med.*, 65 (1937), pp. 787–808.

63 It is not established how Noguchi became infected (deliberate infection has been suggested), but his untidy and harried laboratory methods left open several possibilities, such as handling autopsy and similar materials, the virus entering through skin abrasions. Eight days after Noguchi's death, his assistant, Dr William A. Young, also died of yellow fever. Dr Adrian Stokes, of the Yellow Fever Commission in Lagos, had died of yellow fever the previous year as well. These and other RF deaths showed just how dangerous the yellow fever virus could be.

64 NLM, Ms 359, Soper Papers, Box 51, Folder Yellow Fever and Noguchi. Typed document: 'Noguchi Leptospira Fiasco', dated 3 February 1967. In retirement, Soper made a careful study of Noguchi and the missed opportunities in understanding yellow fever.

65 As late as 1929, Simon Flexner, the director of the Rockefeller Institute, still defended Noguchi's work and held out the possibility that Noguchi's leptospira might yet be found to be the cause of another disease clinically similar to yellow fever: Flexner, 'Hideyo Noguchi: A Biographical Sketch', *Science*, 69 (1800) (28 June 1929), pp. 635–60.

66 Roberto Franco, et al., 'Fiebre amarilla y fiebre espitoquetal; endemias e epidemias en Muzo, de 1907 à 1910', *Academia Nacional de Medicina, Sesiones Cientificas del Centenario, Bogotá*, 1 (1911), pp. 169–228.

67 Sir Rubert Boyce, *Yellow Fever and its Prevention. A Manual for Medical Students and Practitioners* (New York, 1911). Boyce said yellow fever was mild, endemic and often unrecognized in West Africa, and that childhood infections gave immunity to Africans who survived and this was often mistaken for racial immunity.

68 A good account of this period is given by Fred L. Soper, 'Rehabilitation of the Eradication Concept in Prevention of Communicable Disease', *Public Health Reports*, 80 (10) (1965), pp. 855–69.

69 Soper's *Ventures in World Health*, pp. 29–30. See also Soper's interview with Hackett, RAC, RG 3.1, series 908, Box 7H, Folder 86.102, pp. 1–18.

70 Soper, *Ventures in World Health*, p. 30.

71 For example, the *Haemagogus* species. About thirteen species of mosquitoes are implicated today, and perhaps some species of ticks.

72 Fred L. Soper, et al., 'Yellow Fever Without *Aedes aegypti*: Study of a Rural Epidemic in the Valle de Chanaan, Espiritu Santo, Brazil, 1932', *Amer. J. Hyg.*, 18 (1933), pp. 555–87. The term 'jungle yellow fever' was coined to describe the jungle cases in Brazil and before the epidemiology of the form was understood. The cycle involving non-urban vector mosquitoes is better described as 'sylvatic', but 'jungle yellow rever' has stuck as the most usual or preferred term.

73 *Yellow Fever*, ed. Strode, pp. 173–194. The test involved inoculating a mouse with yellow fever virus, together with serum from a human individual; if the mouse survived, it was concluded the human serum had protected the mouse from yellow fever, and proved that the human individual supplying the serum had already acquired immunity, and thus had had a previous infection from the disease. The test was first developed using monkeys as experimental animals, but they were expensive, and the discovery of white mice as experimental animals resulted in a cheaper and more practical test.

74 Fred L. Soper, 'The Geographical Distribution of Immunity to Yellow Fever in Man in South America', *Amer. J. Tropical Med. and Hyg.*, 17 (4) (1937), pp. 457–511; and W. A. Sawyer and Loring Whitman, 'The Yellow Fever Immunity Surveys in North, East and South Africa', *Transactions of the Royal Society of Tropical Medicine and Hygiene*, 29 (4) (25 January 1936), pp. 397–412.

75 Bell, *Frontiers of Medicine in the Anglo-Egyptian Sudan*, pp. 184–186, here: p. 186.

76 Farley, *To Cast Out Disease*, p. 100.

77 In addition to primates, some marsupials have been implicated.

78 On the tangled tale of how jungle yellow fever was discovered, with an emphasis on the unacknowledged contributions of Colombian physicians and Soper's efforts to get credit himself, see Emilio Quevedo V., et al., 'Knowledge and Power: The Asymmetry of Interests of the Colombian and Rockefeller Doctors in the Construction of the Concept of "Jungle Yellow Fever", 1907–1938', *Canadian Bulletin*

of Medical History, 25 (1) (2008), pp. 71–109.

79 Farley, *To Cast Out Disease*, p. 102.

80 Before 1929, the RF agreement allowed the RF to work in only five states of the Brazilian federation, all in the northeast. In 1930, with the federal centralization of power, the remit extended to all the states except São Paulo, thus overriding the principle of states' rights in the field of yellow fever control. Rio de Janeiro was added to the CYFS in 1931, and São Paulo, the powerful state in the southeast, was brought in to the CYFS in 1932. See Soper, *Ventures in World Health*, pp. 97, 106.

81 Soper, *Ventures in World Health*, p. 117.

82 Soper, *Ventures in World Health*, p. 11.

83 NLM, Soper Papers, Box 22, Biographical Information, Document 'Administration is the Essence of Eradication'. Typed notes for Harvard Lecture, 13 May 1965: http://profiles.nlm.nih.gov/ps/access/VVBBDR.pdf

84 Details in this section from Robert M. Levine, *Father of the Poor? Vargas and His Era* (Cambridge, 1998).

85 Levine, *Father of the Poor?*, p. 3.

86 Vargas left the Presidency in 1945; he returned in 1950 in an elected capacity, and died by suicide in 1954 just as he was about to be ousted from office by another *coup d'état*.

87 Soper, *Ventures in World Health*, pp. 112–15 for an account of Soper's relations with Vargas.

88 Soper, in *Building a Health Bridge*, p. 333, from the article, 'Eradication versus Control in Communicable Disease Prevention', first given as a lecture in 1959, and published in 1960.

89 F. Fenner, A. J. Hall and W. R. Dowdle, 'What is Eradication?', in *The Eradication of Infectious Diseases*, ed. Dowdle and D. R. Hopkins (New York, 1998), p. 7.

90 Soper, 'Rehabiliation of the Eradication Concept in Prevention of Communicable Disease'.

91 Williams, *The Plague Killers*, p. 279.

92 Socrates Litsios, 'Rene J. Dubos and Fred L. Soper: Their Contrasting Views on Vector and Disease Eradication', *Perspectives in Biology and Medicine*, 41 (1) (Autumn 1997), pp. 138–149, here: p. 147.

93 Soper, in 'Rehabilitation of the Eradication Concept in the Prevention of Communicable Disease', reprinted in *Building the Health Bridge*, pp. 337–54, here: p. 343.

94 Eventually, the entire system of running an eradication campaign was written up as a practical Manual, first in Portuguese, then in English: Soper, et al., *The Organization of Permanent Nation-Wide Anti-Aedes aegypti Measures in Brazil* (New York, 1943).

95 Soper, 'Rehabilitation of the Eradication Concept in the Prevention of Communicable Diseases', pp. 860–61. Tight central control and an insistence on efficiency allowed Soper to reduce the size of CYFS; when he took over it had some 3,000 employees (down from high of 10,000 in 1929, during the Rio epidemic). Soper was able to further reduce the numbers to 1,200, without loss of efficiency.

96 Ilana Löwy, 'What/Who Should be Controlled? Opposition to Yellow Fever Campaigns in Brazil, 1900–1939', in *Western Medicine as Contested Knowledge*, ed. Andrew Cunningham and Bridie Andrews (Manchester, 1997), pp. 124–46.

97 On the viscerotomy service, see Soper, *Ventures in World Health*, pp. 157–67; and E. R. Rickard, 'The Organization of the Viscerotome Service of the Brazilian Cooperative Yellow Fever Service', *Amer. J. Trop. Med.*, 17 (2) (1937), pp. 163–190. Dr E. R. Rickard, and a Brazilian, Dr Decio Parreiras, both claimed priority for the invention of the viscerotome.

98 Dr Waldemar S. Antunes, 'Field Control in Yellow Fever', in *Proceedings of the Fourth International Congresses on Tropical Medicine and Malaria* (Washington, DC, 1948), pp. 498–505, here: p. 499. Antunes was at this time the Director of the Yellow Fever Service in Brazil.

99 On the agents killed, see the reference by Soper in the interview with Hackett, in 1950, RAC, RG3.1, series 908, Box 17H, Folder 86.102; Rickart in an interview with Hackett said he did not think such a service in the interior of the country could be organized, but Soper insisted on it. On the resistance to the programme, see Löwy, 'What/Who Should be Controlled?'.

100 Soper, 'Rehabitation of the Eradication Concept in Prevention of Communicable Diseases,' p. 859.

101 Soper singled out for praise this term in a book review of Emilio Pampana, A *Textbook of Malaria Eradication* in the *Amer. J. Trop. Med. and Hyg.*, 12 (1963), pp. 936–939.

102 Soper, *Ventures in World Health*, p. 124.

103 The law decree was No. 23434, passed by the federal government in May 1932, giving the Yellow Fever Service authority to employ any sanitary measures deemed necessary for its work. Other South American countries used this law as a model for authorizing similar services.

104 Soper, 'Rehabilitation of the Eradication Concept in Prevention of Communicable Disease', reprinted in *Building the Health Bridge*, p. 343.

105 See Fred L. Soper, Dr Bruce Wilson, Servulo Lima and Waldemar Sá Atunes, *The Organization of Permanent Nationwide Anti-Aedes Aegypti Measures in Brazil* (New York, 1943). The book was based on the work of the Cooperative Yellow Fever Service maintained by the RF and the Brazilian government between 1929 and 1940.

106 Soper, 'Present-Day Methods for the Study and Control of Yellow Fever', *Amer. J. Tropical Med. and Hyg.*, 17 (5) (1937), p. 675.

107 Soper, 'Rehabilitation of the Eradication Concept in the Prevention of Communicable Diseases'.

108 NLM, Ms C 359, Profiles in Science, Soper Papers, 'Administration is the Essence of Eradication'.

109 NLM, Ms C 359, Soper Papers, Box 30.
110 NLM, Ms C 359, Soper Papers, Box 1, Personal and Biographical, 8 May 1974. Typescript. This was first published in *Amer. J. Pub. Health*, 52 (1962), p. 743 and republished in *Building the Health Bridge*, p. 524.
111 NLM, Ms C 359, Soper Papers, Box 8, 1964.
112 Malcolm Gladwell, 'The Mosquito Killer', *New Yorker* (2 July 2001), p. 49, quoting Litsios.
113 John Duffy, Editor's note, in Soper, *Ventures in World Health*, pp. xiii–xiv.
114 Stapleton, 'Lessons of History'. These debates about how to control malaria are treated in more detail in chapter Four of this book.
115 The Medfly had arrived in Florida in spring 1929; it was devastating to crops, and so an intense effort was made to eradicate it. Some 5,000 men were employed in destroying the host plants and products in order to eliminate breeding sites. The Medfly returned in 1956 and was again eradicated.
116 Fred L. Soper and D. Bruce Wilson, 'Eradication: Species Eradication: A Practical Goal of Species Reduction in the Control of Mosquito-borne Disease', *J. Nat. Malaria Soc.*, 1 (1) (1942), pp. 5–24.
117 It was not known in Soper's day that the *A. gambiae* is actually a 'species complex' made up of several variants or races with different malaria-transmitting efficiencies. Scientists have not been able to determine from museum samples which variant Soper's gambiae dealt with.
118 Accounts of the campaign appear in Soper, *Ventures in World Health*, pp. 201–233; and Fred L. Soper and D. Bruce Wilson, *Anopheles Gambiae in Brazil 1930–1940* (New York, 1943).
119 Soper, *Ventures in World Health*, p. 229.
120 R. M. Packard and Paulo Gadelha, 'A Land Filled with Mosquitoes: Fred L. Soper, the Rockefeller Foundation, and the *Anopheles gambiae* Invasion of Brazil', *Medical Anthropology*, 17 (3) (1997), pp. 215–238.
121 Fred L. Soper and D. Bruce Wilson, 'Anopheles gambiae in Brazil, 1930 to 1940', excerpt in Soper, *Building the Health Bridge*, section 'Will Brazilian Anti-Gambiae Measures Succeed in Africa?', pp. 289–91.
122 Soper and Wilson, *Anopheles Gambiae in Brazil*, pp. 233–4.
123 Sir Malcolm Watson, *African Highways: The Battle for Health in Central Africa* (London, 1953), p. 23.
124 Quoted by Paul F. Russell in the Forward to *Ventures in World Health*, p. vii. There are also current admirers of Soper's achievement; see Gerry Killeen, 'Following in Soper's Footsteps: Northeast Brazil 63 years after eradication of *Anopheles gambiae*', *The Lancet Infectious Diseases*, 3 (10) (October 2003), pp. 663–66, and Killeen, et al., 'Eradication of *Anopheles gambiae* from Brazil: Lessons for Malaria Control in Africa?', *The Lancet Infectious Diseases*, 2 (10) (October 2002), pp. 618–27, where the authors propose larviciding (which is hardly used in malaria control today) be re-introduced as part of the Roll Back Malaria project's control tools (they are not, however, talking of species eradication as such).
125 Fred L. Soper and H. H. Smith, 'Vaccination with Virus 17D in the Control of Jungle Yellow Fever in Brazil', and Soper, 'Complications of Yellow Fever Vaccination', reprinted in *Building the Health Bridge*, pp. 231–241, 242–244. A similar result occurred in the United States during the opening year of the Second World War, when human serum was still used, despite the evidence from Brazil of its negative effect. Vaccination of the military had to be stopped until investigations once again identified the human serum as the risk factor, and the vaccine prepared without it. For a detailed account of the Brazilian involvement in the testing, correction and mass use of the yellow fever vaccine, see Jaime Larry Benchimol, ed., *Febre Amarela. A Doença e a Vacina, Uma História Inacabada* (Rio de Janeiro, 2001), especially chaps 3 and 4.
126 Soper, *Building the Health Bridge*, pp. 43–44.
127 'The RF never did accept the program of *Aedes aegypti eradication* from Brazil', wrote Soper in *Ventures in World Health*, p. 130, italics Soper's emphasis.
128 Soper and Wilson, *Anopheles Gambiae in Brazil*, p. 217.
129 Soper, *Ventures in World Health*, p. 133.
130 NLM, Ms C 359, Soper Papers, Box 12, 25 January 1951.
131 Soper's terms in his interview with Hackett, 1950, RAC, RG3.1, Series 908, Box 7H, Folder 86.102, p. 18 of typescript of interview.
132 Farley, *To Cast Out Disease*, p. 90.

4 Post-war: A Capacity for Fanaticism

1 Socrates Litsios, 'Criticism of WHO's Revised Malaria Eradication Strategy', *Parassitologia*, 42 (1–2) (2000), pp. 167–72, here: p. 167.
2 Paul R. Russell, Foreword to Soper, *Ventures in World Health: The Memoirs of Fred Lowe Soper* (Washington, DC, 1977), p. vii.
3 NLM, Ms C 359, Fred L. Soper Papers, Box 30, Document: Eradication, 11 January 1965, typescript from original notes dated 1959: 'Cannot afford to play it too safe. Must have courage of their convictions. Capacity for fanaticism.'
4 Jonathan B. Tucker, *Scourge: The Once and Future Threat of Smallpox* (New York, 2001), p. 44.
5 Soper, *Ventures in World Health*, pp. 257–8.
6 Soper's relations with his military superiors in the US Army Typhus Commission were so unsatisfactory, from his point of view, that Soper refused to accept the medal awarded to all members of the Commission, in recognition of their wartime services. Military members of the Commission found Soper obstreperous; one 'irascible individual' (as Farley describes him), described Soper as 'not only personally

a stinker . . . but . . . just plain dumb'; Farley, *To Cast Out Disease*, p. 130.

7 Soper had in fact anticipated the possibility of an anti-gambiae eradication campaign in the Anglo-Egyptian Sudan around Khartoum, which he mentioned in a report to the RF in 1940, saying gambiae breeding had become an important problem along the Nile and its irrigation system. See Soper, *Building the Health Bridge*, p. 285.

8 See Nancy Elizabeth Gallagher, *Egypt's Other Wars: Epidemics and the Politics of Public Health* (Syracuse, NY, 1990), quotation on p. 30. This book gives a very detailed account of UK-Egyptian political and medical relations during the war years, especially in relation to malaria and the Rockefeller Foundation's involvement.

9 Soper, *Ventures in World Health*, p. 236.

10 M. A. Farid, 'Round Table: The Malaria Programme – from Euphoria to Anarchy', *World Health Forum*, 1 (1, 2) (1980), pp. 8–33. Farid at the time was an Egyptian malariologist working on malaria control. He later joined the WHO. The figure of 180,000 deaths is probably on the high side; a later estimate was 100,000.

11 The original Manual, in Portuguese, amounted to four volumes. Soper gave the English-language version to Shousha on 2 February 1943 in Cairo. See NLM, Ms C 359, Soper Papers, Box 53, Folder: Malaria-Brazil 1966–1975. The book, published by the RF, was Fred L. Soper and D. Bruce Wilson, *Anopheles Gambiae in Brazil, 1930 to 1940* (New York, 1943).

12 When Kerr got to Egypt he found that the Egyptians had already set up the administrative framework for the campaign, having divided the area into 641 serially numbered zones. At its peak, the campaign involved over 4,000 personnel, two thirds of whom were labourers carrying out Paris Greening. Kerr's report (which was never published) can be found in the Soper papers at NLM, Ms C 359, Box 53: Malaria Folder: Egypt, 1943–1969.

13 Farid, 'The Malaria Programme – From Euphoria to Anarchy', p. 10.

14 For the campaign, see Sir Aly Tewfik Shousha, 'Species-Eradication: The Eradication of Anopheles gambiae from Upper Egypt, 1942–1945', *Bull. WHO*, 1 (2) (1948), pp. 309–52.

15 J. Austin Kerr concluded it was enough to aim to reduce the gambiae mosquito sufficiently to interrupt transmission; there was no need to eradicate the species entirely.

16 Mark Harrison, *Medicine and Victory: British Military Medicine in the Second World War* (Oxford and New York, 2004), pp. 133–43.

17 Soper, 'My Lousy Adventure', in *Ventures in World Health*, pp. 279–80. DDT was also used against typhus in Sicily in 1943; see also Frank M. Snowden, *The Conquest of Malaria: Italy, 1900–1962* (New Haven, CT, and London, 2006), p. 199.

18 *Ventures in World Health*, p. 289.

19 Soper, 'The Use of DDT against Malaria Evaluated on a Cost-Benefit Basis', NLM, Ms C 359, Soper Papers, Box 52, 3 December 1970; also cited in Snowden, *The Conquest of Malaria*, p. 199.

20 Russell had been sent first to the Pacific theatre where he served under General Douglas MacArthur and worked to control malaria among US troops. DDT was first tested in Italy in a pilot study of its effects, in Castel Volturno, in the Campania, with a further trial being made in the Delta of the Tiber River and the Pontine Marshes.

21 Snowden, *Conquest of Malaria*, chap. 7, with case and mortality figures on p. 196. The main vector in the area, *A. labranchiae*, preferred brackish water to fresh water as a breeding ground; the drainage system and improved agriculture known as 'bonification', which was used in Italy had reduced the brackish water and successfully kept malaria at bay.

22 Snowden, *Conquest of Malaria*, chap. 8, gives a full account.

23 Wilbur G. Downs, 'A New Look at Yellow Fever and Malaria', *Amer. J. Tropical Med. and Hyg.*, 30 (3) (1981), p. 517. The IHD was merged with the Division of Medicine and Public Health (later renamed the Division of Medical Education and Public Health), so the RF did not in fact immediately quit the public health field.

24 Previously, the director of the League of Nation's Health Organization, Ludwig Rajchman, had proposed a United Nations Health Service.

25 The Universal Declaration of Human Rights, UN General Assembly Resolution 217A, 10 December, 1948.

26 The analysis of WHO that follows in this chapter is based on consultation of the WHO archives in Geneva (in May 2009), and the books and articles that appear in the footnotes. But as the major post-war organization in international health, WHO desperately needs a new, comprehensive and scholarly history. A very useful beginning is the article by Theodore M. Brown, Marcos Cueto and Elizabeth Fee, 'The World Health Organization and the Transition from "International" to "Global" Public Health', *Amer. J. Pub. Health*, 96 (1), (2006), pp. 62–72.

27 In his time, Chisholm was among the best known of Canadians; now he is almost forgotten. For a recent resurrection of his career and role in WHO, as well as a detailed history of the negotiations in the first years of the UN and WHO, see John Farley, *Brock Chisholm, The World Health Organization and the Cold War* (Vancouver, BC, and Toronto, ON, 2008).

28 PAHO underwent numerous changes of names in the course of its history; it began as the International Sanitary Bureau, which in 1925 became the Pan American Sanitary Bureau (PASB); in 1947 the bureau was renamed the Pan American Sanitary

Organization (PASO), with the PASB as its executive arm; and finally, in 1958, PASO's name was changed to the Pan American Health Organization. For simplicity sake I refer to it and PASB documents throughout this book as PAHO.

29 Final ratification by all members was achieved only in 1936. See Myron E. Wegman, 'A Salute to the Pan American Health Organization', *Public Health Then and Now*, 67 (12) (December 1977), pp. 1198–204.

30 A very valuable new history of PAHO is by Marcos Cueto, *The Value of Health: A History of the Pan American Health Organization* (Washington, DC, 2007); it gives considerable attention to the Soper years.

31 Farley, *Brock Chisholm*, p. 152.

32 On the IIAA, see Public Health Service, Dept. of Health, Education and Welfare for the Institute of Inter-American Affairs, *10 Years of Cooperative Health Programs in Latin America: An Evaluation* (Washington, DC, 1953); and Paola Mejia, *Intolerable Burdens: Malaria and Yellow Fever Control in Colombia in the Twentieth Century*. PhD Dissertation, Columbia University (2009), chap. 3.

33 Cueto, *The Value of Health*, pp. 87–8.

34 A similar Latin Americanization occurred in the parent organization, the Pan American Union, at the same time. Renamed the Organization of the American States (OAS), the recruitment of Latin Americans was part of the Cold War strategy of the US to keep Latin America as *its* back yard. A total of 66 per cent of OAS's budget in 1956 was paid by the US ($2.3 million). See Marcos Cueto, *Cold War, Deadly Fevers: Malaria Eradication in Mexico, 1955–1975* (Baltimore, MD, 2007), p. 23.

35 Soper's name was added to a list of potential Director-Generals for tactical reasons, but Soper, perhaps realizing he could not win, was anxious not to run against Candau.

36 Quotes from NLM, Ms C 359, Soper Papers, Box 11, Folder: Diary September–December 1947, entry: 2 September 1947. Farley, in *Brock Chisholm*, takes a very negative view of PAHO's efforts to remain intact as an organization while nonetheless becoming part of WHO; he sees it as negating Chisholm's vision of a world unified in outlook and not divided by the various voting blocs that quickly made their presence felt in WHO affairs. There was also the worry that PAHO would exclude from membership the colonial possessions of European countries in the Caribbean (though eventually they all joined).

37 'Fundamentally, as Director of PASB', wrote Soper, 'I was happy to find that WHO was unable to bail out the Bureau immediately', for had WHO been well funded in 1947 PAHO would have been subordinated to WHO. Soper, *Ventures in World Health*, p. 320.

38 Cueto, *Cold War, Deadly Fevers*, p. 20. The US contributed 31 per cent of the funds of the UN and its ten specialized agencies in 1956, to the tune of $23 million.

39 Fiona Godlee, 'The World Health Organization: The Regions – Too Much Power, Too Little Effect', *Brit. Med. J.*, 309 (10 December 1994), pp. 1566–70, here: p. 1566.

40 NLM, Ms C 359, Soper Papers, Box 12, Typed Diaries, 2 May 1950 – 3 December 1957, Folder 1, May–June 1950, 20 May 1950.

41 Cueto, *The Value of Health*, p. 98.

42 Data from Cueto, *Cold War, Deadly Fevers*, pp. 34 and 41 for the WHO budget, and p. 34 (the US contribution to WHO represented 55 per cent of WHO's entire budget); and Cueto, *The Value of Health*, p. 96 (staff size).

43 Farid, 'The Malaria Programme – From Euphoria to Anarchy', pp. 11–12.

44 Fred L. Soper, 'Address by the Director of PASB', PAHO *Official Document No. 18* [1956] (Washington, DC, 1957), pp. 25–6. The Official Documents of PAHO represent the records of great many different kinds of meetings: of the Directing Council of the Pan American Sanitary Bureau of PAHO, the Regional Committee of WHO, and the Pan American Sanitary Conferences, with regular Annual and Quadrennial Reports by the Directors of PAHO. For simplicity, throughout the book I cite all of the Official Documents as *PAHO Official Documents*, their number and the date of the meetings (plus place and date of publication). This allows unambiguous identification of the documents concerned.

45 *The Boletín de la Oficína Sanitaria Panamericana*, today called the *Revista Panamericana de la Salud Pública.*

46 See especially NLM, Ms C 359, Soper Papers, Box 12.

47 Fred L. Soper, 'Problems to be Solved if the Eradication of Tuberculosis is to be Realized', *Amer. J. Pub. Health*, 52 (5) (1962), pp. 734–45. 'Although the final eradication of TB is many years off, the results of all our efforts for eradication are cumulative from here on', Soper wrote in his files. NLM, Ms C 359, Soper Papers, Box 30, Folder Daily Files, October–December 1964, document called *Tuberculosis Eradication*, 15 December 1964.

48 John Lewis Gaddis, *The Cold War: A New History* (New York, 2005).

49 Robert Service, *Comrades: A World History of Communism* (Oxford, 2007), p. 239.

50 Socrates Litsios, 'Malaria Control, the Cold War, and the Postwar Reorganization of International Assistance', *Medical Anthropology*, 17 (3) (1997), pp. 255–78; Sunil Amrith, *Decolonizing International Health: India and Southeast Asia, 1930–1965* (Basingstoke, 2006), p. 85, makes a similar point about the narrowing of the definitions of public health in Asian countries, as a way to de-politicize it.

51 Javed Siddiqi, *World Health and World Politics: The World Health Organization and the UN System* (Columbus, OH, 1995).

52 Cueto, *Cold War, Deadly Fevers,* especially chap. 2.

53 R. M. Packard, 'Malaria Dreams: Postwar Visions of Health and Development in the Third World', *Medical Anthropology*, 17 (3) (1997), pp. 279–96, and Packard and Peter J. Brown, 'Rethinking Health, Development, and Malaria: Historicizing a Cultural Model in International Health', *Medical Anthropology*, 17 (3) (1997), pp. 181–94. The US was particularly concerned to develop anti-communist strategies. President Truman's Point Four Plan of 1947 had among its objectives the containment of communist expansion. In 1961, two years after the Cuban Revolution led by Castro, President Kennedy announced the Alliance for Progress, which was designed to offer aid to Latin American countries but also bind them to the United States.

54 Williams, *The Plague Killers*, pp. 321–2.

55 Soper certainly understood the connection in this way. In his Annual Report as Director of PAHO in 1957, he refers to Eisenhower's State of the Union address, where the US President referred to the power to eradicate malaria worldwide, and invited the Soviet Union to join the US in 'this great work of humanity'. 'As if in reply', said Soper, 'the government of the USSR is going to present to the 1958 World Health Assembly a proposal for smallpox eradication'. PAHO, *Official Documents no. 25* [1957] (Washington, DC, 1958), p. 18.

56 James A. Gillespie, 'Europe, America, and the Space of International Health', in *Shifting Boundaries of Public Health: Europe in the Twentieth Century*, ed. Susan G. Solomon, Lion Murard, and Patrick Zylberman (Rochester, NY, 2008), pp. 114–37.

57 Amrith, *Decolonizing International Health*, p. 97.

58 NLM, Ms C 359, Soper Papers, Box 12, Diary entry, 16 June 1950.

59 Soper was critical of the wave of McCarthyism and the proposal to make members of international organizations pass loyalty tests, but he did in fact take (and pass) a loyalty test himself: NLM Ms C 359, Soper Papers, Box 30, Folder Daily Files, October–December 1964.

60 Cueto, *Cold War, Deadly Fevers*, p. 36, associates Soper's idea of the obligation states had to eradicate diseases with the Cold War rhetoric of 'loyalty'; but as I have shown in chapter Three, this notion of obligation derived from the so-called 'Soper's law', which argued there was a necessary and logical obligation of contiguous states to eradicate a disease once one state had done so, or else eradication would fail.

61 NLM, Ms C 359, Soper Papers, Box 12, Folder: January–December 1954, Notes from 27 May 1954.

62 'Annual Report', PAHO *Official Documents no. 25*, p. 18.

63 Amrith, *Decolonizing International Health*, chaps 5 and 6; Niels Brimnes, 'BCG Vaccination and WHO's Global Strategy for Tuberculosis Control, 1948–1983', *Social Science and Medicine*, 67 (5) (2008), pp. 863–873; and Christian W. McMillen and Niels Brimnes, 'Medical Modernization and Medical Nationalism: Resistance to Mass Tuberculosis Vaccination in Postcolonial India, 1948–1955', *Comparative Studies in Society and History*, 52 (1) (2010), pp. 180–209.

64 'Quadrennial Report of the Director', *PAHO Official Document no. 25*, pp. 31–7.

65 Fred L. Soper, *Yaws: Its Eradication in the Americas* (May 1956): http://profiles.nlm.nih.gov/VV/B/B/D/H.

66 In fact, the campaign eventually came to use lower doses of penicillin than were used elsewhere against yaws.

67 NLM, Ms C359, Soper Papers, Ms C 359, Box 5. Letter from John C. Cutler, written 27 November 1973, on the occasion of Soper's 80th birthday celebrations.

68 NLM, Ms C 359, Soper Papers, Box 12, Folder 1, May–June 1950.

69 Cueto, *Value of Health*, p. 109.

70 Editorial, 'Campaña de Erradicación del Pian en Haiti', *Boletin de la Oficína Sanit. Panamericana*, 33 (2) (August 1952), pp. 160–1.

71 Donald R. Hopkins, 'Yaws in the Americas, 1950–1975', *The Journal of Infectious Diseases*, 136 (4) (October 1977), pp. 548–55.

72 'New Era in Yaws Control', *The Lancet*, 262 (6778) (25 July 1953), p. 175.

73 Different sources give different figures. A recent WHO document, 'WHO revives efforts to eliminate forgotten disease', dated 25 January 2007, says the Global Yaws Control Programme, fully operational between 1952 and 1964, succeeded in treating 300 million people in 50 countries. The variableness of the data in different sources indicates the inadequate reporting and surveillance mechanisms in place in many poor countries.

74 Stephen L. Walker and Roderick J. Hay, 'Yaws – A Review of the Last 50 Years', *Intern. J. Dermatology*, 39 (4) (2000), pp. 258–60.

75 Donald A. Henderson, 'Eradication: Lessons from the Past', *Morbidity and Mortality Weekly Report*, 48 (suppl.) (31 December 1999), pp. 16–22.

76 C. J. Hackett and T. Guthe, 'Some Important Aspects of Yaws Eradication', *Bull. WHO*, 15 (6) (1956), pp. 869–96, recognized that the social and economic factors were essential to eradication, but seemed to think that in principle, cleanliness, clean water, proper ventilation and improved domestic hygiene could be obtained by 'the inexpensive efforts of the people themselves' (p. 870).

77 R. Duncan Catterall and John C. Hume, 'Summary and Recommendations', in *International Symposium on Yaws and other Endemic Trepenomatoses*, held at PAHO, Washington, 16–18 April 1984, and published in *Reviews of Infect. Diseases*, 7 (suppl. 2) (May–June 1985), pp. 343–51.

78 Andrea Rinaldi, 'Yaws: A Second (and Maybe Last?)

Chance for Eradication', *PLOS Neglected Tropical Diseases*, 2 (8) (August 2008), p. e275. Online journal at: www.plosntds.org.

79 The PAHO conference in Rio de Janeiro in 1942 requested governments to pursue eradication, a decision that most countries were incapable of acting upon at the time.

80 Soper told the Brazilians the proposal would be much more valuable coming from them, than from him. NLM, Ms C 359, Soper Papers, Box 11, Folder Diary, May–Sep 1947, meeting 22 April 1947.

81 Fred L. Soper, 'Editorial: Continental Eradication of Aedes Aegypti', in Soper, *Building the Health Bridge: Selections from the Works of Fred L. Soper, M.D.*, ed. J. Austin Kerr (Bloomington, IN, and London, 1970), pp. 45–6.

82 Fred L. Soper and D. Bruce Wilson, 'Species Eradication: A Practical Goal of Species Reduction in the Control of Mosquito-borne Disease', *J. Nat. Malaria Soc.*, 1 (1) (1942), pp. 5–24, quote from pp. 19–20.

83 Fred L. Soper, D. Bruce Wilson, S. Lima and W. Sá Atunes *The Organization of Permanent Nation-Wide Anti-Aedes Aegypti Measures in Brazil* (New York, 1943).

84 Fred L. Soper, 'International Health in the Americas' (3 May 1948), typescript: http://profiles.nlm.nih.gov/VV/B/B/D/F.

85 Soper, *Ventures in World Health*, p. 340.

86 Quoted in *Smallpox and its Eradication*, ed. F. Fenner, et al. (Geneva, 1988), pp. 593–4.

87 According to Soper, in the early years of the campaign, motor vehicles were also supplied by the Argentine government.

88 NLM, Ms C 359, Soper Papers, Box 12, Folder Diary, September–October 1950, from a meeting in Soper's Washington office on DDT.

89 In what Darwin Stapleton, the then director of the Rockefeller Archive Center, called 'vintage Soper', Soper argued in an (unpublished) letter of 24 July 1946 to Strode, at the time head of the IHD, that the deaths of birds and rabbits reported by a researcher had not been proven to be due to DDT. Letter RAC, RF 1.2, ser 700, box 12, folder 104, two-page letter. Personal communication by Stapleton; I thank him for drawing my attention to this document.

90 NLM, Ms C359, Soper Papers, Box 11, Folder Diary, March–May 1948, entry dated 2 March 1948.

91 NLM, Ms C 359, Soper Papers, Box 12, Folder Diary, January–March 1951, diary notes on conversation in Buenos Aires.

92 NLM, Ms C 359, Soper Papers, Box 12, Folder Diary, January–December 1957, note made during a visit to Buenos Aires, 21 February 1957.

93 *Smallpox and its Eradication*, ed. Fenner, et al., pp. 1104–7.

94 Fred L. Soper, 'The Unfinished Business With Yellow Fever', In *Yellow Fever: A Symposium in Commemoration of Carlos Juan Finlay*, Jefferson Medical College, Philadelphia, Pennsylvania, 22–25 September 1955, pp. 79–88, maps pp. 80 and 81. The maps seem to show an overall increase in yellow fever cases, but this is because immunity surveys had uncovered many jungle yellow fever cases that had been undetected and unknown before the 1930s. See: http://profiles.nlm.gov/ps/access/VVBBDG.pdf.

95 Moreover, the viscerotomy services which had been set up in several countries to detect yellow fever after deaths from fevers, had revealed the continent-wide distribution of otherwise overlooked rural yellow fever cases; unless such systems of surveillance was put in place and actively maintained in all the countries, it was inevitable that yellow fever cases would be overlooked, only to pass along routes of travel into cities wherever the urban vector still remained.

96 NLM, Ms C 359, Soper Papers, Box 34, Folder: Yellow Fever-Americas. Letter from Soper to the Minister of Health in Brazil, 24 August 1967.

97 These were: Argentina, Belize, Bermuda, Bolivia, Chile, Ecuador, the Panama Canal Zone, Paraguay, Peru and Uruguay.

98 Perez Yekutiel, 'Lessons from the Big Eradication Campaigns', *World Health Forum*, 2 (4) (1981), pp. 465–90. The report, prepared for PAHO, was *The Prevention of Diseases Transmitted by Aedes aegypti in the Americas – A Cost-Benefit Study* (Cambridge, 1972).

99 Soper, 'The Unfinished Business With Yellow Fever', p. 87.

100 Between 1937 and 1949, 5,700,000 people in Brazil were vaccinated with the yellow fever vaccine. Figures from *Yellow Fever*, ed. George Strode (New York, 1951), p. 614. By the early 1940s, the RF's 17D yellow fever vaccine was replacing the French 'Dakar' yellow fever vaccine as the vaccine of choice because the French vaccine, which was based on a different strain of the virus than the 17D vaccine, had proved to be less safe than 17D.

101 NLM, Ms C 359, Soper Papers, Box 38, Folder 'Yellow Fever', document 'Aedes a eradication'.

102 Rachel Carson, *Silent Spring* (Boston, MA, 1962).

103 Soper served as a consultant to the Office of International Health in the US Surgeon-General's Office, starting in 1962.

104 NLM, Ms C 359, Soper Papers, Box 38, Yellow Fever, Folder: Yellow Fever USA. Extract from Fred L. Soper's Diary Notes.

105 Soper note in NLM, Ms C 359, Soper Papers, Box 19, Folder on Pesticides.

106 Soper, *Ventures in World Health*, pp. 344–57.

107 PAHO, *Official Document no. 27* [1958] (Washington, DC, 1959), p. 107.

108 NLM, Ms C 359, Soper Papers, Box 30, Daily Files, 11 January 1965, in an essay on eradication.

109 PAHO, *Official Document no. 41* [1961] (Washington, DC, 1962), p. 143.

110 PAHO, *Official Document no. 41* [1961] (Washington, DC, 1962), p. 144.
111 PAHO, *Official Document no. 86* [1967] (Washington, DC, 1968), p. xxi.
112 PAHO, *Official Document no. 89* [1969] (Washington, DC, 1970), pp. 31–2.
113 PAHO, *Official Document no. 100* [1969] (Washington, DC, 1970), p. 58.
114 PAHO, *Official. Document no. 86* [1967] (Washington, DC, 1968), p. xxi.
115 PAHO, *Official Doument no. 108* [1970] (Washington, DC, 1971), p. 238 for French delegate's question.
116 PAHO, *Official Document no. 100* [1969] (Washington, DC, 1970), pp. 57–8.
117 PAHO, *Official Document no. 100*, pp. 115.
118 Wilbur G. Downs, 'The Story of Yellow Fever Since Walter Reed', *Bull. NY Acad. Med.*, 44 (6) (June 1968), pp. 721–7, here: p. 727.
119 Wilbur G. Downs, 'A New Look at Yellow Fever and Malaria', *Amer. J. Trop. Med. and Hyg.*, 30 (3) (1981), pp. 516–22.

5 The End of Malaria in the World?

1 NLM, Ms C 359, Fred Lowe Soper Papers, Box 11, Soper Diaries 1946–1950, Meeting, 4 July 1947.
2 Paul F. Russell and others, *Practical Malariology*, 2nd edn (Oxford and London, 1963), p. 22.
3 Socrates Litsios, 'Malaria Control, the Cold War, and the Postwar Reorganization of International Assistance', *Medical Anthropology*, 17 (3) (1997), pp. 255–78.
4 General accounts of malaria are numerous. Among several valuable older works, see Lewis W. Hackett, *Malaria in Europe: An Ecological Study* (London, 1937); Leonard C. Bruce-Chwatt and Julian de Zulueta, *The Rise and Fall of Malaria in Europe: An Historico-Epidemiological Study* (London, 1980). Among many newer works, I have found especially valuable the following: Socrates Litsios, *The Tomorrow of Malaria* (Wellington, 1996); the three excellent issues of the journal *Parassitologia* (Rome): vol. 36 (1994), vol. 40 (1998) and vol. 42 (2000); Randall M. Packard, *The Making of a Tropical Disease: A Short History of Malaria* (Baltimore, MD, 2007); Sandra M. Sufian, *Healing the Land and the Nation: Malaria and the Zionist Project in Palestine, 1920–1947* (Chicago, IL, and London, 2007); Margaret Humphries, *Malaria: Poverty, Race, and Public Health in the United States* (Baltimore, MD, and London, 2001); Saúl Franco Agudelo, *El Paludismo en América Latina* (Guadalajara, Mexico, 1990); and Sunil Amrith, *Decolonizing International Health: India and Southeast Asia, 1930–1965* (Basingstoke, 2006). A general account of efforts to control many kinds of vector-transmitted diseases, written by a medical entomologist, is also very useful: James R. Busvine, *Disease Transmission by Insects: Its Discovery and 90 Years of Effort to Prevent It* (Berlin and New York, 1993). Recent, excellent country-specific studies by historians are Marcos Cueto's *Cold War, Deadly Fevers: Malaria Eradication in Mexico, 1955–1975* (Baltimore, MD, 2007); Frank M. Snowden's *The Conquest of Malaria: Italy, 1900–1962* (New Haven, CT, and London, 2006) and Paola Mejia's *Intolerable Burdens: Malaria and Yellow Fever Control in Colombia in the Twentieth Century*, PhD Dissertation, Columbia University (2009).
5 Soper denied he was a malaria expert, and did not serve as such on the WHO's Expert Committee on Malaria (he did attend several of its sessions as director of the PAHO). See NLM, Ms C 359, Soper Papers, Box 53, his remarks to this effect on his trip to Africa in 1959 as a consultant.
6 Fred L. Soper, 'The Epidemiology of a Disappearing Disease: Malaria', *Amer. J. Tropical Med. and Hyg.*, 9 (1960), pp. 357–366, where, as was his wont, he explains the story of malaria by analogy to that of yellow fever.
7 Quoted in *Smallpox and its Eradication*, ed. F. Fenner, et al. (Geneva, 1988), p. 381.
8 Viruses are extremely small packets of genetic material that reproduce only by invading host cells and destroying them. Protozoa (meaning animal-like) are larger, single-celled micro-organisms that are visible under the microscope and whose complicated life cycles are often spent in human and non-human hosts (for example, insects) which are necessary to their survival.
9 Packard, *The Making of a Tropical Disease*, pp. 19–24, for a clear account of the biology of the parasites.
10 Nancy Leys Stepan, '"The Only Serious Terror in these Regions": Malaria Control in the Brazilian Amazon', in *Disease in the History of Modern Latin America: From Malaria to AIDS*, ed. Diego Armus (Durham, NC, and London, 2003), pp. 25–50 for a discussion.
11 Packard, *The Making of a Tropical Disease*.
12 Figures from E. J. Pampana and P. F. Russell, *Malaria: A World Problem* (Geneva, 1955), p. 6.
13 J. A. Sinton, writing in 1936, as quoted in Pampana and Russell, *Malaria: A World Problem*, p. 7.
14 Pampana and Russell, *Malaria: A World Problem*, pp. 10–11.
15 Pampana and Russell, *Malaria: A World Problem*, p. 8.
16 Snowden, *The Conquest of Malaria*, chap. 6.
17 The methods used in the TVA are described in *Malaria and Its Control in the Tennessee Valley*, 2nd edn (Chattanooga, 1942).
18 Malcolm Watson, *Prevention of Malaria in the Federated Malay States* (Liverpool, 1911).
19 W. Takken, 'Species Sanitation', and J. P. Verhave, 'Swellengrebel and Species Sanitation, the Design of an Idea', in *Environmental Measures for Malaria Control in Indonesia: An Historical Review on Species*

Sanitation, ed. W. Takken, et al., (Wageningen, 1991), pp. 5–8 and 63–80. See also D. J. Bradley, 'Watson, Swellengrebel and Species Sanitation: Environmental and Ecological Aspects', *Parassitologia*, 36 (1–2) (1994), pp. 137–47.

20 The Brazilian, Dr Carlos Chagas, in 1908 was the first to describe malaria in these terms.

21 G. A. Park Ross, 'Insecticide as a Major Measure in Control of Malaria, being an Account of the Methods and Organization put in force in Natal and Zululand during the past Six Years', *Bull. Health Org. League of Nations*, 5 (1936), pp. 114–33.

22 Fred L. Soper, *Ventures in World Health. The Memoirs of Fred Lowe Soper*, ed. John Duffy (Washington, DC, 1977), p. 145.

23 The results with pyrethrum prepared him, Soper said, to appreciate the value of DDT later, since DDT was used in malaria eradication to spray inside houses to get rid of adult mosquitoes.

24 Quinine, which derived from the bark of the cinchona tree, was indigenous to the western Andes of South America; its properties as a febrifuge were first described in the seventeenth century. The name Jesuit's bark referred to the quasi-monopoly of the supply from the New World obtained by the Jesuits, who learned of the effect of cinchona bark on fevers from the Amerindians.

25 Snowden, *The Conquest of Malaria*, p. 75.

26 Stepan, '"The Only Serious Terror in These Regions"', pp. 38–39.

27 The title given to chap. 1 in Hackett's *Malaria in Europe*.

28 J. Farley, 'Mosquitoes or Malaria? Rockefeller Campaigns in the American South and Sardinia', *Parassitologia*, 36 (1–2) (1994), pp. 165–73.

29 William F. Bynum, 'An Experiment that Failed: Malaria Control at Mian Mir', *Parassitologia*, 36 (1–2) (1994), pp. 107–20. Ross was convinced the experiment was planned to fail by his enemies, notably Captain S. P. James of the India Medical Service who, following Mian Mir, certainly became a sceptic about anti-mosquito measures.

30 As quoted in Bynum, 'An Experiment that Failed', p. 119.

31 Quoted in Hackett, *Malaria in Europe*, pp. 21–22. See also Hughes Evans, 'European Malaria Policy in the 1920s and 1930s: The Epidemiology of Minutiae', *Isis*, 80 (1989), pp. 40–59. The report was written by S. P. James, with the collaboration of Swellengrebel. The conclusion greatly irritated many of the American malaria specialists and the part of the report covering the US was as a result circulated only in mimeographed form.

32 Letter from Strode to F. F. Russell, 25 January 1926, in RG 5, series 1.2, Box 254, Folder 3237, Rockefeller Archive Center (RAC).

33 Hackett, *Malaria in Europe*, pp. 264 and 265.

34 Quoted in Litsios, *The Tomorrow of Malaria*, p. 62.

35 Humphries, *Malaria: Poverty, Race and Public Health in the United States*, pp. 140–54.

36 Marshall A. Barber, *A Malariologist in Many Lands* (Lawrence, KS, 1946), chap. 1.

37 B. Fantini, 'Anopheles Without Malaria: An Ecological and Epidemiological Puzzle', *Parassitologia*, 36 (1–2) (1994), pp. 83–106.

38 Hackett, *Malaria in Europe*, p. 266.

39 See especially the excellent analysis by Helen Tilley, in 'Ecologies of Complexity: Tropical Environments, African Trypanomiasis, and the Science of Disease Control in British Colonial Africa, 1900–1940', in *Landscapes of Exposure: Knowledge and Illness in Modern Environments*, ed. Gregg Mitman, Michelle Murphy and Christopher Sellers, special issue of *Osiris*, 19 (2004), pp. 21–38.

40 According to Evans, in 'European Malaria Policy, in the 1920s and 1930s', Hackett 'remained an eradicationist, and, consequently, he believed that every anopheles capable of biting humans should be exterminated' (p. 57).

41 See the extremely interesting analysis by Eric D. Carter, 'Development Narratives and the Uses of Ecology: Malaria Control in Northwest Argentina, 1890–1940', *J. Hist. Geog.*, 33 (2007), pp. 619–50.

42 Litsios, *The Tomorrow of Malaria*, p. 141.

43 Humphries, *Malaria: Poverty, Race and Public Health in the United States*, p. 147. In fact, by the 1940s, there were so few cases of malaria that success was measured by mosquitoes killed, not the declines in the numbers of malaria patients

44 Figures from Fred L. Soper, 'Report and Recommendations on Malaria: A Summary. International Cooperative Administration Expert Panel on Malaria', *Amer. J. Tropical Med. and Hyg.*, 10 (4) (1961), p. 454.

45 Humphries, *Malaria: Poverty, Race and Public Health in the United States*, pp. 451–502, here: p. 454.

46 P. J. Brown, 'Malaria, Miseria, and Underpopulation in Sardinia: The "Malaria Blocks Development" Cultural Model', *Medical Anthropology*, 17 (3) (1997), pp. 239–54.

47 Quoted by Litsios, *The Tomorrow of Malaria*, p. 144.

48 Darwin H. Stapleton, 'Lessons of History? Anti-Malaria Strategies of the International Health Board and the Rockefeller Foundation from the 1920s to the Era of DDT', *Public Health Reports*, 119 (2) (March–April 2004), pp. 206–15.

49 The concept of epistemic community was introduced by Peter Haas in his 'Introduction: Epistemic Communities and International Policy Coordination', *International Organization*, 46 (1) (Winter 1992), pp. 1–35. J. Jackson employed the concept in relation to the MEP in 'Cognition and the Global Malaria Eradication Programme', *Parassitologia*, 40 (1–2) (1998), pp. 193–216. George Macdonald contributed the concept of the Basic Reproduction Number, or BRN. This is a measure of additional infections each originally infected person will generate in a non-immune population. Malaria can

have a BRN of 100, compared to a BRN of 12 to 14 for measles (considered one of the most contagious of diseases). The infectivity rate of malaria is enhanced by the fact that many mosquitoes can bite the same infected person in the same day, adding to their parasite load and the force of transmission. Mosquito vectors can often fly long distances, and can be quite long lived. The ideal conditions used by Macdonald to work out the BRN are not met in actual circumstances, but the quantitative assessment of the infectivity of diseases has been a very important addition to epidemiology. See Andrew Spielman and Michael D'Antonio, *Mosquito: A Natural History of our Most Persistent and Deadly Foe* (New York, 2001), pp. 96–97.

50 *Proceedings of the Fourth International Congresses on Tropical Medicine and Malaria* (Washington, DC, 1948), vol. I. Hackett made the humorous references to Soper in his Address, pp. 10–15.

51 UNRRA had been set up in 1943 to deal with the chaos facing populations as a result of the war; largely funded by the US, it lasted until 1949, working mainly in Mediterranean countries (Italy and especially Greece).

52 Kerr had run the anti-gambiae project in Egypt. He later edited a collection of Soper's papers. Austin Kerr's doubts are noted by Soper in NLM, Ms C 359, Soper Papers, Box 11, Folder: June–July 1948, entry in his diary, 23 July 1948.

53 John A. Logan, *The Sardinian Project. An Experiment in the Eradication of an Indigenous Malarious Vector.* Written in collaboration with others (Baltimore, MD, 1953). Logan succeeded Kerr as director of the project.

54 On the Sardinia experiment, see John Farley, 'Mosquitoes or Malaria? Rockefeller Campaigns in the American South and Sardinia', *Parassitologia*, 36 (1–2) (1994), pp. 165–173; P. J. Brown, 'Failure-as-Success: Multiple Meanings of Eradication in the Rockefeller Foundation Sardinia Project, 1946–1951', *Parassitologia*, 40 (1–2) (1998), pp. 117–130; Snowden, *The Conquest of Malaria*, pp. 205–208.

55 RAC, RF 1.2, ser 700, box 12, folder 104. 2-page letter from Soper to Strode, dated 24 July 1946(?). I thank Darwin Stapleton, Emeritus Director of the RAC, for drawing my attention to this letter and sending me a transcript.

56 Soper's failure to repeat the success he had in Brazil and Egypt may explain why his Memoirs contain almost no references to malaria except his two gambiae campaigns, in Brazil and Egypt.

57 See, for example, his reference to the eradication of *A. lambranchiae* in his 1959 address, 'Rehabilitation of the Eradication Concept in Prevention of Communicable Disease', *Public Health Reports*, 80 (10) (October 1965), pp. 855–69. The paper was presented on 27 October 1959.

58 Snowden, *The Conquest of Malaria*, p. 207.

59 From Fred L. Soper, 'International Health in the Americas, 1954–1957: Director's Review', in *Building the Health Bridge*, ed. Kerr, pp. 435–462, here: p. 460.

60 NLM, Ms C 359, Soper Papers, Box 11, Diary Entries 1946–1950, entry for 2 July 1948.

61 Wilbur G. Downs, 'A New Look at Yellow Fever and Malaria', *Amer. J. Tropical Med. and Hyg.*, 30 (3) (1981), pp. 516–22, here: p. 520.

62 The shift can be traced in the many malaria textbooks that appeared between 1945 and 1955.

63 Paul F. Russell, *Man's Mastery of Malaria* (London, New York and Toronto, 1955); my emphasis.

64 Pampana and Russell, *Malaria: A World Problem*, p. 17.

65 Russell, *Man's Master of Malaria*, pp. 160–61.

66 Ibid., p. 162.

67 Pampana and Russell, *Malaria: A World Problem*, p. 32.

68 Paul F. Russell, et al., *Practical Malariology*, 2nd edn (London, 1963), pp. 549–50.

69 Russell, et al., *Practical Malariology*, p. 562.

70 The job of the Expert Committee, which was modelled on the similar committee that the League of Nations Health Committee had organized, was to advise the WHO on malaria policy. It was formed on the suggestion of the Venezuelan malaria expert, Gabaldón. Producing reports between 1947 and 1986, the Committee had a rotating membership but for several years included a repeating core that included Gabaldón (who often served as chair), Russell, Macdonald and Pampana. Soper attended the second meeting in 1948 ex-officio, as the director of PAHO, when he presented a paper on species sanitation.

71 'Malaria Control: Survey and Recommendations', *Bull. WHO*, 1 (2) 1948, pp. 213–52; and *WHO Technical Report Series no. 8*, 1950, quote p. 7.

72 An account of this debate is given by Litsios, in *The Tomorrow of Malaria*, pp. 106–22; and by Mary Dobson, M. Malowany and R. W. Snow, 'Malaria Control in East Africa: the Kampala Conference and the Pare-Taveta Scheme: A Meeting of Common and High Ground', *Parassitologia*, 42 (1–2) (2000), pp. 149–66.

73 *Proceedings of the Fourth International Congresses on Tropical Medicine and Malaria*, p. 928.

74 'Malaria Conference in Equatorial Africa. Kampala, Uganda, 27 November – 9 December 1950, *WHO Technical Report Series no. 38* (Geneva, 1951), pp. 22ff.

75 Leonard Bruce-Chwatt was Polish by birth and a naturalized British citizen who served in West Africa during the war; after his years in Nigeria, in 1958 he became director of research and intelligence in the Division of Malaria at WHO, and following his retirement, Director of the Ross Institute of the London School of Hygiene and Tropical Medicine. While at WHO he became deeply involved with the problems of malaria eradication.

76 P.C.C. Garnham, 'Professor L. J. Bruce-Chwatt's

80th Birthday', *Amer. J. Tropical Med. and Hyg.*, 92 (2) (1989), p. 68. Bruce-Chwatt went on to test the new insecticides in the control of malaria in holo-endemic (high transmission area) Nigeria. After four years of work, the main vector in the area had virtually disappeared, parasite rates in children had been reduced by 30 per cent, and there was a decrease in the number of actual malaria cases. There was, however, little change in the older population. These results were reported at the Fifth International Congress of Tropical Medicine and Malaria, held in Istanbul in 1953.

77 Leonard J. Bruce-Chwatt, 'Lessons Learned from Applied Field Research Activities in Africa during the Malaria Eradication Era', *Bull. WHO*, 62 (suppl.) (1984), pp. 19–29. The most important of the pilot projects was in highly malarial Kenya, in an effort known as the Pare-Taveta Malaria Scheme led by D. B. Wilson; see Dobson, Malowany, and Snow, 'Malaria Control in East Africa'.

78 'Expert Committee on Malaria Eighth Report', *WHO Technical Report Series no. 205* (Geneva, 1961).

79 Listios, *The Tomorrow of Malaria*, quote from p. 122.

80 The results of a later control experiment in the 1970s, carried in a number of highly endemic African villages in northern Nigeria, near the town of Garki, showed that insecticide spraying was ineffective in reducing local populations of *A. gambiae*, but the regular and preventive use of anti-malarial drugs greatly reduced falciparum malaria. The fact that in the villages targeted, parasitemia declined to below 1 per cent, was viewed at the time as less important than the failure to stop transmission, the latter indicating that, even using the best tools available, eradication was impossible. See L. Molineux and G. Gramiccia, *The Garki Project: Research on the Epidemiology and Control of Malaria in the Sudan Savanna of West Africa* (Geneva, 1980).

81 DDT had been tested on animals by the British and the US Army during the war; though the tests showed DDT could damage the animals' nervous systems, and even result in their deaths, the recommendation at the time was that wartime necessity dictated the rapid application of the insecticide. It was decided to restrict its use for civilian purposes until it could be properly evaluated. But at war's end, DDT was seen to be so exceptional that it was rapidly released for civilian use, in public health and of course, in agriculture.

82 G. Davidson, 'Studies on Insecticide Resistance in Anopheline Mosquitoes', *Bull. WHO*, 18 (4) (1958), pp. 579–621.

83 George Macdonald, 'Eradication of Malaria', *Public Health Reports*, 80 (10) (1965), pp. 870–9.

84 For a history of the regulation of DDT in the US, see Thomas R. Dunlap, *DDT: Scientists, Citizens, and Public Policy* (Princeton, NJ, 1981).

85 The results in Ceylon (now Sri Lanka) were particularly striking, as reported at the time, for instance, by W. A. Karunaratne, 'The Influence of Malaria Control on Vital Statistics in Ceylon', *J. Trop. Med. and Hyg.*, 62 (4) (April 1959), pp. 79–85.

86 'Expert Committee on Malaria Sixth Report', *WHO Technical Report Series no. 123* (Geneva, 1957). The plan was added to and adjusted in subsequent seventh, eighth, ninth and tenth meetings (*Technical Report Series Nos. 162, 205, 243, 272*).

87 The plan is laid out clearly in Russell's *Practical Malariology* [1963], pp. 551–2. A glossary of the terms being used in malaria eradication appeared in Arnoldo Gabaldón, P.C.C. Garnham, George Macdonald and E. J. Pampana, eds, *Terminology of Malaria and Malaria Eradication* (New York, 1963).

88 Sunil S. Amrith, *Decolonizing International Health: India and Southeast Asia, 1930–1965* (Basingstoke and New York, 2006), p. 102, citing the estimate by Jeffery.

89 Amrith, *Decolonizing International Health*, p. 99.

90 Chile was apparently the first country in Latin America to get rid of malaria, but its temperate climate made eradication easier. Before 1944, a combination of drugs, anti-larval measures (drainage, filling of pools, covering of drains and gambusia larvae eating fish) were used; DDT was introduced in late 1944, with house spraying every three months, and some use as a larvicide. Aircraft, trains and automobiles were sprayed every month. By April 1945, both malaria and anopheles mosquitoes had disappeared. See comments by Dr Neghme in the *Proceedings of the Fourth International Congresses of Tropical Medicine and Malaria*, pp. 929–30. The speaker saw success as the result of a ten-year effort, meaning not everything was due to DDT.

91 Gabaldón served on the Interim Commission of WHO, and chaired the first and second meetings of the Expert Committee on Malaria, and participated in several of the later meetings as well.

92 Socrates Litsios, 'Arnoldo Gabaldón's Independent Path for Malaria Control and Public Health in the Tropics: A Lost "Paradigm" for WHO', *Parassitologia*, 40 (1–2) (1998), pp. 231–38. Litsios also covers aspects of the Venezuelan case in his book, *The Tomorrow of Malaria* (1996), pp. 94–101.

93 Sources used for this section, in addition to Gabaldón's own publications, include Ana Teresa Gutierrez, *Tiempos de Guerra y Paz: Arnaldo Gabaldón y la Investigación sobre Malaria en Venezuela (1936–1990)* (Caracas, 1998); Tulio López Ramírez, *Historia de la Escuela de Malariologia y Saneamiento Ambiental de Venezuela* (Caracas, 1987); and Arturo Luis Berti, *Arnoldo Gabaldón: Testimonios Sobre Una Vida al Servicio de la Gente* (Caracas, 1997).

94 H. Micheal Tarver and Julia C. Frederick, *The History of Venezuela* (New York, 2001), especially chap. 7.

95 Arnoldo Gabaldón, 'The Nation-Wide Campaign Against Malaria in Venezuela', *Trans. Roy. Soc. Trop. Med. and Hyg.*, 43 (2) (September 1949), pp. 113–64.

96 Gutierez, *Tiempos de Guerra y Paz*, pp. 1–18, gives a good account of the various RF activities in Venezuela in the 1920s and '30s.

97 The IIAA participated in seventeen of the nineteen malarious countries of the Americas in malaria control efforts. See Soper, 'Report and Recommendations on Malaria: A Survey. International Cooperation Administration Expert Panel on Malaria', *Amer. J. Tropical Med. and Hyg.*, 10 (4) (1961), pp. 451–502, here: p. 453. The main technique used in the Amazon regions of Venezuela was the distribution of the anti-malarial drug, atebrin, but the overall results of the effort were relatively meagre. See Stepan, '"The Only Serious Terror in These Regions"', p. 44.

98 Arnoldo Gabaldón, *Una Política Sanitaria* (Caracas, Venezuela, 1965), vol. I, pp. 437–50 on 'sanidad mínima y elemental' (minimal and basic sanitation), another way of referring to integral sanitation.

99 According to Gutierrez, in the late 1930s Gabaldón read Chagas's paper on the domiciliary character of malaria and Chagas's success in using sulphur fumigation in houses to get rid of mosquitoes; he also read about the experiences with pyrethrum in South Africa and India, and began to use pyrethrum diluted with kerosene: Gutierrez, *Tiempos de Guerra y Paz*, p. 61.

100 Gutierrez, *Tiempos de Guerra y Paz*, p. 35.

101 Arnoldo Gabaldón and Arturo Luis Berti, 'The First Large Area in the Tropical Zone to Report Malaria Eradication: North-Central Venezuela', *Amer. J. Trop. Med. and Hyg.*, 3 (5) (September 1954), pp. 793–807, here: p. 793.

102 Arnoldo Gabaldón, 'The Nation-Wide Campaign Against Malaria in Venezuela'.

103 These were 1) a zone in the northwest of the country, made up of a costal plain (including Lake Maracaibo, the largest lake in Latin America), backed by mountains; this was the smallest of the three zones, but contained the majority (77 per cent) of the population; it was the least hospitable to anopheles breeding but had most of the oil; 2) the vast highland grasslands in the interior, known as the *llanos*, which represented 36 per cent of the territory but only 20 per cent of the population; criss-crossed by rivers and lagoons, it offered many opportunities for anopheline breeding and was occupied by vast herds of cattle; and 3) the vast region of Guayana south of the Orinoco, comprising 46 per cent of the country but only 3 per cent of the population, an area whose many rivers were too acidic to allow the breeding of the most efficient vector, with the result that much of the area was non-malarious.

104 Gabaldón, 'The Nation-Wide Campaign Against Malaria in Venezuela', pp. 156–157.

105 Arnoldo Gabaldón, 'Progress of the Malaria Campaign in Venezuela', in the special issue, *Nation-Wide Malaria Eradication Projects in the Americas* of the *J. Nat. Malaria Soc.*, 10 (2) (1951), pp. 124–41.

106 Gabaldón, 'Nation-wide Campaign Against Malaria in Venezuela', p. 146.

107 Berti, *Arnoldo Gabaldón*, p. 69.

108 In his 1949 presentations, Gabaldón spoke in terms of malaria control. See, for example, his 'Malaria Incidence in the West Indies and South America', in *Malariology: A Comprehensive Survey of all Aspects of this Group of Diseases from a Global Standpoint*, ed. Mark F. Boyd (Philadelphia, PA, and London, 1949), vol. I, pp. 764–87; and Gabaldón, 'The Malaria Problem in the Neotropical Region', in *Proc. Fourth Inter. Congresses of Trop. Med. and Malaria*, pp. 913–27.

109 Gabaldón, 'The Nation-Wide Campaign Against Malaria in Venezuela', p. 159.

110 Gabaldon and Berti, 'The First Large Area in the Tropical Zone'.

111 Farid, 'The Malaria Programme – From Euphoria to Anarchy', pp. 11–12.

112 Litsios, 'Arnoldo Gabaldon's Independent Path', p. 231.

113 'Expert Committee on Malaria Thirteenth Report', *WHO Technical Report Series no. 357* (1967), p. 12. The criteria used were those of the National Malaria Society, as laid out in 'Criteria of Malaria Eradication', *J. Nat. Malaria Soc.*, 10 (2) (1951), pp. 195–6. To receive certification, a region or a country had to have three years without a single indigenous case of malaria. See also Gabaldón, 'Malaria Eradication in Venezuela: Doctrine, Practice, and Achievements after Twenty Years', *Amer. J. Trop. Med. and Hyg.*, 32 (2) (1983), pp. 203–11.

114 Amrith, *Decolonizing International Health*, pp. 165–71 reviews this period in India's malaria eradication programme.

115 PAHO, *Official. Document no. 18* [1956] (Washington, DC, 1957), p. 67.

116 Gilberto Hochman, 'From Autonomy to Partial Alignment: National Malaria Programs in the Time of Global Eradication, Brazil, 1941–1961', *Canadian Bulletin of Medical History*, 15 (1) (2008), pp. 161–92.

117 Packard, *The Making of a Tropical Disease*, p. 184.

118 Cueto, *Cold War, Deadly Fevers*.

119 PAHO, *Official Document no. 69* [1965] (Washington, DC, 1966), p. 31.

120 Soper, 'Eradication versus Control in Communicable Disease Prevention', in *Building the Health Bridge* (originally given as a lecture in 1960), p. 336.

121 See Marcus Hall, 'Today Sardinia, Tomorrow the World: Malaria, the Rockefeller Foundation, and Mosquito Eradication': www.rockarch.org/publications/resrep/hall.pdf (accessed 10 February 2011) for a good account. Hall notes that ever since the Sardinia experiment, the island population has been tested for the long-term effects of DDT, but the end result shows no evidence that the massive use of DDT caused health problems in humans. 'And so DDT opponents have more grounds to focus on disruptions to ecosystems than on disruptions to human health', he writes.

122 Rachel Carson, *Silent Spring* (Boston, MA, 1962), p. 22. Quoted in Dunlap, *DDT: Scientists, Citizens, and Public Policy*, p. 3.

123 NLM, Ms C 359, Soper Papers, Box 19, handwritten document, December 1970. Thirteen pages of notes, abbreviated, document called 'DDT Cost Benefit'.

124 NLM, Ms C 359, Soper Papers, Box 19, letter from Dr Joseph W. Still, 14 December 1970, reply by Soper, 30 December 1970.

125 Proceedings of the 22nd World Health Assembly, *Official Records no. 176* (Geneva, 1969).

126 J. A. Nájera, 'The Control of Tropical Diseases and Socioeconomic Development (with special reference to malaria and its control)', *Parassitologia*, 36 (1–2) (1994), pp. 17–34.

127 Arnoldo Gabaldón, 'Global Eradication of Malaria: Changes of Strategy and Outlook', *Amer. J. Tropical Med. and Hyg.*, 18 (5) (1969), pp. 641–56, see pp. 655 and 641.

128 Arnoldo Gabaldón, 'Global Eradication of Malaria: Changes in Strategy and Future Outlook', p. 655.

129 Arnoldo Gabaldón, 'Duration of Attack Measures in a Malaria-Eradication Campaign', *Amer. J. Trop. Med. and Hyg.*, 17 (1) (1968), pp. 1–12.

130 Gabaldón, 'Malaria Eradication in Venezuela: Doctrine, Practice and Achievements after Twenty Years', *Amer. J. Trop. Med. and Hyg.*, 32 (2) 1983, pp. 203–11.

131 A Programa Nacional de la Vivienda Rural (National Rural Housing Programme) had been initiated in 1958. This gave loans to house owners to improve their houses, especially against Chagas disease, by replacing palm roofs with zinc, and replacing mud walls and earth floors with concrete. By 1966, the Minister of Health was diverting part of the malaria control budget and expertise to set up a national Chagas disease control programme with domestic spraying.

132 Gabaldón, 'Malaria Eradication in Venezuela: Doctrine, Practice, and Achievements After Twenty Years', p. 208.

133 Paul F. Russell, quoting Bruce-Chwatt, in *Bull. NY Acad. Med.*, 45 (10) (1969), pp. 1013–15, here: p. 1015.

134 S. Litsios, 'Criticism of WHO's Revised Malaria Eradication Strategy', *Parassitologia*, 42 (1–2) (2000), pp. 167–72, suggests that the absence of comment in Soper's memoirs, *Ventures in Public Health*, was due to Soper's lack of direct responsibility for the MEPs (compared to his direct responsibility in Brazil and Egypt); Litsios also suggests that if malaria eradication had been achieved in the Americas, Soper would have written more about malaria. Soper did, in fact, present and publish many papers on malaria eradication as a general proposition.

135 Fred L. Soper, 'The Epidemiology of a Disappearing Disease: Malaria', *Amer. J. Trop. Med. and Hyg.*, 9 (4) (1960), pp. 357–66.

136 Amrith, *Decolonizing International Health*, pp. 171–175.

137 Amrith, p. 168. See also V. P. Sharma, 'Re-emergence of Malaria in India', *Indian J. Med. Research*, 103 (January 1996), pp. 26–45.

138 Arnoldo Gabaldón, 'Assignment Report on Malaria Eradication in Ceylon'. 16 February – 20 March 1966. Unpublished document: WHO/SEA/Mal/59–12.7.66 (restricted).

139 Among historians and epidemiologists Sri Lanka has been somewhat of a test case of malaria eradication and DDT's effects. As an island, Sri Lanka was in theory (but not in fact) protected from the invasion of vectors from surrounding countries; like Venezuela, malaria declines post-DDT were a continuation, if dramatic continuation, of declines already achieved by pre-Second World War malaria control efforts. See P. J. Brown, 'Socioeconomic and Demographic Effects of Malaria Eradication: A Comparison of Sri Lanka and Sardinia', *Social Science and Medicine*, 22 (8) (1986), pp. 847–59.

140 Farley, *To Cast Out Disease*, pp. 284–5.

141 Claire Wallenstein, 'Malaria Epidemics Seize Venezuela', *Brit. Med. J.*, 320 (7249) (10 June 2000), p. 1562.

142 Editorial: 'Epitaph for Global Malaria Eradication?', *The Lancet*, 306 (7923) (July 1975), pp. 15–16. Data on mortality and morbidity in 1974 taken from this source.

143 Downs, 'A New Look at Yellow Fever and Malaria', p. 516.

6 The Last Inch: Smallpox Eradication

1 Any account of smallpox eradication has to start with the following: first, the enormous and very detailed compilation that was produced by WHO after smallpox eradication was achieved, called *Smallpox and its Eradication*, ed. F. Fenner, D. A. Henderson, I. Arita, Z. Ježek and I. D. Ladnyi (Geneva, 1988); and second, two books by participants in eradication, Donald R. Hopkins's, *The Greatest Killer: Smallpox in History* (Chicago, IL, 2002), which is a history of the disease rather than eradication; and Donald A. Henderson's, *Smallpox – The Death of a Disease. The Inside Story of a World-wide Killer* (Amherst, NY, 2009), an account by the person who led WHO's Intensified Smallpox Eradication Programme to success between 1967 and 1977.

2 *Smallpox and its Eradication*, chap. 30, pp. 1321–33.

3 The exact origins of *Variola minor* are not known; according to Hopkins, *The Greatest Killer*, pp. 227, 230, the first 'unequivocal description' of variola minor was in an outbreak in Jamaica in 1863.

4 *Smallpox and its Eradication*, p. 622.

5 Donald A. Henderson, 'Eradication: Lessons from the Past', *Morbidity and Mortality Weekly Report*, suppl. 48 (1) (31 December 1999), pp. 16–22, here: p. 16.

6 Hopkins, *The Greatest Killer*, p. 42.
7 Both China and India have been claimed as the original source of the procedure.
8 Quarantine and/or isolation could be combined with variolation, and usually were; variolation was also often connected to worship of various smallpox deities and religious rituals.
9 Edward Jenner, *An Inquiry into the Causes and Effects of the Variolae Vaccinae, a Disease Discovered in Some Western Counties of England* (London, 1798). Other publications by Jenner were: *Further Observations on the Variolae Vaccinae, or Cow Pox* (London, 1799); and *A Continuation of Facts and Observations Relative to the Variolae Vaccinae, or Cow Pox* (London, 1800). Jenner was not the first to use cowpox as a preventive against smallpox; the procedure had been known since the 1770s. A Benjamin Jesty inoculated his wife and his two sons in this fashion; later his two sons were variolated (exposed to smallpox virus) and did not get smallpox. The difference between Jesty and Jenner is that Jesty did not publish his result, promote the procedure, or go on to test the procedure in the way Jenner did. Nor was he rewarded with large grants (Jenner received £30,000 from Parliament) and fame. Thus smallpox vaccination is rightly associated with Jenner's name. See Cary P. Gross, and Kent A. Sepkowitz, 'The Myth of the Medical Breakthrough: Smallpox, Vaccination, and Jenner Reconsidered', *Intern. J. Infect. Diseases*, 3 (1) (July–September 1998), pp. 54–60.
10 Andrea Rusnock, 'Catching Cowpox: The Early Spread of Smallpox Vaccination, 1798–1810', *Bull. Hist. Med.*, 83 (1) (2009), pp. 17–36.
11 Rusnock, 'Catching Cowpox'.
12 Quoted in Hopkins, *The Greatest Killer*, p. 310.
13 For a good review, see Anne Hardy, 'Smallpox in London: Factors in the Decline of the Disease in the Nineteenth Century', *Med. Hist.*, 27 (2) (1983), pp. 111–38.
14 The origin of Jenner's vaccine is not clear. Jenner believed that his cowpox derived originally from a horse disease known as 'grease'. What is generally accepted is that many different kinds of viruses were used in vaccination. One hypothesis is that variola virus (the causative pathogen of smallpox itself), variola vaccinae (Jenner's cowpox), and vaccinia virus (which is the basis of today's vaccine) all had a common ancestor.
15 By 1888, 50 per cent of all vaccinations in Germany were based on glycinerated calf lymph; by 1897 the figure was 99.95 per cent. The shift from arm-to-arm methods to glycinerated lymph took longer in England.
16 Even today, when vaccination is generally accepted, that trust can be lost and people opt-out of vaccination regimes that ensure herd immunity. The decline in MMR (measles, mumps and rubella) vaccination rates in the UK following a paper suggesting an association between MMR vaccination and autism, is a recent example. More generally, on the topic of anti-vaccinationism, see Stuart Blume, 'Anti-Vaccination Movements and Their Interpretations', *Social Science and Medicine*, 62 (3) (February 2006), pp. 628–42; Robert M. Wolfe and Lisa K. Sharp, 'Anti-Vaccinationists Past and Present', *Brit. Med. J.*, 325 (24 August 2002), pp. 430–2.
17 See Peter Baldwin, *Contagion and the State in Europe 1830–1930* (Cambridge, 1999), on the great divergence in public health policies in Europe in relation to smallpox, cholera and syphilis.
18 Nadja Durbach, *Bodily Matters: The Anti-Vaccination Movement in England, 1853–1907* (Durham and London, 2005); Stanley Williamson, *The Vaccination Controversy: The Rise, Reign and Fall of Compulsory Vaccination for Smallpox* (Liverpool, 2007). Today, historians tend to treat the opposition to vaccination with a great deal more sympathy than in earlier accounts, which tended to view anti-vaccinationism as a sign of irrational opposition to modern science.
19 Naomi Williams, 'The Implementation of Compulsory Vaccination Health Legislation: Infant Smallpox Vaccination in England and Wales, 1840–1890', *J. Hist. Geog.*, 20 (4) (1994), pp. 396–412; and E. P. Hennock, 'Vaccination Policy Against Smallpox, 1853–1914: A Comparison of England with Prussia and Imperial Germany', *Social History of Medicine*, 11 (1) (1998), pp. 49–71.
20 Stuart F. Frazer, 'Leicester and Smallpox: The Leicester Method', *Med. Hist.*, 24 (3) (1980), pp. 315–32. Most of the doctors and nurses treating smallpox patients in Leicester did, however, get vaccinated.
21 Between 1896 and 1905, England had much higher death rates from smallpox than Germany, a fact that allowed the German authorities, says Hennock, to argue against Germany's own anti-vaccination movement and resist giving up compulsion. Hennock, 'Vaccination Policy Against Smallpox'.
22 See James Colgrove, *States of Immunity: The Politics of Vaccination in Twentieth-Century America* (Berkeley, CA, 2006). Similar stories of resistance to vaccination could be told of many other countries and places, for example, the 'Vaccination Revolt' in Rio de Janeiro in 1904 that paralysed the city and was followed in 1908 by a major epidemic. See Teresa A. Meade, 'Civilizing Rio de Janeiro: The Public Health Campaign and the Riot of 1904', *J. Soc. Hist.*, 20 (2) (1986), pp. 301–22.
23 José Rigau-Pérez, 'Strategies that Led to the Eradication of Smallpox in Puerto Rico, 1882–1921', *Bull. Hist. Med.*, 59 (1) (1985), pp. 75–88; on Cuba, see P. Villoldo, 'Smallpox and Vaccination in Cuba' (1911), reprinted in *Public Health Reports*, 121 (suppl. 1) (2006), pp. 46–9, with a Commentary by Stephen Morse.
24 *Smallpox and its Eradication*, p. 259.
25 *Smallpox and its Eradication*, pp. 390–391; Kent A. Sepkowitz, 'The 1947 Smallpox Vaccination Campaign in New York City, Revisited', *Emerging*

Infectious Diseases, 10 (5) (2004), pp. 960–1, shows that daily reported tallies of the numbers vaccinated do not tally with the usual claim that five to six million were vaccinated. In any event, it was a large number, and carried out in a hasty and disorganized way.

26 The fatality rate today would be about one death per million smallpox vaccinations.

27 *PAHO Official Document no. 69* [1965] (Washington, DC, 1966), pp. 102–3.

28 Scott Barrett, 'The Smallpox Eradication Game', *Public Choice*, 130 (1–2) (January 2007), pp. 179–207.

29 Henderson, 'Eradication: Lessons from the Past', p. 16.

30 Tucker, *Scourge*, p. 44. The delegates first referred the proposal back to the Director-General for further study and consideration, voting it down two years later in 1955.

31 Tucker, *Scourge*, pp. 45–6.

32 Quote from *Smallpox and its Eradication*, p. 366.

33 D. A. Henderson, 'Smallpox Eradication – A Cold War Victory', *World Health Forum*, 19 (2) (1998), pp. 113–19.

34 Tucker, *Scourge*, p. 47. The main interest of the author in this book is on the future threat, that is, on smallpox as a potential bioterrorist weapon.

35 'WHO Expert Committee on Smallpox', *WHO Technical Report Series no. 283* (Geneva, 1964).

36 Henderson, 'Eradication: Lessons from the Past'.

37 Fred L. Soper, 'Smallpox – World Changes and Implications for Eradication', *Amer. J. Pub. Health*, 56 (10) (October 1966), pp. 1652–6, here: p. 1653.

38 Sanjoy Bhattacharya, *Expunging Variola: The Control and Eradication of Smallpox in India 1947–1977* (New Delhi, 2006), pp. 7–11.

39 Henderson's recent book, *Smallpox – The Death of a Disease*, chap. 4, is particularly severe; the same complaints had already appeared in chap. 12 of *Smallpox and its Eradication*.

40 Hennock, 'Vaccination Policy Against Smallpox, 1853–1914', p. 69.

41 *Smallpox and its Eradication*, p. 484.

42 *Smallpox and its Eradication*, pp. 390–1.

43 Fred L. Soper, 'Smallpox – World Changes', p. 1654. In tests, children were vaccinated with freeze-dried vaccine in one arm, and glycinerated vaccine in the other, and take rates compared – 94 per cent in the first, and only 35 per cent in the second. The tests were conducted by Dr Abraham Horwitz, who ten years later succeeded Soper at the head of PAHO.

44 Soper, 'Smallpox – World Changes'.

45 *PAHO Official Document no. 36*, Meeting of the Directing Council, Havana, Cuba, 14–26 August 1960, p. 133–4. A project in 1955 to re-vaccinate the island, using vaccine and equipment supplied by PAHO, was not put into effect when money from the government was not forthcoming; at a 1960 meeting in Havana, a year after the 1959 Cuban Revolution, the country was planning a mass immunization programme.

46 'Expert Committee on Smallpox First Report', *WHO Technical Report Series no. 283* (Geneva, 1964).

47 *Smallpox and its Eradication*, p. 484.

48 *PAHO Official Document no. 36* [1960] (Washington, DC, 1961), pp. 129–30.

49 To ensure proper identification, and reliable reporting of every case, photographic identification cards were later employed in India to help vaccinators distinguish smallpox from other rash-like infections.

50 Bichat de Rodrigues, 'Smallpox Eradication in the Americas', *PAHO Bull.*, 9 (1) (1975), p. 59.

51 *Smallpox and its Eradication*, p. 623.

52 *PAHO Official Documents no. 25* [1975], data from Annual Report of the Director, p. 16.

53 Paul Greenough, 'Intimidation, Coercion and Resistance in the Final Stages of the South Asian Smallpox Eradication Campaign, 1973–1975', *Social Science and Medicine*, 41 (5) (September 1995), pp. 633–45.

54 *Smallpox and its Eradication*, p. 473.

55 *PAHO Official Document no. 27* [1958], p. 473.

56 Fiona Godlee, 'WHO in Retreat: Is it Losing its Influence?', *Brit. Med. J.*, 309 (3 December 1994), pp. 1491–5.

57 'Quadrennial Report of the Director', *PAHO Official Document no. 43* (Washington, DC, 1962), pp. 3–17. The entire Charter has been reprinted in: http://avalon.law.yale.edu/20th_century/intam16.asp (accessed 21 February 2011).

58 Leonard J. Bruce-Chwatt, 'Lessons Learned from Applied Field Research Activities in Africa During the Malaria Eradication Era', *Bull. WHO*, 62 (suppl.) (1984), pp. 19–29.

59 NLM, Ms C 359, Soper Papers, Box 42, Folder, Mass Campaigns and General Public Health. 32-page typed document, pp. 5 and 23.

60 One of the few articles to analyse the differences between Dubos and Soper is Socrates Litsios, 'Rene J. Dubos and Fred L. Soper: Their Contrasting Views on Vector and Disease Eradication', *Perspectives in Biology and Medicine*, 41 (1) (Autumn 1997), pp. 138–49. Litsios notes there was no direct communication between the two men.

61 Warwick Anderson, 'Natural Histories of Infectious Diseases: Ecological Vision in Twentieth-Century Biomedical Science', in *Landscapes of Exposure: Knowledge and Illness in Modern Environments*, ed. Gregg Mitman, et al., special issue of *Osiris*, 19 (2004), pp. 39–61, reviews Dubos in the context of several ecologically informed epidemiologists; the quote from Dubos appears on p. 56.

62 For example, Charles Elton, one of the founders of modern animal ecology, with his book, *Animal Ecology* (London, 1926), devoted chap. 1 of his *The Ecology of Invasions by Animals and Plants* (London, 1958) to a discussion of Soper's eradication of the invading *gambiae* mosquito in Brazil; other eradi-

cation stories (for example, the Mediterranean fruit fly in Florida) gave similarly satisfactory results from the human point of view, he argued. Similarly, Frank Fenner, an ecologist who had worked in Dubos' laboratory, though dubious about yellow fever and malaria eradication, thought the smallpox virus could be eradicated, and later served as chairman of the WHO commission in charge of the global certification of smallpox eradication. On Fenner, see again Anderson, 'Natural Histories of Infectious Disease', pp. 39–61.

63 Quote from Richard Preston, *The Demon in the Freezer* (New York, 2003), p. 73.

64 NLM, Ms C 359, Soper Papers, Box 5, Letter, 4 December 1973, sent to Soper by Davis, on the occasion of the celebrations of Soper's 80th birthday in Washington.

65 Quoted by Marcus Hall, 'Today Sardinia, Tomorrow the World: Malaria, the RF, and Mosquito Eradication': www.rockarch.org/publications/resrep/hall.pdf (accessed 19 April 2011).

66 *PAHO Official Document no. 86* [1967] (Washington, DC, 1968), p. xxi.

67 Horwitz, 'Status of Smallpox Eradication in the Americas', *PAHO Official Document no. 36* [1960] (Washington, DC, 1961), pp. 129–30.

68 *PAHO Official Document no. 63* [1964] (Washington, DC, 1965), p. 12.

69 *PAHO Official Document no. 36* [1960] (Washington, DC, 1961), p. 135.

70 *PAHO Official Document no. 63* [1964] (Washington, DC, 1966), pp. 12–13.

71 *PAHO Official Document no. 69* [1965] (Washington, DC, 1966), p. 31.

72 Ibid., p. 96.

73 *PAHO Official Document no. 77* [1966] (Washington, DC, 1967), p. 248.

74 PAHO, *Official Document no. 63* [1964] (Washington, DC, 1965), p. 101.

75 *Smallpox and its Eradication*, p. 417.

76 Ibid., p. 395.

77 Donald R. Hopkins, 'Smallpox: Ten Years Gone', *Amer. J. Pub. Health*, 78 (12) (1988), pp. 1589–95.

78 Quoted in Jack Hopkins, The *Eradication of Smallpox: Organizational Learning and Innovation in International Health* (Boulder, CO, 1989), pp. 73–4.

79 Barrett, 'The Smallpox Eradication Game', p. 186.

80 Horace G. Ogden, *The CDC and the Smallpox Crusade* (Washington, DC, 1987), pp. 23–4.

81 NLM, Ms C 359, Soper Papers, Box 19, Letter from Soper to President Johnson, 24 June 1965.

82 Ogden, *The Center for Disease Control and the Smallpox Crusade*, p. 16.

83 NLM, Ms C 359, Soper Papers, Box 19, Letter to President Johnson.

84 *Smallpox and its Eradication*, p. 413.

85 Ogden, *The CDC and the Smallpox Crusade*, p. 39.

86 *Smallpox and its Eradication*, p. 479.

87 *Smallpox and its Eradication*, pp. 479–80. Several labs participated in this work; they found that the smallpox virus does not survive long outside humans.

88 In French West Africa the French colonial authorities had vaccinated African populations routinely against smallpox, and had continued to supply vaccine in the years following independence from colonial rule. Vaccination rates there were considerably higher than in British West Africa.

89 China did not become a member of the WHO until 1972, and it was not until then that the west began to learn that the People's Republic had eliminated smallpox on its own by 1960, along with many other diseases, through nationally organized campaigns.

90 Battacharya, *Expunging Variola*, chap. 4 gives an excellent and detailed account of the final phase of smallpox eradication in India.

91 Hopkins, *The Eradication of Smallpox*, p. 3.

92 Battacharya, *Expunging Variola*, p. 153. See also Henry M. Gelfand, 'A Critical Examination of the Indian Smallpox Eradication Campaign', *Amer. J. Pub. Health*, 56 (10) (1966), pp. 1634–51.

93 Battacharya, *Expunging Variola*, pp. 8–9.

94 Battacharya, *Expunging Variola*, p. 210.

95 Greenough, 'Intimidation, Coercion and Resistance'.

96 John F. Wickett, 'The Final Inch: The Eradication of Smallpox and Beyond', *Social Scientist*, 30 (5–6) (May–June 2002), pp. 62–78. Solzhenitzyn's actual phrase was 'the rule of the final inch'.

97 Epidemiological studies in Pakistan were also important to the new strategy.

98 See William H. Foege, J. Donald Millar and J. Michael Lane, 'Selected Epidemiologic Control in Smallpox Eradication', *Amer. J. Epid.*, 94 (4) (1971), pp. 311–15. The method was originally referred to as 'Eradication Escalation' or E2. See also William H. Foege, J. D. Millar and D.A. Henderson, 'Smallpox Eradication in West and Central Africa', *Bull. WHO*, 52 (2) (1975), pp. 209–22.

99 Ogden, *The CDC and the Smallpox Crusade*, p. 47.

100 Henderson, *Smallpox – The Death of a Disease*, p. 110.

101 See for example the rather different account by Gilberto Hochman, who places smallpox eradication in the context of Brazil's political history: 'Priority, Invisibility, and Eradication: The History of Smallpox and the Brazilian Public Health Agenda', *Med. Hist.*, 53 (2) (2009), pp. 229–52.

102 Eurico Suzart de Carvalho Filho, et al., 'Smallpox Eradication in Brazil, 1967–1969', *Bull. WHO*, 43 (1970), pp. 797–808.

103 Henderson, *Smallpox – The Death of a Disease*, p. 111.

104 *Smallpox and its Eradication*, p. 522.

105 *Smallpox and its Eradication*, Box on p. 625.

106 Tucker, *Scourge*, pp. 126–30. In addition, the victim's father died of a heart attack.

107 Tucker's *Scourge* devotes several chapters to the impact of the Soviet weaponization programme on the debates over what to do with the smallpox virus.

108 Henderson, *Smallpox – The Death of a Disease*, chap.

10, 'Smallpox as a Biological Weapon', for his very valuable account of these developments.

7 Controversies: Eradication Today

1 Held in Washington in 1973. Soper died 9 February 1977; the last naturally occurring case of smallpox was found in Somalia on 31 October 1977, but absolute certainty about smallpox eradication was not assured until two years later in 1979.

2 Walter R. Dowdle and Stephen L. Cochi, 'Global Eradication of Poliovirus: History and Rationale', in *Molecular Biology of Picornaviruses*, ed. B. L. Semler and E. Wimmer (Washington, DC, 2002), pp. 473–8, here: p. 473.

3 From the 'Recommendations of the International Task Force for Disease Eradication': http://wonder.cdc.gov/wonder/prevguid/m0025967/m0025967.asp (accessed 11 February 2011) and from A. Hinman, 'Eradication of Vaccine-Preventable Diseases', *Annual Rev. Pub. Health*, 20 (May 1999), pp. 211–29, here: p. 211.

4 I. Arita, Miyuki Nakane and Frank Fenner, 'Is Polio Eradication Realistic?', *Science*, 312 (5775) (12 May 2006), pp. 852–54. See also Leslie L. Roberts, 'Polio Eradication: Is it Time to Give Up?', *Science*, 312 (5775) (12 May 2006), pp. 832–35.

5 Donald A. Henderson 'Eradication: Lessons from the Past', *Morbidity and Mortality Weekly Reports (MMWR)*, suppl. 48 (1) (31 December 1999), pp. 16–22.

6 Ivan Illich's book was *Medical Nemesis: The Expropriation of Health* (New York, 1976); John H. Bryant's book, *Health and the Developing World* (Ithaca, New York, 1969), was the result of a Rockefeller Foundation-funded study.

7 Socrates Litsios, 'The Long and Difficult Road to Alma-Ata: A Personal Reflection', *Intern. J. of Health Services*, 32 (4) (2002), pp. 709–32; Marcos Cueto, 'The Origins of Primary Health Care and Selective Primary Health Care', *Amer. J. Pub. Health*, 94 (11) (November 2004), pp. 1864–74, and his 'The Promise of Primary Health Care', *Bull. WHO*, 83 (5) (May 2005), pp. 322–3.

8 Cueto, 'The Origins of Primary Health Care and Selective Primary Health Care'.

9 'Expert Committee on Malaria Tenth Report', *WHO Technical Report Series no. 272* (Geneva, 1964).

10 The Declaration of Alma-Ata can be accessed online at: http://who.int/hpr/NPH/docs/declaration_almaata.pdf (accessed 19 April 2011).

11 Laurie Garrett, *Betrayal of Trust: The Collapse of Public Health* (New York, 2000).

12 J. Walsh and J. K. Warren, 'Selective Primary Health Care, an Interim Strategy for Disease Control in Developing Countries', *NE J. Med.*, 301 (18) (1979), pp. 967–74; and Cueto, 'The Origins of Primary Health Care and Selective Primary Health Care'.

13 Later, family spacing (or planning), female education and food supplementation were added to GOBI to give the acronym GOBI-FFF.

14 The opposition to many of the GOBI goals by Western, largely US private agencies and pharmaceutical companies helped to torpedo PHC further. Breastfeeding, for example, ran up against the massive marketing of powdered milk, which WHO and other organizations found themselves powerless to stop.

15 WHO later established a standardized vaccination schedule for the original six vaccines; other vaccines were added to the list later, such as Hepatitis B vaccine, and the yellow fever vaccine in countries where yellow fever was endemic. In 1999, the Global Alliance for Vaccines and Immunology (GAVI), a coalition that included the UN agencies (WHO, UNICEF), the World Bank, and various private philanthropies (for example, The Rockefeller Foundation, The Bill and Melinda Gates Foundation, and other NGOs) worked to improve and expand the vaccination initiative.

16 R. Kim-Farley, et al., 'Global Immunization', *Annual Rev. Pub. Health*, 13 (1992), p. 223.

17 Donald A. Henderson, 'The Miracle of Vaccination', *Notes and Records of the Roy. Soc. London*, 51 (2) (July 1997), pp. 235–45, here: p. 240.

18 Peter F. Wright, 'Global Immunization – A Medical Perspective', *Social Sci. Med.*, 41 (5) (1995), pp. 609–16; see also Alfred S. Evans, 'The Eradication of Communicable Diseases: Myth or Reality?', *Amer. J. Epid.*, 122 (2) (August 1985), pp. 199–207.

19 Henderson, 'Eradication: Lessons from the Past'.

20 Ibid.

21 Donald A. Henderson, 'Smallpox Eradication', *Public Health Reports*, 95 (5) (September–October 1980), pp. 422–26.

22 Donald R. Hopkins, 'After Smallpox Eradication: Yaws?', *Amer. J. Trop. Med. and Hyg.*, 25 (6) (1976), pp. 860–65. He argued that the new surveillance-containment methods developed in smallpox eradication could be used complete the yaws eradication campaigns of the 1950s and '60s, using penicillin as before. The campaigns had brought prevalence rates to very low levels but not to the point of eradication.

23 'Guinea Worm Disease', Letter from Donald R. Hopkins and William H. Foege in *Science*, 212 (4494) (1 May 1981), p. 495.

24 The conference papers were published as 'The International Conference on Eradication of Infectious Diseases: Can Infectious Diseases be Eradicated?', in *Reviews of Infect. Diseases*, 4 (5) 1982, entire issue.

25 An account of the ITFDE meetings and the final conclusions appear in 'Recommendations of the International Task Force for Disease Eradication', *Morbidity and Mortality Weekly Report*, 42 (RR16) (31 December 1993), pp. 1–25 and at www.cdc.gov/preview/mmwrhtml/00025967/htm. On Dalhem,

see *The Eradication of Infectious Diseases*, ed. W. R. Dowdle and D. R. Hopkins (Chichester, West Sussex, 1998). The workshop was held from 16–22 March 1997.

26 Earlier discussions are found in the Report of a WHO Study, 'Integration of Mass Campaigns Against Specific Diseases into General Health Services', *WHO Technical Report Series no. 294* (Geneva, 1965). Another appeared in a short chapter in E. H. Hinman's *World Eradication of Infectious Diseases* (Springfield, IL, 1966), pp. 194–8. Written at the height of enthusiasm for eradication and reflecting the Cold War political context of the times, Hinman divided the criteria into the technical, the economic, the political and the professional.

27 A good early review was by Perez Yekutiel, 'Lessons from the Big Eradication Campaigns', *World Health Forum*, 2 (4) (1981), pp. 465–90.

28 'The International Conference on the Eradication of Infectious Diseases', p. 913.

29 'Introduction', *The Eradication of Infectious Diseases*, ed. Dowdle and Hopkins, p. 1.

30 David H. Molyneux, Donald R. Hopkins and Nevio Zagara, 'Disease Eradication, Elimination and Control: The Need for Accurate and Consistent Usage', *Trends in Parasitology*, 20 (8) (1 August 2004), pp. 347–51.

31 Author's telephone interviews with Dr Donald R. Hopkins, 15 April and 11 June 2009.

32 This refers to its *Basic Reproduction Number*, a measure of the infectivity of a disease.

33 Box 1, 'Criteria for Targeting a Disease for Eradication', in David H. Molyneux, Donald A. Hopkins and Nevio Zagaria, 'Disease Eradication, Elimination and Control: The Need for Accurate and Consistent Usage', p. 349.

34 Hinman, *World Eradication of Infectious Diseases*, p. 194.

35 The first cost-benefit analysis of the eradication of the *Aedes aegypti* mosquito was calculated belatedly in 1972; see PAHO, *The Prevention of Diseases Transmitted by Aedes aegypti. A Cost-Benefit Study* (Cambridge, MA, 1972).

36 Peter J. Hotez, *Forgotten People, Forgotten Diseases: The Neglected Tropical Diseases and their Impact on Global Health and Development* (Washington, DC, 2008).

37 'Global Disease Elimination and Eradication as Public Health Strategies', *Bull. WHO*, 76 (suppl. 2) (1998). Entire issue.

38 Dowdle and Cochi, 'Global Eradication of Poliovirus', p. 473.

39 Some of the sources on which I have drawn for this section of the book are: Walter E. Dowdle and Stephen L. Cochi, 'Global Eradication of Poliovirus: History and Rationale', pp. 473–8; Ciro A. de Quadros, et al., 'Polio Eradication from the Western Hemisphere', *Annual Rev. Pub. Health*, 13 (1992), pp. 239–52; Ciro A. de Quadros and Donald A. Henderson, 'Disease Eradication and Control in the Americas', *Biologicals*, 21 (4) (1993), pp. 335–43; Ciro de Quadros, 'Global Eradication of Poliomyelitis and Measles: Another Quiet Revolution', *Annals of Internal Medicine*, 127 (2) (15 July 1997), pp. 156–158; and William Muraskin, *The Politics of International Health: The Children's Vaccine Initiative and the Struggle to Develop Vaccines for the Third World* (New York, 1998), especially chap. 1. I would also like to thank Sara Sievers, who was working in the Policy Advocacy Section of the Gates Foundation, when I interviewed her on aspects of the polio eradication efforts, especially in Nigeria. Interview 3 March 2009, New York City.

40 One million children in the USA were tested in double blind tests with the inactivated Salk vaccine in 1952; the Sabin oral vaccine was tested in the USSR in the early 1960s, and eventually replaced the IPV. More recently, however, the IPV has come back into favour for routine maintenance of polio immunization, largely in industrialized countries. The rivalry between Salk and Sabin was intense. See Arthur Allen, *Vaccine: The Controversial Story of Medicine's Greatest Life Saver* (New York, 2007), chap. 5.

41 De Quadros was an epidemiologist who had worked in the smallpox eradication campaign as the director of field operations in Ethiopia.

42 André Luiz Vieira de Campos, Dilene Raimundo do Nascimento and Eduardo Maranhão, 'A História da poliomielite no Brasil e seu controle por imunização', *História, Ciência, Saúde-Manguinhos*, 10 (suppl. 2) (2003), pp. 573–600. WHO certified polio eradication in Brazil in 1994.

43 Ciro A. de Quadros, et al., 'Polio Eradication from the Western Hemisphere', *Annual Rev. Pub. Health*, 13 (1992), pp. 239–52. Only the year before, in 1984, an International Symposium on Polio Control, held in Washington at the Fogarty International Center of the NIH, concluded that the world health community should aim for control and not eradication. Frederick C. Robbins, 'Summary and Recommendations', *Reviews of Infect. Diseases*, 6 (suppl. 2) May–June 1984, p. S600.

44 Walter R. Dowdle and Stephen L. Cochi, 'Global Eradication of Poliovirus: History and Rationale', p. 473.

45 Leslie Roberts, 'Polio Eradication: The Final Assault?', *Science*, 303 (5666) (March 2004), pp. 1960–8, here: p. 1962.

46 Rotary International originally pledged to raise $120 million, a sum that was later doubled. The RI had already been involved in overseas immunization efforts when it was persuaded by Sabin to put its resources, its huge membership, clubs, organizational skills, advocacy and fund-raising abilities into polio eradication. See Jonathan Majiyagbe, 'The Volunteers' Contribution to Polio Eradication', *Bull. WHO*, 82 (1) (January 2004), p. 2. Subsequently, the campaign

has received financial and other help from the CDC, UNICEF, the World Bank, national governments (for example, Denmark, Canada, the UK, Germany, Finland, Italy, Japan, Belgium and the USA), and from private foundations, including in the later phases, from The Bill and Melinda Gates Foundation.

47 Henderson, at the time, was unconvinced that the existing polio vaccine was adequate to the task of eradicating polio in very heavily populated and poor places, like India, and in this he has so far been proven right.

48 Stephen L. Cochi, 'Polio Today: Are We on the Verge of Global Eradication?', *J. Amer. Med. Assn*, 300 (7) (2008), pp. 839–41.

49 Albert B. Sabin, 'Vaccination Against Polio in Economically Underdeveloped Countries', *Bull. WHO*, 58 (1) (1980), pp. 141–57; and 'Strategies for Elimination of Poliomyelitis in Different Parts of the World with the Use of Oral Poliovirus Vaccine', *Reviews of Infect. Diseases*, 6 (suppl. 2) 1984, pp. S391–S396.

50 WHO, *Global Polio Eradication Initiative Strategic Plan 2004–2008* (Geneva, 2003), p. 7.

51 Atul Gawande, *Better: A Surgeon's Notes on Performance* (New York, 2007), p. 37.

52 Cochi, 'Polio Today', pp. 839–41.

53 Figures from www.polioeradication.org/datamonitoringpoliothisweek/aspx (accessed 19 May 2010).

54 Ciro de Quadros and Donald A. Henderson, 'Disease Eradication and Control in the Americas', and C. de Guerra Macedo and B. Melgaard, 'The Legacies of Polio Eradication', *Bull. WHO*, 78 (3) (March 2000), pp. 283–4.

55 *The Impact of the Expanded Program on Immunization and the Polio Eradication Initiative on Health Systems in the Americas. Final Report of the Taylor Commission* (Washington, DC, 1995).

56 See Carl Taylor, Felicity Cutts, Mary E. Taylor, 'Ethical Dilemmas in Current Planning for Polio Eradication', *Amer. J. Pub. Health*, 87 (6) (June 1997), pp. 922–5.

57 Andrew L. Creese, 'Priorities in Health Care: A Discussion', *Reviews of Infect. Diseases*, 6 (suppl. 2), International Symposium on Poliomyelitis Control (May–June 1984), pp. S589–S590, here: p. S589.

58 Roland Sutter and Stephen L. Cochi replied in an Editorial, giving a positive account of polio eradication's contributions: 'Comment: Ethical Dilemmas in Worldwide Polio Eradication Programs', *Amer. J. Pub. Health*, 87 (6) (June 1997), pp. 913–16.

59 Gawande, *Better*, p. 31.

60 For this section on GW eradication, I have drawn on the numerous reports by Hopkins and his colleagues at TCC, as well as the following accounts and evaluations: D. R. Hopkins and E. Ruiz-Tiben, 'Strategies for Dracunculiasis Eradication', *Bull. WHO*, 69 (5) (1991), pp. 533–40; Hopkins, et al., 'Dracunculiasis Eradication: Beginning of the End', *Amer. J. Trop. Med. and Hyg.*, 49 (3) (1993), pp. 281–9; Hopkins, et al., 'Dracunculiasis Eradication: March 1994 Update', *Amer. J. Trop. Med. and Hyg.*, 52 (1) 1995, pp. 14–20; Hopkins, et al., 'Dracunculiasis Eradication: Almost a Reality', *Amer. J. Trop. Med. and Hyg.*, 57 (3) (1997), pp. 252–9; D. R. Hopkins, 'Perspectives from the Dracunculiasis Eradication Programme', *Bull. WHO*, 76 (suppl. 2) (1998), pp. 38–41; Hopkins, et al., 'Dracunculiasis Eradication: Delayed, Not Denied', *Amer. J. Trop. Med. and Hyg.*, 62 (2) (2000), pp. 163–8; Hopkins, et al., 'Dracunculiasis Eradication: And Now, Sudan', *Amer. J. Trop. Med. and Hyg.*, 67 (4) (2002), pp. 415–22; Hopkins, et al., 'Dracunculiasis Eradication: The Final Inch', *Amer. J. Trop. Med. and Hyg.*, 73 (4) (2005), pp. 669–75; Hopkins, et al., 'Dracunculiasis: Neglected No More', *Amer. J. Trop. Med. and Hyg.*, 79 (4) (2008), pp. 474–9. A very useful overall assessment of GWD eradication is given by Sandy Cairncross, Ralph Muller and Nevio Zagaria, 'Dracunculiasis (Guinea Worm Disease) and the Eradication Initiative', *Clinical Microbiology Reviews*, 15 (2) (April 2002), pp. 223–46.

61 Neglected Tropical Diseases (NTDs) only began to get attention at WHO in the 1990s. Hotez, *Forgotten People, Forgotten Diseases*, lists thirteen NTDs.

62 Hopkins and Foege, 'Guinea Worm Disease'. The first to suggest GW for eradication was the Indian medical scientist, Dr M.I.D. Sharma, in 'Lessons Learned from the Intensified Campaign Against Smallpox in India and Their Possible Applicability to Other Health Programmes, with Particular Reference to Eradication of Dracunculiasis', *J. Communicable Diseases*, 12 (2) (1980), pp. 59–64.

63 Hopkins was in Geneva for an epidemiological meeting at WHO when a discussion with a French doctor led him to read an article on the International Drinking Water and Sanitation Decade which mentioned its potential effect in reducing various waterborne diseases. Hopkins immediately thought that though clean water would reduce many diseases, it could actually eradicate GW disease. Phone interview with Dr Donald R. Hopkins, 15 April 2009.

64 Hopkins became the Senior Consultant on Health Programs at The Carter Center in 1987, where he leads The Center's programmes to eradicate GW disease and river blindness (onchocerciasis). Previously he had served as deputy director (1984–1987) and acting director (1985) of the Centers for Disease Control. William H. Foege, Director of the CDC from 1977 to 1983, then served as the Executive Director of The Carter Center from 1986–1992. The institutional and intellectual links between the CDC and TCC, both based in Atlanta, Georgia, are strong.

65 Resolution WHA44.5, 13 May 1991.

66 Michele Barry, 'Editorial: Slaying Little Dragons: Lessons from the Dracunculiasis Eradication Program', *Amer. J. Trop. Med. and Hyg.*, 75 (1) (2006),

pp. 1–2.

67 www.who.int/neglected_diseases/integrated_media/index.html (accessed 19 April 2011).

68 Sandy Cairncross, Ralph Muller and Nevio Zagaria, 'Dracunculiasis (Guinea Worm Disease) and the Eradication Initiative'. The Ivory Coast built 12,500 new bore wells in rural areas between 1973 and 1985. GW cases plummeted from above 67,000 in 1966 to only 1,889 in 1985. But a 1991 national survey found an estimated 12,690 cases; plus it discovered that a large number of the hand pumps were out of order.

69 In some countries, the volunteers were paid.

70 D. R. Hopkins and E. Ruiz-Tiben, 'Strategies for Dracunculiasis Eradication'. They felt the use of chemicals like Abate to kill Cyclops in the water sources should only be used sparingly, for example in epidemic control in highly endemic villages.

71 In the case of Sudan, President Carter managed to help broker a six-month GW-ceasefire in 1995, which allowed health workers to reach populations cut off by the armed conflict in the country.

72 Donald R. Hopkins, Frank O. Richards Jr, Ernesto Ruiz-Tiben, Paul Emerson and P. Craig Withers Jr, 'Dracunculiasis, Onchocerciasis, Schistosomiasis, and Trachoma', *Ann. NY Acad. Sci.*, 1136 (2008), pp. 45–52. There are other examples of such 'piggy backing'; in Ghana, for example, there are pilot projects in which Insecticide Treated Bednets are distributed to every family with a child under the age of five during measles vaccination. In Ethiopia, The Carter Center is involved in a combined GW and trachoma elimination effort. The latter involves mass distribution of antibiotics for the treatment of active cases, health education to promote facial cleanliness, and environmental hygiene.

73 The following section is based on a series of interviews I had with the core group of experts at The Carter Center, starting with two hour-long telephone interviews with Dr Donald R. Hopkins, on 15 April 2009 and 11 June 2009; and then interviews lasting about two hours each and in person, with 1) Dr Frank O. Richards Jr, at The Carter Center, Atlanta, 11 May 2009; 2) with Dr P. Craig Withers Jr, at The Carter Center, 12 May 2009; and 3) with Dr Ernesto Ruiz-Tiben, at The Carter Center on 12 May 2009.

74 Hopkins in *Bull. WHO*, 76 (suppl. 2) (1998), pp. 38–41, here: p. 41.

75 Soper, 'Problems to be Solved if the Eradication of Tuberculosis is to be Realized', in *Building the Health Bridge*, pp. 513–27, here: p. 516. Paper first published in *Amer. J. Pub. Health*, 52 (1962), pp. 734–48.

76 Hopkins quoted in the *Financial Times*, Weekend Edition (23–24 August 2008), Life and Arts Section, p. 2.

77 As reported in the Op-Ed by Nicholas D. Kristoff, 'Winning the Worm War', *New York Times* (29 April 2010), p. A31.

78 In the most persistent pockets of polio in India (in the poorest states of Uttar Pradesh and Bihar in the northern Hindi-speaking belt of the country), monovalent polio vaccine is being used to target type-I polio, instead of the multivalent form.

79 Gawande, *Better*, p. 46.

80 A. Tayeh and S. Cairncross, 'Dracunculiasis Eradication by 2009: Will Endemic Countries Meet the Target?', *Trop. Med. and Internat. Health*, 12 (12) (2007), pp. 1403–8.

81 Muraskin, *The Politics of International Health*, p. 12.

82 Henderson, 'Eradication: Lessons from the Past'.

83 Leslie Roberts, 'Polio Eradication: Is it Time to Give Up?'.

84 Arita, et al., 'Is Polio Eradication Realistic?'.

85 Donald G. McNeil Jr, 'Can Polio be Eradicated? A Skeptic Now Thinks So', *New York Times* (15 February 2011), p. D4.

86 Theodore M. Brown, Marcos Cueto and Elizabeth Fee, 'Public Health Then and Now: The World Health Organization and the Transition from "International" to "Global" Public Health', *Amer. J. Pub. Health*, 96 (1) (January 2006), pp. 62–72.

87 Lauric Garrett, 'The Challenge of Global Health', *Foreign Affairs*, 86 (1) (2007), pp. 14–38, here: p. 14.

88 Jeffrey D. Sachs *The End of Poverty: Economic Possibilities for Our Time* (New York, 2005); and John Luke Gallup and Jeffrey D. Sachs, 'The Economic Burden of Malaria', *Amer. J. Trop. Med. Hyg.*, 64 (1–2) (2001), pp. 85–96. See Garrett, *Betrayal of Trust*, p. 4. Sachs is responsible for the idea of Millenium Villages in Africa, which try to show- case what large resources, directed at many fronts at the same time, from agriculture, to health, to education can do to lift people out of poverty. Some fourteen to fifteen such villages complexes, each comprising several small villages, have thus far been organized (data from 2010).

89 Amir Attaran, 'An Immeasurable Crisis? A Criticism of the Millenium Development Goals and Why They Cannot be Measured', *PLoS Med.*, 2 (10) (2005), p. e318, doi:10.1371/journal.pmed.0020318. The funds needed to meet the goals have also not been forthcoming.

90 It is impossible to list here all the organizations that are involved in international or global health programmes. One of the most important is The Global Fund to Fight AIDS, TB and Malaria, which is WHO-based but funded by individual governments and philanthropies; it is a fund, not an operating organization. Between 2001 and 2007, the fund had collected $4.7 billion (but by 2010 the Global Fund's commitments were already not being met). Then there is the Global Alliance for Vaccine and Immunization, President Bush's Malaria Initiative, the many programmes of The Carter Center, the foreign aid programmes of national governments, and huge numbers of non-governmental organizations.

91 Matthew Bishop and Michael Green, *Philanthro-*

Capitalism: How the Rich Can Save the World (New York, 2008), especially chap. 4, 'Billanthropy'.

92 Data from Brown, Cueto, and Fee, 'Public Health Then and Now', pp. 66–7.

93 The first Gates foundation was set up in 1994 as the William G. Gates Foundation, named after Bill Gates's father. In 1999 this was renamed The Bill and Melinda Gates Foundation. In addition to its health missions, the Gates Foundation is involved in funding programmes to improve American education, improving libraries, and various other causes. In 2008 Bill Gates left Microsoft to direct his foundation on a fulltime basis. Data from www.gatesfoundation.org (accessed 19 May 19 2010)

94 William Easterly, *The White Man 's Burden: Why the West's Efforts to Aid the Rest Have done so Much Ill and So Little Good* (New York, 2007), pp. 241–2. He classifies health workers as 'searchers', people who act locally and on specific problems, as opposed to the 'planners', who have grandiose schemes for getting rid of poverty and other world problems by technical means.

95 Anne-Emmanuelle Birn, 'Gates's Grandest Challenge: Transcending Technology as Public Health Ideology', *The Lancet*, 366 (9484) (6–12 August 2005), pp. 514–19.

96 The Gates Foundation, as the foundation with the greatest resources, has been the target of numerous criticisms, ranging from its bias in channelling the bulk of its research funding to US-based recipients, its lack of transparency in its grant-making procedures, and its neglect of child health, maternal health and nutrition. Among many articles, see 'Editorial: What Has the Gates Foundation Done for Global Health?', *The Lancet*, 373 (9695) (9 May 2009). p. 1577; David McCoy, Gayatri Kembhavi, Jinesh Patel and Akish Luintel, 'The Bill and Melinda Gates Foundation's Grant-Making Programme for Global Health', *The Lancet*, 373 (9695) (9 May 2009), pp. 1645–53; 'Health Policy: Misfinancing Global Health: A Case for Transparency in Disbursements and Decision-Making', *The Lancet*, 372 (9644) (27 September 2008), pp. 1185–91; and 'Editorial: Governance Questions at the Gates Foundation', *The Lancet*, 369 (9557) (20–26 January 2007), p. 163.

97 Meri Koivusalo, 'The Shaping of Global Health Policy', in *Morbid Symptoms: Health Under Capitalism*, ed. Leo Panitch and Colin Leys, *Socialist Register 2010* (London, 2009), pp. 279–94.

98 According to Packard, *The Making of a Tropical Disease*, p. 200, a recent study shows that 'HIV-1 increased malaria incidence in 41 African countries by between .20 and 28%. The impact of HIV infection on malaria mortality ranged from .65 to 114%', depending on the nature of the malaria transmission (stable or unstable).

99 Telephone interview with Dr Regina Rabinovich, Director, Infectious Diseases Development, Global Health Programs, 10 April 2009.

100 These comments are based on a telephone interview with Dr Regina Rabinovich, Director, Infectious Diseases Development, Global Health Program, and Dr David Brandling-Bennett, Senior Program Officer in the same Infectious Diseases Development section, Bill and Melinda Gates Foundation, on 10 April 2009.

101 Artemisinin-based combination therapies (ACTs) are considered the best anti-malarial drugs available right now. Use of artemisinin as a single therapy is discouraged by WHO in order to delay development of resistance. Originally derived from the plant, *Artemisia annu*, research into synthetic forms are underway, but steady resistance has already been detected.

102 The vaccine RTS,S, has gone through three trials, but gives only partial protection.

103 The words are those of Bruce Aylward and refer to polio eradication (Alyward being the GF's top person on polio), as quoted in the article, 'So Near, and Yet so Far', *The Economist* (24 January 2009), p. 66.

104 Packard, *The Making of a Tropical Disease,* gives a very interesting assessment of the pluses and minuses of the RBM programme thus far; see his chap. 8.

105 Leslie Roberts and Martin Enserink, 'Malaria: Did They Really Say . . . Eradication?', *Science*, 318 (5856) (7 December 2007), pp. 1544–5. A recent discovery adds further caution to the idea of eradication: the discovery of *Plasmodium falciparum* parasites, the most dangerous form of malaria parasites, in gorillas. This suggests a potential animal reservoir of malaria parasites and would mean that malaria could not, in principle, be eradicated. See Sonia Shah, 'Learning to Live With Malaria', *New York Times* (8 October 2010): www/nytimes.com/2010/10/09/opinion/09iht-edshah.html (accessed 20 April 2011).

106 Gerry F. Killeen, Ulrike Fillinger, Ibrahim Kiche, Louis C. Gouagana and Bart G. J. Knols, 'Eradication of *Anopheles gambiae* from Brazil: Lessons for Malaria Control in Africa?', *The Lancet Infectious Diseases*, 2 (10) (2002), pp. 618–27.

107 Unfortunately, the 17D yellow fever vaccine is not as safe as it once was, being associated in some circumstances with fatal viscerotropic multiple organ failure and death. Nevertheless, yellow fever vaccine is widely used as a protection for people at risk of yellow fever infection.

108 João Bosco Siqueira, et al., 'Dengue and Dengue Hemorrhagic Fever, Brazil, 1981–2002', *Emerging Infectious Diseases*, 11 (1) (January 2005), pp. 48–53.

109 These interviews took place in June and July 2009 in Brazil, and involved officials at the mayoral (Rio) level, state level and federal level (Brasilia): 1) Interview with Dr Hans Fernando Rocha Dohman, Secretary of Health and Civil Defence of the City of Rio de Janeiro, and his assistant, Dr Betina Durovni,

in Rio de Janeiro, at the Prefeitura, Rio de Janeiro, on 30 June 2009; 2) Interviews with a team at the Secretaria de Saúde Pública of Rio de Janeiro (Secretariat of Public Health for the State of Rio de Janeiro): Drs Victor Augusto Louro Benbara, Superintendent de Vigilância Epidemiologica; Mario Sergio Ribeiro, Coordinator Vigilância Ambiental (Coordinator of Environmental Preparedness); Monica Machado, Coordinatora Centro Informações Estrategicas e Vigilância de Saúde (Coordinator of the Centre for Strategic Information in Health Preparedeness); and Ana Paula Araújo Liberal, Assistente em Tecnica Saúde Geral (Technical Assistant in Health), on Thursday, 2 July 2009; and 3) Dr Giovannini Coelho, Coordinator-Geral, Ministerio da Saúde, Secretaria de Vigilância em Saúde, Coordinação Geral do Programa Nacional de Controle de Dengue (General Coordinator, Ministry of Health, Department of Health Preparedness, and General Coordinator of the National Programme for the Control of Dengue), at the Ministry of Health in Brasilía, on 9 July 2009.

110 Duane J. Gubler, in '*Aedes aegypti* and *Aedes aegypti*-borne Disease Control in the 1990s: Top Down or Bottom Up', *Amer. J. Trop. Med. and Hyg.*, 40 (6) (1989), pp. 571–8, drew attention to Soper's methods and to a CDC-based programme of dengue control in Puerto Rico in the 1980s that relied on targeted larviciding, as Soper did (and not on the general spraying of ultra-low volume insecticides, which did not work). A new method being tried is the release of genetically-altered mosquitoes.

111 Hotez, *Forgotten People, Forgotten Diseases*, p. 3.

112 Soper knew Chagas in Brazil, but for many years uncertainty about the extent of Chagas disease prevented measures for its control from being devised (the triatomas are not vulnerable to DDT so other insecticides have to be used). Serious assessment and research into Chagas disease did not really develop until the 1960s. On the strange history of Chagas disease, see Nancy Leys Stepan, *Picturing Tropical Nature* (London, 2001), chap. 6, and Simone Petraglia Kropf, *Doença de Chagas, Doença do Brasil: Ciência, Saúde e Naçäo, 1909–1962* (Rio de Janeiro, 2009).

113 Chagas disease itself is far from being eradicated; but other mechanisms, such as the screening of donated blood to detect potential trypanosomes, which is now established in all the endemic countries (including the United States in at-risk areas such as California, where there is a large Hispanic population that is possibly infected by the trypanosome), are helping reduce the possibility of new infections.

114 In 1999 a rather similar effort, the Pan-African Trypanosomiasis and Tsetse Eradication campaign, was launched against African trypanosomiasis (African sleeping sickness) by the WHO, the UN's Food and Agriculture Organization (FAO), the African Union and the International Atomic Energy Agency. The campaign is not actually an eradication campaign, but an effort at control of both the animal and human forms of the disease, which have been on the upswing in recent years. The use of 'eradication' in this campaign is another example of the 'sponginess' of the term, as it is currently being employed in WHO and related organizations. See Jean Maurice, 'Continent-wide Attack Launched on African Trypanosomiasis', *Bull. WHO*, 79 (11) (2001), p. 1087.

115 Similar initiatives against Chagas disease transmission are underway in the Andean countries and those in Central America.

116 Dr Margaret Chan, 'Director-General's Message', *Primary Health Care (Now More than Ever) The World Health Report* 2008, on the 30th anniversary of Alma-Ata.

117 Alan Berkman, J. Garcia, M. Muñoz-Laboy, Vera Paiva and Richard Parker, 'A Critical Analysis of the Brazilian Response to HIV/AIDS: Lessons Learned for Controlling and Mitigating the Epidemic in Developing Countries', *Amer. J. Pub. Health*, 95 (7) (July 2005), pp. 1162–72.

118 Paulo Eduardo M. Elias and Amelia Cohn, 'Health Reform in Brazil: Lessons to Consider', *Amer. J. Pub. Health*, 93 (1) (2003), pp. 44–8. SUS is based on four key principles: universal access, integral care, social control (meaning by this, control by civil society) and public funding. Nationwide, about 80 per cent of Brazilians depend on SUS for their medical needs; the other roughly 20 per cent of the richer citizens rely on various forms of private insurance. An innovative feature of SUS is its Health Councils (Conselhos de Saude), of which there are over 5,000 in the country, in addition to a national Health Council at the federal level; the councils are representative, elected bodies made up of citizens and doctors, whose job it is to supervise and evaluate the operations of SUS. A rather similar argument about how HIV/AIDS activism has contributed to a public health movement with a wider scope is made about India by Sanjay Basu, 'Building a Comprehensive Public Health Movement: Learning from HIV/AIDS Mobilization', *Socialist Register* (2010), pp. 295–314.

119 For a critique of SUS, see Celia Almeida, Claudia Travassos, Silvia Porto and Maria Eliana Labra, 'Health Sector Reform in Brazil: A Case Study of Inequity', *International Journal of Health Services*, 30 (1) (2000), pp. 129–62.

Select Bibliography

Allen, Arthur, *Vaccine: The Controversial Story of Medicine's Greatest Life Saver* (New York, 2007)

Amrith, Sunil, *Decolonizing International Health: India and Southeast Asia, 1930–1965* (Basingstoke, Hampshire, 2006)

Anderson, Warwick, 'Natural Histories of Infectious Diseases: Ecological Vision in Twentieth-Century Biomedical Science', in *Landscapes of Exposure: Knowledge and Illness in Modern Environments*, eds Gregg Mitman, et al., special issue of *Osiris*, 19 (2004), pp. 39–61

Arita, I., Miyuki Nakane and Frank Fenner, 'Is Polio Eradication Realistic?', *Science*, 312 (5775) (12 May 2006), pp. 852–54

Aylward, Bruce, et al., 'When is a Disease Eradicable?: 100 Years of Lessons Learned', *Amer. J. Public Health*, 90 (10) (October 2000), pp. 1515–20

Baldwin, Peter, *Contagion and the State in Europe, 1830–1930* (Cambridge, 1999)

Barber, Marshall A., *A Malariologist in Many Lands* (Lawrence, KS, 1946)

Barrett, Scott, 'The Smallpox Eradication Game', *Public Choice*, 130 (1–2) (January 2007), pp. 179–207

Bhattacharya, Sanjoy, *Expunging Variola: The Control and Eradication of Smallpox in India, 1947–1977* (New Delhi, 2006)

Birn, Anne-Emannuelle, 'Gates's Grandest Challenge: Transcending Technology as Public Health Ideology', *The Lancet*, 366 (9484) (6–12 August 2005), pp. 514–19

——, *Marriage of Convenience: Rockefeller International Health and Revolutionary Mexico* (Rochester, NY, 2006)

Bishop, Matthew, and Michael Green, *Philanthro-Capitalism: How the Rich Can Save the World* (New York, 2008)

Blume, Stuart, 'Anti-Vaccination Movements and their Interpretations', *Social Science and Medicine*, 62 (3) (February 2006), pp. 628–42

Brown, P. J., 'Failure-as-Success: Multiple Meanings of Eradication in the Rockefeller Foundation Sardinia Project, 1946–1951', *Parassitologia*, 40 (1–2) (1998), pp. 117–30

Brown, Theodore M., Marcos Cueto and Elizabeth Fee, 'The World Health Organization and the Transition from "International" to "Global" Public Health', *American Journal of Public Health*, 96 (1) (January 2006), pp. 62–72

Bruce-Chwatt, Leonard C., and Julian de Zulueta, *The Rise and Fall of Malaria in Europe: An Historico-Epidemiological Study* (London, 1980)

Busvine, James R., *Disease Transmission By Insects: Its Discovery and 90 Years of Effort to Prevent It* (Berlin and New York, 1993)

Bynum, William F., 'An Experiment that Failed: Malaria Control at Mian Mir', *Parassitologia*, 36 (1–2) (1994), pp. 107–20

Cairncross, Sandy, Ralph Muller and Nevio Zagaria, 'Dracunculiasis (Guinea Worm Disease) and the Eradication Initiative', *Clinical Microbiology Reviews*, 15 (2) (April 2002), pp. 223–46

Caldwell, John C., 'Health Transition: The Cultural, Social and Behavioural Determinants of Health in the Third World', *Social Science and Medicine*, 36 (2) (1993), pp. 125–35

——, 'Routes to Low Mortality in Poor Countries', *Population and Development Review*, 12 (2) (June 1986), pp. 171–220

Carson, Rachel, *Silent Spring* (Boston, MA, 1962)

Carter, Eric, 'Development Narratives and the Uses of Ecology: Malaria Control in Northwest Argentina, 1890–1940', *Journal of Historical Geography*, 33 (2007), pp. 619–50

Casman, Elizabeth A., and Hadi Dowlatabadi, eds, *The Contextual Determinants of Malaria* (Washington, DC, 2002)

Cirollo, Vincent J., *Bullets and Bacilli: The Spanish–American War and Military Medicine* (New Brunswick, NJ, 2004)

Cochi, Stephen L., 'Polio Today: Are We on the Verge of Global Eradication?', *Journal of the American Medical Association*, 300 (7) (2008), pp. 839–41

Colgrove, James, 'The McKeown Thesis: A Historical Controversy and its Enduring Influence', *American Journal of Public Health*, 92 (5) (1 May 2002), pp. 725–29

——, *States of Immunity: The Politics of Vaccination in Twentieth-Century America* (Berkeley, CA, 2006)

Cueto, Marcos, *Cold War, Deadly Fevers: Malaria Eradication in Mexico, 1955–1975* (Baltimore, MD, 2007)

——, 'The Origins of Primary Health Care and Selective Primary Health Care', *American Journal of Public Health*, 94 (11) (November 2004), pp. 1864–74

——, *The Return of the Epidemics: Health and Society in Peru During the Twentieth Century* (Aldershot, 2001)

——, *The Value of Health: A History of the Pan American Health Organization* (Washington, DC, 2007)

——, ed., *Missionaries of Science: The Rockefeller Foundation in Latin America* (Bloomington, IN, 1994)

Dowdle, Walter R., and Stephen L. Cochi, 'Global Eradication of Poliovirus: History and Rationale', in *Molecular Biology of Picornaviruses*, ed. B. L. Semler and E. Wimmer (Washington, DC, 2002), pp. 473–78

——, and D. R. Hopkins, eds, *The Eradication of Infectious Diseases* (Chichester, West Sussex, and New York, 1998)
Dubos, Rene, *Man Adapting* (New Haven, CT, 1980)
Durbach, D. N., *Bodily Matters: The Anti-Vaccination Movement in England, 1853–1907* (Durham and London, 2005)
Easterly, William, *The White Man's Burden: Why the West's Efforts to Aid the Rest Have done so Much Ill and So Little Good* (New York, 2007)
Espinosa, Mariela, *Epidemic Invasions: Yellow Fever and the Limits of Cuban Independence, 1898–1930* (Chicago, IL, 2009)
Fantini, B., 'Anopheles Without Malaria: An Ecological and Epidemiological Puzzle', *Parassitologia*, 36 (1–2) (1994), pp. 83–106
Farid, M. A., 'Round Table: The Malaria Programme – from Euphoria to Anarchy', *World Health Forum*, 1 (1–2) (1980), pp. 8–33
Farley, John, *Brock Chisholm, the World Health Organization, and the Cold War* (Vancouver, BC, and Toronto, ON, 2008)
——, 'Mosquitoes or Malaria? Rockefeller Campaigns in the American South and Sardinia', *Parassitologia*, 36 (1–2) (1994), pp. 165–73
——, *To Cast Out Disease: A History of the International Health Division of the Rockefeller Foundation, 1913–1951* (Oxford and New York, 2004)
Fenner, F., D. A. Henderson, I. Aritya, Z. Jezek and E. D. Ladnyi, *Smallpox and Its Eradication* (Geneva, 1988)
Franco Agudelo, Saúl, *El Paludismo en América Latina* (Guadalajara, Mexico, 1990)
Frazer, Stuart M., 'Leicester and Smallpox: The Leicester Method', *Medical History*, 24 (3) (1980), pp. 315–32
Gabaldón, Arnoldo, 'Malaria Eradication in Venezuela: Doctrine, Practice and Achievements after Twenty Years', *American Journal of Tropical Medicine and Hygiene*, 32(2) 1983, pp. 203–11
——, 'The Nation-Wide Campaign Against Malaria in Venezuela', *Transactions of the Royal Society of Tropical Medicine and Hygiene*, 43 (2) (September 1949), pp. 113–64
——, *Una Política Sanitaria* (Caracas, Venezuela, 1965)
Gallup, John Luke, and Jeffrey D. Sachs, 'The Economic Burden of Malaria', *American Journal of Tropical Medicine and Hygiene*, 64 (1–2) (2001), pp. 85–96
Garrett, Laurie, *Betrayal of Trust: The Collapse of Public Health* (New York, 2000)
——, 'The Challenge of Global Health', *Foreign Affairs*, 14 (2007), pp. 14–38
Gladwell, Malcolm, Annals of Public Health, 'The Mosquito Killer', *New Yorker* (2 July 2001), pp. 42–51
Godlee, Fiona, 'WHO in Retreat: Is it Losing its Influence?', *British Medical Journal*, 309 (3 December 1994), pp. 1491–95
Greenough, Paul, 'Intimidation, Coercion and Resistance in the Final Stages of the South Asian Smallpox Eradication Campaign, 1973–1975', *Social Science and Medicine*, 41 (5) (September 1995), pp. 633–45
Hackett, Lewis W., *Malaria in Europe: An Ecological Study* (London, 1937)
Hardy, Anne, *The Epidemic Streets: Infectious Disease and the Rise of Preventive Medicine, 1866–1900* (Oxford, 1993)
Harrison, Gordon, *Mosquitoes, Malaria and Man: A History of the Hostilities Since 1880* (London, 1978)
Henderson, Donald A., 'Eradication: Lessons from the Past', *Morbidity and Mortality Weekly Report*, 48 (1) (31 December 1999) (supp. SU01), pp. 16–22
——, *Smallpox – The Death of a Disease. The Inside Story of Eradicating a Worldwide Killer* (Amherst, NY, 2009)
Hinman, E. H., *World Eradication of Infectious Diseases* (Springfield, IL, 1966)
Hochman, Gilberto, 'From Autonomy to Partial Alignment: National Malaria Programs in the Time of Global Eradication, Brazil, 1941–1961', *Canadian Bulletin of Medical History*, 15 (1) (2008), pp. 161–92
——, 'Priority, Invisibility, and Eradication: The History of Smallpox and the Brazilian Public Health Agenda', *Medical History*, 53 (2) (2009), pp. 229–52
Hopkins, Donald R., *The Greatest Killer: Smallpox in History* (Chicago, IL, 2002)
——, 'Perspectives from the Dracunculiasis Eradication Programme', *Bulletin of the WHO*, 76 (suppl. 2) 1998, pp. 38–41
——, 'Yaws in the Americas, 1950–1975', *The Journal of Infectious Diseases*, 136 (4) (October 1977), pp. 548–54
——, and E. Ruiz-Tiben, 'Strategies for Dracunculiasis Eradication', *Bulletin of the WHO*, 69 (5) (1991), pp. 523–40
Hotez, Peter J., *Forgotten People, Forgotten Diseases: The Neglected Tropical Diseases and their Impact on Global Health and Development* (Washington, DC, 2008)
Humphries, Margaret, *Malaria: Poverty, Race, and Public Health in the United States* (Baltimore, MD, and London, 2001)
——, *Yellow Fever and the South* (Baltimore, MD, 1992)
Jackson, J., 'Cognition and the Global Malaria Eradication Programme', *Parassitologia*, 40 (1–2) (1998), pp. 193–216
Jeffery, Geoffrey M., 'Malaria Control in the Twentieth Century', *American Journal of Tropical Medicine and Hygiene*, 25 (3) (1976), pp. 361–71
Jenner, Edward, *An Inquiry into the Causes and Effects of the Variolae Vaccinae, a Disease Discovered in Some Western Counties of England* (London, 1798)

Kunitz, Stephen J., *The Health of Populations: General Theories and Particular Realities* (Oxford, 2007)
Litsios, Socrates, 'Arnoldo Gabaldón's Independent Path for Malaria Control and Public Health in the Tropics: A Lost "Paradigm" for WHO', *Parassitologia*, 40 (1998), pp. 231–38
——, 'Criticism of WHO's Revised Malaria Eradication Strategy', *Parassitologia*, 42 (1–2) (2000), pp. 167–72
——, 'The Long and Difficult Road to Alma-Ata: A Personal Reflection', *International Journal of Health Services*, 32 (4) (2002), pp. 709–42
——, 'Malaria Control, the Cold War, and the Postwar Reorganization of International Assistance', *Medical Anthropology*, 17 (3) (1997), pp. 255–78
——, 'Rene J. Dubos and Fred L. Soper: Their Contrasting Views on Vector and Disease Eradication', *Perspectives in Biology and Medicine*, 41 (1) (Autumn 1997), pp. 138–49
——, *The Tomorrow of Malaria* (Wellington, 1996)
Löwy, Ilana, 'Epidemiology, Immunology and Yellow Fever: The Rockefeller Foundation in Brazil, 1923–1939', *Journal of the History of Biology*, 30 (1997), pp. 397–417
——, *Virus, Moustiques et Modernité: La Fièvre Jaune au Brésil entre Science et Politique* (Paris, 2001)
——, 'What/Who should be Controlled? Opposition to Yellow Fever Campaigns in Brazil, 1900–1939', in *Western Medicine as Contested Knowledge*, ed. Andrew Cunningham and Bridie Andrews, (Manchester, 1997), pp. 124–46
McKeown, Thomas, *The Modern Rise of Population* (New York, 1976)
——, *The Role of Medicine: Dream, Mirage or Nemesis?* (London, 1976)
Mitman, Greg, et al., *Landscapes of Exposure: Knowledge and Illness in Modern Environments*, Special Issue of *Osiris* (19) (2004)
Montgomery, Scott L., *The Scientific Voice* (New York and London, 1996)
Muraskin, William, *The Politics of International Health: The Children's Vaccine Initiative and the Struggle to Develop Vaccines for the Third World* (New York, 1998)
Needham, Cynthia A., and Richard Canning, *Global Disease Eradication: The Race for the Last Child* (Washington, DC, 2003)
Ogden, Horace G., *The CDC and the Smallpox Crusade* (Washington, DC, 1987)
Packard, Randall M., *The Making of a Tropical Disease: A Short History of Malaria* (Baltimore, MD, 2007)
——, 'Malaria Dreams: Postwar Visions of Health and Development in the Third World', *Medical Anthropology*, 17 (3) (1997), pp. 279–96
——, and Paulo Gadelha, '"A Land Filled with Mosquitoes": Fred L. Soper, the Rockefeller Foundation, and the *Anopheles gambiae* Invasion of Brazil', *Medical Anthropology*, 17 (3) (1997), pp. 215–38
Palmer, Steven, *Launching Global Health: The Caribbean Odyssey of the Rockefeller Foundation* (Ann Arbor, MI, 2010)
——, 'Migrant Clinics and Hookworm Science: Peripheral Origins of International Health, 1840–1920', *Bulletin of the History of Medicine*, 83 (4) (2009), pp. 676–709
Pampana, E. J., and P. F. Russell, *Malaria: A World Problem* (Geneva, 1955)
Riley, James C., *Rising Life Expectancy: A Global History* (Cambridge, UK and New York, 2001)
Roberts, Leslie L., 'Polio Eradication: Is it Time to Give Up?', *Science*, 312 (5775) (2006), pp. 832–35
——, and Martin Enserink, 'Malaria: Did They Really Say . . . Eradication?', *Science*, 318 (5856) (7 December 2007), pp. 1544–5
Russell, Edmund, *War and Nature: Fighting Humans and Insects with Chemicals from World War I to Silent Spring* (Cambridge and New York, 2001)
Russell, Paul F., *Man's Mastery of Malaria* (London and New York, 1955)
Sachs, Jeffrey D., *The End of Poverty: Economic Possibilities for Our Time* (London and New York, 2005)
Siddiqi, Javed, *World Health and World Politics: The World Health Organization and the UN System* (Columbus, SC, 1995)
Snowden, Frank M., *The Conquest of Malaria: Italy, 1900–1962* (New Haven, CT, and London, 2006)
Solomon, Susan G., Lion Murard and Patricl Zylberman, eds, *Shifting Boundaries of Public Health: Europe in the Twentieth Century*, (Rochester, NY, 2008)
Soper, Fred L., *Building the Health Bridge: Selections from the Works of Fred L. Soper*, ed. J. Austin Kerr (Ann Arbor, IN, 1970)
——, 'The Epidemiology of a Disappearing Disease: Malaria', *American Journal of Tropical Medicine and Hygiene*, 9 (1960), pp. 357–66
——, 'Problems to be Solved if the Eradication of Tuberculosis is to be Realized', *American Journal of Public Health*, 52 (5) (1 May 1962), pp. 734–45
——, 'Rehabilitation of the Eradication Concept in the Prevention of Communicable Diseases', *Public Health Reports*, 80 (10) (October 1965), pp. 855–69
——, *Ventures in World Health: The Memoirs of Fred Lowe Soper*, ed. John Duffy (Washington, DC, 1977)
——, and D. Bruce Wilson, *Anopheles Gambiae in Brazil, 1930 to 1940* (New York, 1943)
——, et al., *The Organization of Permanent Nation-Wide Anti-Aedes aegypti Measures in Brazil* (New York, 1943)
Spielman, Andrew, and Michael D'Antonio, *Mosquito: A Natural History of our Most Persistent and Deadly Foe* (New York, 2001)
Stapleton, Darwin H., 'Lessons of History? Anti-Malaria Strategies of the International Health Board and the Rockefeller Foundation from the

1920s to the Era of DDT', *Public Health Reports*, 119 (2) (March–April 2004), pp. 206–15
Stepan, Nancy Leys, *Beginnings of Brazilian Science: Oswaldo Cruz, Medical Research and Policy, 1890–1920* (New York, 1976)
——, 'The Interplay between Socio-Economic Factors and Medical Science: Yellow Fever Research, Cuba, and the United States', *Social Studies of Science*, 8 (4) (1978), pp. 397–423
——, '"The Only Serious Terror in these Regions": Malaria Control in the Brazilian Amazon', in *Disease in the History of Modern Latin America: From Malaria to AIDS*, ed. Diego Armus (Durham and London, 2003), pp. 25–50
——, *Picturing Tropical Nature* (London, 2001)
Strode, George, ed., *Yellow Fever* (New York, 1951)
Szreter, Simon R., *Health and Wealth: Studies in History and Policy* (Rochester, NY, 2005)
——, 'The Importance of Social Intervention in Britain's Mortality Decline *c.* 1850–1914: A Re-interpretation of the Role of Public Health', *Social History of Medicine*, 1 (1) (1988), pp. 1–38.
Tayeh, A., and S. Cairncross, 'Dracunculiasis Eradication by 2009: Will Endemic Countries Meet the Target?', *Tropical Medicine and International Health*, 12 (12) (2007), pp. 1403–8
Tucker, Jonathan B., *Scourge: The Once and Future Threat of Smallpox* (New York, 2001)
Weindling, Paul, ed., *International Health Organisations and Movements, 1918–1939* (Cambridge, 1995)
Wickett, John F., 'The Final Inch: The Eradication of Smallpox', *Social Scientist*, 30 (5–6) (May–June 2002), pp. 62–78
Wilkinson, Richard G., *Unhealthy Societies: The Afflictions of Inequality* (London and New York, 1996)
——, and Kate Pickett, *The Spirit Level: Why More Equal Societies Almost Always do Better* (London and New York, 2009)
Williams, Greer, *The Plague Killers* (New York, 1969)
Williamson, Stanley, *The Vaccination Controversy: The Rise, Reign and Fall of Compulsory Vaccination for Smallpox* (Liverpool, 2007)
Worboys, Michael, *Spreading Germs: Diseases, Theories, and Medical Practice in Britain, 1865–1900* (Cambridge, 2000)
World Health Organization, *The Global Eradication of Smallpox: The Final Report of the Global Commission for the Certification of Smallpox Eradication* (Geneva, 1980)
——, *The Declaration of Alma-Ata*: http://who.int/hpr/NPH/docs/declaration_almaata.pdf (accessed 10 April 2011)
——, 'Malaria Control: Survey and Recommendations', *Bulletin of the World Health Organization*, 1(2) 1948, pp. 215–52
Yekutiel, Perez, 'Lessons from the Big Eradication Campaigns', *World Health Forum*, 2(4) (1981), pp. 465–90

Acknowledgements

This book began as a lecture in a series I organized on the subject of disease eradication for the Forum in the History of Public Health in International Contexts, at the Center for the History and Ethics of Public Health, Division of Sociomedical Sciences, Mailman School of Public Health, Columbia University, in 2003, and I am grateful to Professor David Rothman and others at the Center for providing an intellectually stimulating place to discuss ideas about public health.

From that experience there came the idea of writing a book on the topic of disease eradication. I knew that one of the chief architects of the eradication idea, Dr Fred Lowe Soper, had given his large archive, consisting of diaries, letters and papers, to the National Library of Medicine in Washington, DC, and that the papers had been carefully organized. I thought that by using the life and career of Soper I could give a narrative shape and chronological order to a book that would take on the broad sweep of the eradication idea, from its early twentieth-century origins to the present. In this regard, I would like to acknowledge the extraordinary resources of the National Library of Medicine, and the assistance many people there gave me, starting with Dr Elizabeth Fee, Chief, History of Medicine Division, whose many contributions to the history of the institutions of public health, national and international, are well known. I thank Stephen Greenberg and Crystal Smith, for help with accessing the Soper Papers; for general advice, Dr David Cantor, historian at the History of Medicine Division and Deputy Director and Senior Research Historian in the Office of National Institutes of Health History, NIH, Bethesda, and Susan Speaker, who was responsible for preparing the splendid online selections of documents from the Soper archive in the Profiles in Science series. Michael Sappol, also a historian in the History of Medicine Division, and Ginny Roth, Collection Manager, Prints and Photographs, were extremely kind in helping me select images from the collections for use as illustrations.

Also in the United States, at the Rockefeller Archive Center, where a number of materials related to eradication can be found, Thomas Rosenbaum, Archivist, was immensely helpful in steering me through the rich collections, and Dr Darwin H. Stapleton, at the time Executive Director of the RAC, took the time to discuss Rockefeller Foundation matters with me and gave me several very useful insights into the Foundation's work in international health. Another valuable resource was the library of The World Health Organization in Geneva, where I spent two weeks consulting the archives concerning WHO involvement in various eradication campaigns. My research home in Brazil has always been the Casa Oswaldo Cruz in Rio de Janeiro, where so much good historical work in the history of medicine is done, and where Gilberto Hochman, Jaime Larry Benchimol, Magali Romero Sá and Simone Petraglia Kropf, among others, have been valued colleagues.

I am extremely grateful to The Mellon Foundation, whose support between 2008 and 2011 made many of the visits to these libraries and archives possible.

Mellon support also allowed me to get a feel for current debates about eradication by funding my travels to interview some of the key 'players' in current eradication campaigns and global health initiatives at The Bill and Melinda Gates Foundation and at The Carter Center. In Brazil, I was able to discuss dengue control and related matters with officials at the mayoral (Rio) level, state level and federal level (Brasilia). The dates of all these interviews, the names, titles, and the relevance of the interviews to the arguments about eradication, are given in the references at the appropriate points in the book.

Books owe their life and animation most of all to the people who, in the writer's mind at least, form an invisible college or critical circle – people whose ideas and written works on international aspects of health have been extremely significant to me, ever-present interlocutors, even when they may not be aware of it. In this circle I put Anne-Emmanuelle Birn, Marcos Cueto, Colin Leys, Steven Palmer, Simon Szreter, Helen Tilley, Anisa Khadem Nwachuku and Paola Mejia. The last-named two people served at crucial moments as my research assistants. I thank them for their efficiency and for the discussions their collaboration prompted.

Above all, I want to acknowledge the help of Colin Leys and Carole Satyamurti, two experienced writers themselves, who took the time to make a close reading of the book while in manuscript, offered gentle but necessary criticism, improved my prose, saved me, I hope, from errors, and generally gave me the encouragement necessary to finish the book. Finally, I come to Alfred Stepan; in addition to being the author of many books, he is known as a brilliant editor and critic, as well as a generous encourager of others, and so it is with my own writing. All I can say, after so many years of sharing ideas and many other things in life, is a heartfelt but inadequate 'thank you'.

Photo Acknowledgements

Introduction, p. 6: *Aedes (stegomyia) aegypti*. Courtesy of the National Library of Medicine.

Chapter One, p. 18: 'Filling the Vaccine bottles before freeze-drying, one of the final steps in smallpox vaccine production'. Courtesy the National Library of Medicine and the WHO, Photographer Jean Mohr.

Chapter Two, p. 34: 'Yellow Fever Santiago de Cuba'. Houses prepared for mosquito fumigation'. Courtesy of the National Library of Medicine.

Chapter Three, p. 66: 'Fred L. Soper on a Donkey in the 1920s in Latin America'. Courtesy of the National Library of Medicine, The Fred Lowe Soper Papers, Ms C 359, Box 28, folder 54.

Chapter Four, p. 104: 'Environmental Sanitation Spraying, Caracas, Venezuela. Spraying *Aedes aegypti* mosquitoes'. Courtesy of the National Library of Medicine, The Fred Lowe Soper Papers, Ms C 359, Box 28, folder 8.

Chapter Five, p. 140: 'Aeroplane Insecticide Drops. The fixed wing aeroplane can make accurate insecticide drops at 60 mph over open stretches of river'. Courtesy of the National Library of Medicine and the WHO.

Chapter Six, p. 184: 'Smallpox Africa. The eradication campaign transcended all language barriers and local traditions'. Courtesy of the National Library of Medicine and the WHO. Photo by J. Ryst.

Chapter Seven, p. 224: 'Immunize and Protect Your Child. Prevention is essential to protect life and there is no substitute for vaccination and immunization.' Courtesy of the National Library of Medicine, and WHO / UNICEF.

Index